MEDICAL
MEANINGS

MEDICAL
MEANINGS

A Glossary of Word Origins

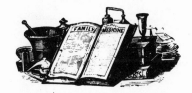

William S. Haubrich, M.D.

HARCOURT BRACE JOVANOVICH, PUBLISHERS

San Diego   New York   London

Requests for permission to make copies of any part of the
work should be mailed to: Permissions, Harcourt Brace
Jovanovich, Publishers, Orlando, Florida 32887

Library of Congress Cataloging in Publication Data
Haubrich, William S.
Medical meanings.
Includes index.
1. Medicine—Terminology. 2. English language—
Etymology—Dictionaries. I. Title. [DNLM: 1. Dic-
tionaries, Medical. 2. Nomenclature. W 15 H368m]
R123.H29   1984   610'.14   83-22614
ISBN 0-15-658572-3

Designed by Lucy Albanese

Printed in the United States of America
First edition
A B C D E

*Dedicated to
the curiosity of all students
of medicine
young and old*

PREFACE

That prodigious 18th-century savant Dr. Samuel Johnson, in compiling his *Dictionary of the English Language,* archly defined a lexicographer as "a harmless drudge." Whether one who compiles a medical etymology can flatter himself as a lexicographer is arguable, but I can honestly say I have meant no harm in putting together this book and at no time have I thought of the task as drudgery. Rather, the work has been fun, and often illuminating into the bargain. I hope the reader, too, will be entertained as well as enlightened by the work.

A Word of Caution

Although the title of this book is *Medical Meanings,* the etymology of a word should never be confused with its current definition. Nevertheless, it comes as a surprise, in some instances, that the origin of a word and its current usage so closely coincide, considering the centuries that have elapsed since the word was coined.

An example is the Greek *amnēstia,* which to the ancients meant forgetfulness and, with only slight modification as "amnesia," means a loss of memory to modern psychiatrists. Moreover, both the Greek word and its English derivative "amnesty" can convey a sense of "forgive and forget." In contrast, "artery" is known to us as a word for a vessel serving to transport blood away from the heart. But its Greek predecessor was derived from a combination of *aer-,* "air," + *tērēo,* "I carry," and to the Greeks *artēria* was the windpipe or trachea. It goes without saying that no one would contend that "artery" really means an air duct simply because of its etymology.

Moreover, there is such a thing as "folk etymology." This is a mistaken attribution, seemingly logical but false nonetheless. "Tip," a commonly used word for a gratuity given to one who performs a personal service, is sometimes said to have been derived as an acronym for "to insure promptness." Sound reasonable? Well, not really. A tip, when it is bestowed, customarily follows, not precedes, the service. It is more a reward than a stimulus. The truth is that the real origin of "tip" is not known, a circumstance pertaining in most instances of folk etymology. The *Oxford English Dictionary* suggests that "tip" may have survived from rogues' cant, or it may come from the use of the word in a sense of touching lightly. But "to insure promptness" it is not (and does not).

How to Use This Book

This volume is not intended to be read from cover-to-cover, front-to-back—although a few brave souls may try. It is intended for reference, to help answer the question: "Now where did *that* word come from?" Entries pertaining to principal words (and important prefixes and suffixes) appear alphabetically. Riffling through the pages, using the guide words, is the easiest way to begin a search.

But the publisher has also provided an index of those subentries which appear in **boldface** type. Thus when a word being sought does not have an entry of its own, it may be found in the index. Second, the word in which you are interested may appear in more than one entry because of uses relating to other words. Multiple citations will be listed in the index. It might be a good idea to look in the index even when you have found your word at a principal entry by thumbing through the pages. Third, some categories of words, such as colors, numbers,

and phobias, are grouped together. Descriptions of these words can be located by consulting the index.

An Explanation of How Words Appear

Principal words for which derivations are given are printed in **boldface** type. Words from languages other than English, particularly foreign words from which English words are derived, are printed in *italic* type. Greek words, which figure prominently in etymology, are composed of letters originating in the Greek alphabet: alpha, beta, gamma, delta, and so on, for a total of twenty-four. (Yes, "alphabet" is a slightly contracted combination of the first two letters, as if we referred to our set of letters as "AB's.") To be quite proper, Greek words should be printed in Greek letters. Purists would so insist. But for many of us, Greek letters are difficult to recognize at a glance, and most lend themselves to an easy transliteration. So Greek words in this book are printed in letters corresponding to the Roman alphabet:

A,α	(alpha)	= a
B,β	(beta)	= b
Γ,γ	(gamma)	= g
Δ,δ	(delta)	= d
E,ϵ	(epsilon)	= e
Z,ζ	(zeta)	= z
H,η	(eta)	= ē
Θ,θ	(theta)	= th
I,ι	(iota)	= i
K,κ	(kappa)	= k
Λ,λ	(lambda)	= l
M,μ	(mu)	= m
N,ν	(nu)	= n

Ξ,ξ	(xi)	= x or z (both pronounced as "z")	
O,o	(omicron)	= o	
Π,π	(pi)	= p	
P,ρ	(rho)	= r or rh	
Σ,σ,ς	(sigma)	= s	
Τ,τ	(tau)	= t	
Υ,υ	(upsilon)	= y or u	
Φ,φ	(phi)	= ph (pronounced as "f")	
Χ,χ	(chi)	= ch (pronounced as "k")	
Ψ,ψ	(psi)	= ps	
Ω,ω	(omega)	= ō	

Note that there are two distinct Greek letters equivalent to the Roman "e" and two distinct Greek letters equivalent to the Roman "o." These have been distinguished by using a macron (a horizontal line placed over the vowel). Thus the Greek ϵ (epsilon) is represented as e, and the Greek η (eta) is represented as ē; the Greek o (omicron) is represented as o, and the Greek ω (omega) is represented as ō.

Still another explanation: the Greek γ (gamma) becomes an "n" when it precedes another gamma, a kappa, a xi, or a chi. Where this is necessary to understanding a connection between the original Greek word and the derived word, the "n" has been inserted as [n].

How to Improve This Book

While the publisher has provided highly expert and much appreciated editorial help in readying my typescript for the press, there may still be pockets of controversy here and there. The publisher and editorial consultants have joined me in trying to assure accuracy, but where errors remain the responsibility is ultimately mine. Readers who wish to dispute points that are made in this book or who can suggest additions, amendments (or perhaps deletions) are invited to write to me forthwith. Your advice will be welcomed and most kindly considered.

William S. Haubrich, M.D.

The Scripps Clinic & Research Foundation
10666 North Torrey Pines Road
La Jolla, California 92037

ACKNOWLEDGMENTS

Throughout this work I have noted my debt to Professor Henry Alan Skinner (1899–1967) and his seminal book *The Origin of Medical Terms,* published by The Williams & Wilkins Company in 1949 and followed by a second edition in 1961. Professor Skinner's book, preeminent among former glossaries of medical etymology, unfortunately is no longer in print. With *Medical Meanings* I hope to fill this gap in medical source material, covering somewhat different ground in a currently relevant way. Meanings of terms are updated, new words are described, and origins tangential to those more commonly associated with the terms are freely explored. However, I do owe much to the scholarship of my worthy predecessor.

Anyone seeking to learn about medical words must have access to various sources. A shelf full of dictionaries, in English and other languages, comes in handy. The *Oxford English Dictionary* will be most frequently thumbed. *Dorland's Illustrated Medical Dictionary,* in my opinion, is the most authoritative source of precise definitions. For background information, Skeat's *Etymological Dictionary of the English Language, Brewer's Dictionary of Phrase and Fable,* and *Bulfinch's Mythology* are indispensable.

A fascination with words, how they came to be, and how they are used is not a genetically determined trait. It must be instilled. I am mindful that my early interest was prompted by exacting schoolteachers and by my preceptors at Franklin & Marshall College, particularly James M. Darlington in biology and W. Nelson Francis in English. My professor of pathology at Western Reserve University, the late Howard T. Karsner, was a demanding, erudite, and inspiring taskmaster when it came to a precise description of disease.

I must mention, too, the help generously

Acknowledgments

given by my medical and professorial colleagues, at home and abroad, who advised me on words peculiar to their special fields. Howard Sandum, Paul McCluskey, and Johanna Jordahl carefully shepherded this work through its phase of publication. My thanks go to my keen-eyed editorial assistants, Mrs. Ellen Shannon and Mrs. Helen Cundiff. And to Eila, for her forbearance.

W. S. H.

MEDICAL
MEANINGS

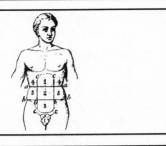

A

aa is an abbreviation formerly used in writing prescriptions and meaning "of each." The pharmacist thereby was instructed to use equal parts of the several ingredients listed. The use of "aa" was more a disguise than a time saver. It stands for the Greek *ana,* a preposition meaning "up, again, or throughout." This is not the same *-ana* as derived from the Latin suffixes *-anus, -ana, -anum,* meaning "of or belonging to" and used to indicate a collection of items or observations as, for example, in "Americana."

abdomen probably comes from the Latin verb *abdere,* "to hide," the inference being that the viscera are hidden or tucked away in the abdomen. While for us "abdomen" encompasses all structures between the diaphragm and the pelvis, the ancients probably used the term in a more restrictive sense to refer to the ventral or belly wall. **Belly,** incidentally, comes from an Anglo-Saxon word meaning "bag or sack." This is yet another instance in which the Anglo-Saxon term has become somewhat vulgar while the Latin is considered more delicate. The patient says, "I got kicked in the belly!" while the doctor says, "This man sustained a non-penetrating injury to the abdomen." They are both describing the same event, but the patient's account is more vivid.

abduct comes from the Latin *abducere* (*ab-,* "from," + *ducere,* "to draw or lead"), hence "to draw away from." The **abducens,** or sixth cranial, nerve is so called because it supplies the lateral rectus muscle that "draws away" the eyeball to the side of the head.

ablation is from the Latin *ablatum,* the past participle of *auferre,* "to carry away," and represents a combination of *ab-,* "from, away," + *latum,* the past participle of *ferre,* "to carry or bear." The French *ablation* means "a removal or excision." In surgery, to ablate is to remove, especially by cutting.

1

Ablatio placentae refers to a detachment, or "carrying away," of the placenta. When this occurs because of a precipitous tear, it is an **abruptio placentae** (from the Latin *abrumpere*, "to sever").

abortus is the Latin word for miscarriage. The Latin verb *aboriri* means "to miscarry or fail," particularly in the sense of not completing a full course. This, in turn, is a combination of *ab-*, "away, from," + *oriri*, "to descend from or to be born."

abrasion comes from the Latin *abradere, abrasum*, "to scrape off, to shave." The Indo-European root is postulated to have been *rēd, rōd*, "to scratch." This is presumably related to the Latin verb *radere*, "to scrape," of which the past participle is *rasum*. From this come such familiar words as "rash" and "razor." The advertisement that warns against "razor rash" unwittingly combines two words of common origin. Medically, an abrasion is an area of skin or other surface where the covering membrane has been scraped off.

abscess might be thought to come from the Latin *abscedere*, "to depart or go away." Not really, says Professor H. A. Skinner, who suggests rather that it began with the Greek *apostēma*, "a throwing off or drawing off," as of "bad humors." The Greek *apostēma* was then rendered as the Latin *abscessus*, both terms referring to a suppurative collection anywhere in the body.

absorb comes from the Latin *absorbere*, "to devour." This, in turn, is a combination of *ab-*, "away or from," + *sorbere*, "to suck, swallow, or gulp." This is in keeping with the sense of the process whereby, for example, the intestinal epithelial cells take in nutritive fluids. "Absorb" and its congeners have a puzzling resemblance, perhaps accidental, to the Arabic *sharaba*, "to drink," from which our word "sherbet" is derived.

a.c. are the initials representing *ante cibum*, Latin for "before a meal." When written in a prescription, this is a convenient shorthand way of directing that a medication is to be given before eating. The initials **"p.c."** represent the Latin *post cibum*, "after a meal."

acanthosis comes from the Greek *akantha*, "thorn," and refers to any thorny, spiny, or prickly surface. **Acanthosis nigricans** is a black roughening of the skin, usually in the axilla or other skin folds, which, in some cases, may be a harbinger of visceral cancer.

acapnia is derived from the Greek *a-*, "without," + *kapnos*, "smoke." The word was devised not to mean "smokeless" but rather to refer to a diminution of carbon dioxide in the blood. Insofar as carbon dioxide is a major component of the common smoke produced by the combustion of carbon-containing fuels, and recognizing the lack of a classical term for carbon dioxide, the contrivance makes sense. **Hypercapnia** is an excess of carbon dioxide in the blood.

accident comes from the Latin *accidere*, "to happen, occur, or befall." The root verb is *cadere*, "to fall." This implies, in a remote sense, that unlikely happenings result from a "falling out" of the heavenly bodies. Ancient writers occasionally used the term *ac-*

cidentia to mean symptoms, the implication being that such were unexpected and extraordinary departures from a state of health.

accommodation comes from the Latin *accommodare,* "to adjust or adapt," and fits nicely with the ophthalmic reference to adjustment of the eyes, particularly of the lenses through contraction of the ciliary fibers, to varying visual distances.

accoucheur is the French word for a male obstetrician and was first used in the 17th century. An **accoucheuse** could be either a female obstetrician or a midwife. The word literally means "one who attends at a couch or bed," the bed, of course, being the bed of confinement for labor (even the French would eschew any double entendre here). The word would be of only passing interest to English-speaking physicians were it not for the term **accoucheur hand,** used to describe the posture of the hand in tetany wherein the metacarpophalangeal joints are flexed and the fingers are extended. Presumably the allusion is to the manner in which an obstetrician holds his hand when delivering a baby.

acetate is derived from the Latin *acetum,* "sour wine." In French this is *vin aigre* (*aigre* being the French word for "sour or bitter"). By only a slight change in spelling and pronunciation, this becomes our word "vinegar." The acid in vinegar is, then, acetic acid. Acetic acid was the earliest known, and until the late 18th century was thought to be the only, organic acid. An acetate is any salt of acetic acid. **Acetone**

was concocted from the Latin root *acet-* and the Greek ending *-ōne,* denoting a female descendant or a weaker derivative. One might conclude that acetone was first thought to be a "weak sister" of acetic acid.

achalasia is a combination of the Greek *a-,* designating "absence or failure," + *chalasis,* "relaxation," and we use the word in its literal sense, "a failure of relaxation." The condition known as achalasia is most commonly found in the esophagus, where it is specifically a failure in relaxation of the lower esophageal sphincter as distinguished from diffuse esophageal spasm. There is a nice distinction between achalasia and spasm, the difference being immediately clear to one who knows the derivation of "achalasia."

ache has, curiously, two origins, one for the verb and the other for the noun. The verb "to ache" comes from the Anglo-Saxon *acun* and should be spelled "ake" and not "ache." For the derived noun, however, the "k" becomes "ch," as in "to speak" and "speech" or "to bake" and "batch." The Oxford English Dictionary blames Dr. Samuel Johnson for confusing the origin of the verb "ake" with the Greek noun *achos,* meaning "a pain or distress." The esteemed lexicographer decreed that henceforth the verb should be spelled with "ch," i.e., "my heart aches" and not "my heart akes." All of this is an etymologic tempest in a teapot. Aching is miserable no matter how it is spelled. The exclamation "Ouch!" or the German "Ach!" may be distantly related to the Greek *achos.*

achondroplasia is a cause of dwarfism wherein the long bones fail to grow as a consequence of an epiphyseal defect. The word is derived from the Greek *a-,* "absence," + *chondros,* "cartilage," + *plassein,* "to form."

achromatic applied to an optical lens means it is free of the disturbing aura of colors that tends to distort microscopic or telescopic images. The construction of such lenses was achieved as early as the 18th century by combining elements of flint and crown glass. The word combines the Greek *a-,* "absence of," + *chroma,* "color."

acid comes from the Latin adjective *acidus,* meaning "sour, tart," and doubtless was used to describe the taste of acidic substances. *Acidus,* in turn, may have come from the Greek *akidos,* meaning "pointed or sharp." **Acid test** can mean a test for acid, but in common parlance an acid test refers to any critical or decisive examination. The expression comes from the old method of testing for gold: nitric acid was poured on the substance in question. Iron pyrite, or "fool's gold," would promptly dissolve. True gold, being a "noble metal," would remain inert and thus would pass the "acid test."

acinus is a Latin word meaning "berry," and a round cluster of epithelial cells, as in the salivary glands or the pancreas, does closely resemble a knobby berry.

acne is of uncertain origin. According to Professor H. A. Skinner, Hippocrates used the Greek word *achnē* "in the sense of 'lint' " to describe scaly lesions. Also, it has been considered a corruption of the Greek word *akmē,* meaning "the highest or critical point," the allusion presumably being to that stage of life when acne usually occurs. But this would seem a highly contrived derivation. "Acne" usually is accompanied by a modifying term, the commonest being the teenager's **acne vulgaris,** which is just that, the Latin *vulgaris* meaning "common or usual."

acoustic comes from the Greek *akoustikos,* "pertaining to hearing," the root verb being *akouein,* "to hear." Thus the acoustic, or eighth cranial, nerve is the "hearing nerve."

acrodynia comes from the Greek *akron,* in the sense of "the end or extremity," + *odynē,* "pain," and is literally a pain in an extremity, usually the foot or hand.

acromegaly is a pituitary disorder that leads to enlargement of the nose, jaw, hands, and feet. The term was introduced in 1886 by the French clinician Pierre Marie (1853–1940), aptly chosen from the Greek *akron,* "extremity," + *megas,* "large."

acromion refers to the point of the shoulder and derives from the Greek *akron,* in the sense of "peak," + *ōmos,* "shoulder." More specifically, the acromion is the lateral process of the spine of the scapula and not a part of the shoulder joint.

actinic is from the Greek *aktis,* "ray," and refers to the ultraviolet rays, as in sunlight, that can cause reaction in skin; sunburn is thus an actinic burn. An **actinic keratosis** (from the Greek *keras,* "horn") is a focal, scaly excrescence on the scalp, face, neck, or other exposed surface of skin resulting, at least in part, from the ultraviolet rays of the sun.

actinomycosis is an infection by the "ray fungus," the common name for the genus *Actinomyces.* The *-myces* comes from the Greek *mykēs,* "fungus." *Actinomyces* is descriptive of the organisms which grow as yellow granules made up of mycelia (again, *myk-* + *ēlos,* Greek for "ornamental nail"), typically in a radiate array. The "radiate fungus" in German is the *Strahlenpilz,* which translates exactly the same.

acumen describes a talent for penetrating analysis and diagnosis. The same word in Latin means "sharpness, shrewdness, ingenuity." It is a derivative of the Latin verb *acuere,* "to make sharp or pointed."

acupuncture combines the Latin *acus,* "needle," + *punctum,* "a prick or puncture." The procedure of acupuncture could easily be called by the simple Anglo-Saxon "needle-stick," but as such it would probably lose much of whatever efficacy it is purported to have. Acupuncture is not new to the Western scene, having been first introduced to European practice in the late 17th century by a Dutch surgeon.

acute is from the Latin adjective *acutus,* meaning "sharp or pointed." There is an ancient precedent for the use of the term in the medical sense of "intense for a short period."

adamantinoma is from the Greek *adamas,* "untamed," + *-ōma,* "tumor." *Adamas* is used here in the sense of being unmalleable or unyielding, hence "hard." *Adamas dentis* is an old term for the enamel of teeth. An adamantinoma is a hard tumor of the jaw, more specifically an **ameloblastoma** (*amel* being an obsolete word for enamel), a neoplasm of the primordial cells that produce dental enamel. Incidentally, "diamond," the name of the hardest of gems, and "adamant," meaning stubborn, are both derived from *adamas.*

Adam's apple, the anterior protuberance of the thyroid cartilage, usually seen in men, is so called, according to *Brewer's Dictionary of Phrase and Fable,* from the superstition that a piece of the forbidden fruit which Adam ate stuck in his throat and occasioned the swelling. There is no mention in the biblical account that the fruit was, in fact, an apple. Professor Alexander Gode points out (*JAMA* 206:1058, 1968) that the Latin term *pomum Adami* ("Adam's apple") is really an early mistranslation of the Hebrew *tappūach ha ādām,* "male bump." Whoever made the mistake might be excused on the grounds that a single Hebrew word means both "bump" and "apple," and that the Hebrew word for "man" came to be the proper name "Adam."

addleheaded means to be confused or muddled. "Addle" comes from the Middle English *adel,* which meant "urine." At that time it was believed that liquid excrement was the result of internal decomposition. An "adel egg" was a rotten egg. Muddled or confused thinking was thought to be a sign of something rotten in the brain, hence "addleheaded" or "addlepated."

adduct is from the Latin *ad-,* "toward," + *ducere,* "to draw or lead." Hence an adductor muscle draws toward a point of reference, usually the axis of the body.

adeno- is a frequently used prefix and represents the Greek *adēn,* originally "an acorn" and, later, "a gland" shaped like an acorn.

Adenitis, then, is an inflammation of a gland, and **adenoid** means "like a gland," while **adenoma** is a benign tumor wherein the glandular elements closely resemble their normal counterparts.

adiadochokinesia is a highly contrived word and a dandy to dissect for its origin. It is composed of the Greek *a-*, "without," + *diadochos,* "successive," + *kinēsis,* "motion." So, adiadochokinesia is a neurologic sign of inability to perform rapid alternating movements, such as pronation and supination of the hands.

adipose is derived from the Latin *adeps,* "fat, particularly lard." "Adipose" usually is used to refer to tissue laden with fat; **obese** (from the Latin *obesus,* "whatever has eaten itself fat," the root verb being *obedere,* "to eat away") is used to refer to the person or animal so burdened. The distinction between "adipose" and "obese" is a nice one. **Adiposis dolorosa** (from the Latin *dolor,* "pain or grief") is a condition marked by painful, fatty swellings, typically in menopausal women.

adrenal is the name for the small endocrine glands that sit atop the kidneys, so called from the Latin *ad-*, "toward," + *renes,* "kidneys." Occasionally they are referred to as the **suprarenal** glands (from the Latin *supra,* "on top"). **Adrenalin** is a registered trademark for epinephrine held by the Parke-Davis company. The pressor effect of extracts from the suprarenal, or adrenal, glands was demonstrated by G. Oliver and E. A. Schäfer in 1895 and reported in the London *Journal of Physiology.* John J. Abel, a professor at the Johns Hopkins University, and Jokichi Takamine, a consultant to Parke-Davis, independently and simultaneously isolated the active pressor principle from the medullary portion of the adrenal gland. Professor Abel conferred on this substance the name **epinephrine** in 1899. The name "adrenalin" was given by Dr. Takamine in 1901. We can also be grateful to him as the donor of the celebrated Japanese cherry trees that adorn the boulevards of Washington, D.C.

adroit is from the French phrase *à droit,* "rightly," and has come to mean skillful or nimble. Conversely, the French word *gauche,* "left," has been taken into English to mean awkward or lacking in grace. The common adjective "gawky" is uncertainly attributed to *gauche* (the obsolete English "gawk-handed" meant left-handed), and "to gawk" is to stare stupidly. The Latin *dexter,* "right," is the origin of the English **dexterity,** meaning skill or agility, while the Latin *sinister,* "left," has been taken directly into English to mean ominous or portending evil. The allusion, obviously, is that most people are more facile with the right hand than the left hand. To those good and graceful folk who happen to be left-handed, this is a prime example of the tyranny of the majority.

adulterate shares the same Latin root as "adultery." The root verb is *adulterare,* "to defile or corrupt," from *ad-*, "to," + *alter,* "other." A substance that has been adversely changed by the admixture of a "corrupting" addition is said to be adulterated. While adultery is usually perpetrated by adults, the two words are quite unrelated in origin. **Adult** is from the Latin *adultus,* "one who has grown up," which in turn is derived from *adolescere,* "to grow up." This is also the source of our word for the period of growing up, **adolescence.**

adventitia is derived from the Latin adjective *adventicius,* meaning "foreign, strange, or extraneous." The connective tissue surrounding an artery is called "the adventitia" because it is looked upon as extraneous to the principal structure itself. At auscultation, **adventitious** sounds are those not normally heard to emanate from the healthy heart or lung.

aerobe is a combination of the Greek *aēr,* "air," + *bios,* "life," and describes organisms dependent on free air or oxygen to live. **Anaerobe** describes a microorganism that flourishes and, indeed, lives only in the absence of oxygen. The word comes from the Greek *an-,* "without," + aerobe. The terms "aerobe" and "anaerobe" were conceived in 1863 by Louis Pasteur (1822–1895), the famed French chemist and bacteriologist.

Aesculapius is the Latin form of Asklēpios, the name of the legendary Greek god of medicine, and Aesculapians are his followers. The mythical Asklēpios was the son of Apollo and the nymph Coronis. His wife was Epiome, and a celebrated issue came from this union, including Panaceia, goddess of healing; Hygieia, goddess of health; and the Homeric heroes Machaon, a surgeon of Peloponnesus, and Podaleiros, a physician of Asia Minor, both of whom are mentioned in the Iliad. Myths aside, there may have been an actual person known by the name Asklēpios who was celebrated for

his gentle and humane remedies, such as the treatment of fevers by fasting. His disciples established temples throughout the Greek world, the most famous being at Kos, Knidos, Epidaurus, and Pergamum. The modern medical fraternity known by the Greek initials Alpha Kappa Kappa takes its name from "*A*esculapians of *K*os and *K*nidos."

afferent comes from the Latin *ad,* "toward," + *ferre,* "to carry." Afferent nerves carry impulses toward the central nervous system; an afferent limb of gut carries its contents toward an anastomosis. **Efferent** is the opposite (*e-* or *ex-,* "away or out").

agar is a Malay word and in its native haunts is usually doubly sounded, as *agar-agar.* The substance was originally prepared from seaweed and was found to form a mucilaginous jelly when mixed with water, heated, then allowed to cool. It is a basic ingredient of many bacterial culture media, hence the reference to "agar plates." Agar also has been used to support emulsions and as a bulk laxative. Its use in the bacteriology laboratory is said to have been suggested by the wife of Walther Hesse, one of Robert Koch's (1843–1910) early associates. Frau Hesse had obtained samples of *agar-agar* from Dutch friends in Batavia.

agglutination is from the Latin *ad,* "to," + *glutinare,* "to glue." Particles that agglutinate are said to be stuck together, as if by glue. Incidentally, our word "glue" is derived from the Latin *gluten,* which means the same thing. But **gluten** for us has come to mean something else again, the sticky substance in certain cereal flours that causes diarrhea in persons afflicted with celiac disease.

agony comes from the Greek *agōn,* "a struggle or contest." The Greek *agōnia* also means "anguish," and this is the nonmedical sense in which our word "agony" usually is used. The medical adjective **agonal** describes pathologic changes occurring just before or at the moment of death, implying a death struggle. When referring to muscles, an **agonist** is a prime mover, and its **antagonist** is a muscle having the opposite effect. In physiological terms, an agonist is a stimulant to a specific action, while an antagonist blocks or counteracts the stimulus. Histamine, for example, is an agonist when it stimulates the secretion of hydrochloric acid by the parietal or oxyntic cells of the stomach; cimetidine, acting as an H_2-receptor antagonist, blocks this action. "Protagonist," incidentally, has a quite distinct meaning, and that is to designate the leading character in a drama or the foremost exponent of a movement or cause.

ague is an archaic word from Old French which, in turn, was derived from the Latin *acutus,* meaning "sharp or pointed." A *fièvre aiguë* was an "acute fever." Often this was shortened to merely "ague," and typically was used to describe an attack of malaria. Professor H. A. Skinner has pointed out that "ague" also may be connected with the Gothic word *agis,* meaning "trembling." Indeed, rigorous shivering often attends an acute fever.

AIDS is the acronym for "acquired immune deficiency syndrome." Often when a medical condition is poorly understood, it is described rather than specifically named, and it is called a syndrome when its status as an entity is uncertain. Because descriptions often are lengthy and cumbersome, ways are sought to shorten them. Forming an acronym by taking the initial letters of a phrase is a clever means, especially useful if it seems to form a short word. Sometimes an acronym eventually becomes a word itself, though its meaning may change in the process. An example is "flak" which originated in the German *Flieger Abwehr Kanone,* "aircraft defense cannon." "Acronym," by the way, comes from the Greek *akros,* "outermost," + *-onym,* the combining form of *ōnoma,* "name."

ala is the Latin word for "wing" and also "armpit." In medicine, it is almost always used in the sense of "wing" and in combination with other terms, as in **ala nasi,** the flaring, winglike outer extension of the nostril. An old term for the mesosalpinx was *ala vespertilionis,* or "bat's wing" (the *vespertilionis* referring to a creature that flies at vesper or "in the evening").

albino is a derivative of the Latin *albus,* "white," but the name "albino" was first given by the Portuguese traders to mottled or white Negroes encountered on the west coast of Africa. Medically, **albinism** refers to a partial or total lack of pigment in the eyes, skin, and hair. Persons so affected are sometimes called albinos.

albumen spelled with an "e" is the white of an egg; when spelled with an "i" before the final "n," it refers to a protein substance, found in almost all animal and many plant tissues, that is soluble in water and coagula-

8

ble by heat. Both words obviously come from the Latin *albus,* "white." "Albumen" is the older word for the simple reason that egg white was known long before biochemistry became a science. The distinctive spelling of "albumin" probably started as "albumine," indicating a substance derived from albumen.

alcohol traces its origin to the Arabic *al,* "the," + *koh l,* "fine, impalpable powder." The first *al koh l* was a preparation of finely powdered antimony used by Arab women to tint their eyelids. Later, the term was applied to any substance that could be pulverized to exceeding fineness. In this sense, a "perfect fineness" would be no powder residue at all, and gradually the concept of *al koh l* as a spiritous substance evolved. Once this idea was conceived, probably it didn't take long to discover that the "spirit" of wine was its alcohol content.

aldehyde is a word contrived to convey the nature of a substance that was recognized as dehydrogenated alcohol. It was Justus Liebig (1803–1873), a pioneer German organic chemist, who coined the word in 1835. Lucky for us he did; otherwise, we might be burdened with "*al*cohol *dehyd*rogenatus."

alexia is from the Greek *a-,* "without," + *lexis,* "word," and means an impaired ability to read or to understand the written word.

alexin was the name given in 1889 by Hans Buchner (1850–1902) to a bacteriolytic substance recognized in blood serum. The name was suggested by the Greek *alexein,* "to ward off." The substance was later renamed **complement.**

alexithymia is a word concocted from a combination of the Greek *a-,* "without," + *lexis,* "a word or expression," + *thymos,* "the mental state or mood." Thus, alexithymia is a condition wherein a person is unable to express his emotions in words. Such a condition is prevalent among patients seeking medical help because of socalled functional disorders. Not being aware of, or unable to express his condition as "depression," the patient complains of loss of appetite, constipation, and inability to sleep soundly.

algorithm is being used today to designate a particular procedure for solving a problem. For example, in medical instruction a branched diagram may be used to graphically illustrate the proper sequence of tests needed to arrive at a correct diagnosis. The Oxford English Dictionary calls "algorithm" an erroneous refashioning of "algorism." Originally, algorism referred simply to the Arabic or decimal system of numeration, which was obviously a much better means of solving mathematical problems than the Greek or Latin numerations. The term "algorism" came from *al Khowarazmi,* the surname of the 9th-century Arab mathematician whose translation of an early work on algebra led to the general use of Arabic numerals in Europe. Incidentally, **algebra,** as one might guess, also is of Arabic origin; it began as *al jebr,* meaning "the reunion of broken parts", and specifically referred to the art of bone-setting. Even as late as the 17th century, "algebra" kept its original Arabic surgical meaning. Gradually, the "reuniting what is broken" shifted to the sense of mathematical equations.

alienist formerly was used to designate a physician who specialized in the diagnosis and treatment of mental disorders, particularly one who advised courts of law in judgments of insanity. The insane were thought to suffer "mental alienation," the term being derived from the Latin verb *alienare,* "to make strange or set at variance." Psychiatrists probably are as glad as anyone that they are no longer referred to as alienists.

alimentary is an adjective derived from the Latin noun *alimentum,* meaning "food or nourishment." "Aliment" is an old word for any nourishing foodstuff, and "alimentation" refers to the process of feeding. Lately, **hyperalimentation** has come to mean the provision of nourishment over and above that which can be handled by the alimentary tract, namely, that introduced through a central venous catheter. The Indo-European root has been postulated as *al,* "to grow, to nurture." This led to the Latin *alere,* "to feed or nourish." From this we have a number of words, such as alma mater (nourishing mother), coalesce (to grow together), abolish (to do away with sustenance), alimony (allowance for sustenance), and adult (grown up, the "-ul-" being equivalent to "al").

alkali suggests its Arabic origin by its beginning with *al-.* The original word was the same: *al-,* "the," + *kali,* a plant from which a basic ash was made. The water-soluble extract of plant ashes was, for many years, referred to as "potash," presumably because the ashes were collected in pots. When the principal base metal of potash was identified, a more dignified, Latinized term was required, and so **potassium** was contrived. The ancient Romans had no such word. But in choosing a symbol for the newly discovered element, "K" was selected to stand for **kalium,** which went back again to the kali plant.

alkaptonuria signifies a metabolic disorder wherein an intermediate product of the catabolism of tyrosine and phenylalanine, namely, homogentisic acid, is excreted in the urine. All of this was not known in 1861 when the word **alkapton** was coined by Karl Bödeker, a German chemist. What he did know was that urine of patients with this condition turned dark brown when allowed to stand or when an alkaline solution was added. In fact, he had difficulty analyzing the substance in urine because of its avidity for oxidation in an alkaline medium. So, to name the substance, he contrived to link *alk-,* referring to alkali, to the Greek word *kaptein,* meaning "to gulp down or to avidly consume." In bygone days it was not unusual for a chemist to know Greek.

allele comes from the Greek *allelon,* "of one another," in the sense of counterparts. An allele is one of two or more contrasting genes, occupying the same locus in homologous chromosomes, that determine alternative characteristics by inheritance.

allergy is derived from the Greek *allo-,* "other or different," + *ergon,* "work." In this sense, an allergy is something that "works differently" from the normal. The word was first used in 1906 by the Austrian pediatrician Clemens von Pirquet (1874–1929) to designate what he conceived as an altered power to react. Specifically, "allergy" should be reserved for abnormal conditions arising from the interaction between a sensitizing substance (an **allergen**) and a peculiarly induced capacity to respond to that substance. The consequence of the interaction between an antigen and an uncommon antibody represents an allergy. However, the observation that a minority of people complain of gas when they eat coleslaw does not mean that such persons are allergic to cabbage. Unfortunately, the term "allergy" has come to be used loosely by pseudosophisticated patients, and such loose use has not always been discouraged by their doctors.

alopecia refers to a pathologic loss of hair, as from the scalp, but distinct from the pattern of "normal" baldness in men. The word seems to be derived from the Greek *alopēx*, "a fox." Here the story becomes murky. Is the allusion to the observation that mangy foxes lose their hair? Is it because the urine of a fox was said to make grass disappear, thus rendering turf barren in patches?

alveolus in Latin means "a small tray or basin" and was also applied to a game board containing small depressions to hold pebbles or other markers. By extension, "alveolus" came to mean any small cavity or compartment. Vesalius (1514–1564), the Flemish anatomist, is said to have first applied the word to anatomy as a term for the socket of a tooth, and we still refer to the dental alveoli of the maxilla and mandible. It was not until the 19th century that "alveolus" was used in reference to the tiny air sac that is the terminus of the finest bronchial channels in the lungs.

amalgam is a malleable alloy such as that used in filling dental cavities. The word was a Medieval Latin term used by alchemists to designate a combination of mercury and another metal. "Amalgam" is said by some to derive from the Greek *malagma*, "an emollient or poultice," the assertion being that "amalgam" was an alchemist's anagram for *malagma*. That sounds devious and not a little farfetched. Others have suggested an Arabic origin wherein *al-*, "the," was simply tacked on as a prefix to form *al-malagma*, which then became "amalgam" in a manner analogous to the formation of the word "alchemy."

amaurosis is taken directly from the Greek word meaning "dark or obscure." The ancients used *amaurosis* to describe dullness or dimness of sight occurring without any apparent lesion in the eye. Later, the word referred to impaired vision consequent to disease in the retina, optic nerve, or brain. Amaurotic family idiocy, also known as Tay-Sachs' disease, is a neuropathy characterized by blindness, muscular atrophy, and intellectual deficiency. It results from lipid degeneration in the brain and occurs as a recessive genetic trait, usually in infants of Jewish parents. **Amblyopia** is another word for diminished vision, being derived from a combination of the Greek *ambly-*, "dull," + *ōps*, "eye." It is interesting to note that the currently understood meaning of "amblyopia" has reverted to the ancient meaning of "amaurosis," i.e., deficient or absent vision in an intrinsically normal eye. The amblyopic eye, sometimes called a "lazy eye," does not see because the image it transmits is suppressed by the cerebral cortex. This happens in the case of marked strabismus so as to avoid diplopia; it happens, too, in the case of a severely disparate refractory error wherein the blurred image from one eye is suppressed in favor of the clearer image transmitted by the other eye.

ambidextrous comes from a combination of the Latin *ambo,* "both," + *dexter,* "the right hand." It means that a person can use his two hands as if both were right hands, referring to the **dexterity** possessed by most people in the right hand. A left-handed person who is equally facile with both hands would properly be ambisinistrous, but that word has never caught on and probably never will.

ambulance comes from the French and began as *hôpital ambulant,* literally "a walking hospital." During Napoleon's campaigns, to bring medical aid directly to soldiers in the field, portable units were devised that contained dressings and medicines and provided for evacuation of the wounded as well. When later introduced into the British army, the name was shortened to simply "ambulance." This was the germ of an idea that was effectively fulfilled by the U.S. Army Medical Corps in the Korean War with the establishment of the celebrated M.A.S.H. (*M*obile *A*rmy *S*urgical *H*ospital) units.

ameba is a single-celled organism that, in its live trophozoite form, is observed to constantly change shape by the extension and retraction of its cell wall. The name, which is classically spelled "amoeba," comes from the Greek *amoibe,* "change." The genus is now called *Entamoeba,* implying that the organisms typically inhabit the intestine.

amethyst is the name for a semiprecious gemstone that ranges in color from purple to violet and is a variety of quartz. While the stone has no present-day medical significance, its name has. It comes from the Greek *amethystos,* meaning "a remedy against drunkenness"; this, in turn, is derived from *a*-, "negative or against," + *methyein,* "to be drunk." Presumably the ancient Greeks attributed to the stone a power to deter wine-bibbers.

amino acids are the organic compounds that, when linked together in various sequences, comprise proteins. **Amine** was contrived to designate a derivative of ammonia. Many of the amino acids were discovered and named individually during the early 19th century, but it was not until about 1848 that the collective term "amino acids" was introduced by Jöns Jakob Berzelius (1779–1848), a Swedish chemist. Another thirty years passed before Albrecht Kossel (1853–1927) originated the German term *Bausteine,* "building stones," for amino acids that Emil Fischer (1852–1919), another German chemist, proved to be the primary components of protein. Professor H. A. Skinner has compiled the explanations for the names of certain of the amino acids. **Cystine** was first obtained from urinary calculi by Wollaston in 1810. Braconnot in 1820 found a breakdown product of protein which had a sweet taste and called it **glycine.** In 1846 Liebig isolated a substance from casein and called it **tyrosine** (from the Greek *tyros,* "cheese"). **Leucine,** discovered by Proust in 1818, was later named by Braconnot because of the whiteness of its crystals. Hopkins and Cole in 1901 isolated **tryptophane,** so called because it was a product of tryptic digestion and gave a bright violet color reaction (the Greek *phanos,* "bright").

ammonia in one form or another is a long-lived word and has been traced by some authorities to a temple at the ancient town of Ammon, in Libya. The name of the town may have come from the Greek *ammos,* "sandy," Ammon being located at the edge of the Libyan desert. How the pungent odor of ammonia became associated with a temple at Ammon is not entirely clear. The ancients knew of *gum ammoniac* (the Greek *ammoniakos* means "of or from Ammon"), a plant resin used as a counterirritant and as an expectorant in the treatment of bronchitis. Possibly it was this substance that was processed for healing purposes at the temple of Ammon.

amnesia is a loss of memory. The word is easy to remember because it comes from the Greek *a-,* "without", + *mnēsis,* "memory." Because amnesia can occur in dramatic circumstances, it has been a favorite motif for storytellers.

amnion is the thin, tough membrane surrounding the fetus during gestation. Contained within the amnion is the **amniotic fluid,** in which the fetus is immersed. The Greek *amnion* was the bowl in which blood of sacrificial sheep was collected. The derivation of this word is uncertain, but it may have come from the Greek *amnos,* "lamb." A connection, if there is one, between a lamb and the fetal membrane could well be that newborn lambs were objects that were intimately familiar to shepherding people. **Amniocentesis** is compounded of *amnio-* + the Greek *kentēsis,* "a puncture."

amphoric describes the sound made by blowing across the small mouth of a bottle. Amphoric breath sounds are low-pitched and hollow, and may signify consolidation in the lungs. The Latin *amphora,* "a jar," comes in turn from the Greek *amphi,* "on both sides," + *phoroi,* "handles." The common, narrow-necked jar in those days had handles at both sides.

amphoteric is borrowed from the Greek *amphoteros,* "in both ways." An amphoteric substance is one having opposite properties, for example, being capable of acting both as an acid and as a base.

ampule is known to us as a small, sealed glass container used to preserve medicines in a sterile, stable condition. The word comes from the Latin *ampulla,* "flask." **Ampulla** also refers in anatomy to a dilated segment in a tubular structure. Interestingly, the Latin word also means bombast or inflated discourse, as a "blowing out." Glass flasks were and are made by "blowing out."

amputation is borrowed from the Latin *amputatio,* "a pruning," which, in turn, derives from *ambi-,* "around," + *putatio,* "cutting short, as in pruning." This is not to be confused with the Latin verb *putare,* "to think or reckon," from which we derive our words putative, impute, compute, and computer.

amulet is an almost direct borrowing of the Latin *amuletum,* "a talisman," usually worn about the neck to ward off evil influences. One version is that this is related to the Arabic *himāla,* "a carrier," especially as a cord bearing a small Koran or prayer book and worn about the neck. The early Christians wore amulets in the shape of a fish and bearing the Greek word *ichthus,* "fish." This was an acronym for "*I*esos *Ch*ristos *Th*eou *U*ios *S*otēr" (Jesus Christ, Son of God, Savior). In former years it was not unusual to find children wearing cords carrying little bags of asafetida about their necks. These were intended to ward off infections. Today one occasionally finds a patient presenting himself for a reassuring physical examination and wearing a necklace bearing a saintly image. This is known as hedging a bet.

amygdaloid usually is thought of in connection with the amygdaloid nucleus of the brain, an almond-shaped mass at the tail end of the caudate nucleus. Its shape suggested its name from the Greek *amygdalē,* "almond," + *-eidos,* "like."

amyl- is a combining form coming from the Greek *amylos,* "starch." This, in turn, is a combination of *a-,* "without," + *mylē,* "mill," and taken to mean "not processed by milling." The explanation is that starch was originally obtained from unground wheat. **Amyloid** is a glycoprotein substance that when first found in certain diseased tissues was observed to react by forming a blue color when treated with iodine. Hence, it was thought to resemble starch and was called "amyloid" from the Greek *amylos,* "starch," + *-eidos,* "like."

anabolism means "building up" in the sense of constructive metabolism, i.e., the formation of complex substances from simpler components, as in the building of tissues. The term is derived from the Greek *anabolē,* "that which is thrown up, a mound of earth." The Greek word combines *ana-,* "up," + *ballein,* "to hurl or throw." Anabolism is the opposite of **catabolism,** a destructive metabolic process.

analgesia is an insensitivity to pain or a suppression of the sense of pain, but with the subject in a conscious state. It comes from the Greek *an-,* "without," + *algēsis,* "sense of pain." An analgesic is a medication that suppresses pain without inducing a loss of consciousness.

analysis is a Greek word that combines *ana-,* "up," + *lysis,* "loosening." We use the word to mean breaking up a whole, either material or abstract, into its components, the usual purpose being to gain an understanding of that which is analyzed. This is what analysis meant to the Greeks, too, though they added the sense of dissolution, even death. It has been suggested that the use of the term might have begun with the practice of loosening up earth so as to discover bits of gold or precious stones. In medicine, an analysis can apply either to a substance or to thoughts. **Urinalysis** (a contraction of urine analysis) is the determination of the various constituents of urine. **Psychoanalysis** (Greek *psychē,* "the mind or soul") is an exploration of psychic content, including that which may not be readily evident in the conscious mind.

14

anamnesis is an archaic term for a patient's history. Occasionally the word will be encountered in old medical writings. It comes directly from the Greek *anamnēsis,* "a recalling." The Greek opposite is *amnēsia,* "forgetfulness or lack of recall," and this has become our term for loss of memory.

anaphylaxis is an unusual or exaggerated reaction of an organism to foreign protein or other immunoreactive substance. The word was contrived by combining the Greek *an-,* "without," + "a" + *phylaxis,* "protection." Charles Robert Richet (1850–1935), the French physiologist, first used the term in 1902 when he observed that a dog previously injected with a noxious substance would, on being given a second small injection of the same substance, react violently, often with bronchial spasm. The original concept was that the first injection had so reduced the dog's immunity to the noxious substance that the dog was left without protection against the second dose. It was later learned that the opposite occurred. The first dose actually heightened the animal's immune reaction to the second injection. Nevertheless, a word was born (and Richet was awarded the Nobel prize for medicine and physiology in 1913).

anasarca is a condition of generalized, massive edema. The term is said to have originated as the Greek *hydrops ana sarka,* literally "dropsy throughout the flesh."

anastomosis is a borrowing from the Greek word of similar spelling which referred to an opening or a junction through a mouth, as of one body of water in relation to another.

The word is a compound of *ana-,* "through," + *stoma,* "a mouth." Galen is said to have used the term to describe interconnections of blood vessels in the body. Today, "anastomosis" is used to refer both to a natural opening between conduits (as in arteriovenous anastomosis) and to an artificially constructed connection (as in gastrojejunal anastomosis).

anatomy is an almost direct borrowing of the Greek *anatomē,* the Greeks being among the first to systematically dissect the human body. The Greek word is a compound of *ana-,* "up or through," + *tomē,* "a cutting." Thus, the earlier anatomy was a "cutting up," and dissection remains to this day the essential means of learning the structure of the body. The study of the human body fell into disrepute during the Dark Ages. Andreas Vesalius (1514–1564), the Flemish anatomist, is generally credited with being the "father of modern anatomy," as the study was revived with his publication of *De Humani Corporis Fabrica,* in 1543 (when Vesalius was only twenty-nine).

androgen designates a sex hormone that occurs naturally in both men and women but, when present in excess from either an endogenous or exogenous source, tends to stimulate the development of male characteristics. The term was contrived from the Greek *andros,* "man," + *gennaō,* "I produce." Thus, an androgen is a "man maker."

anemia is from the Greek *an-,* "without," + *haima,* "blood." Hence, a patient who is anemic is lacking in blood. There is a genus of plants called *Anemone,* but this is of quite a different origin. The plants were popularly known as wind flowers, and the name presumably comes from the Greek *anemos,* "wind." Sea anemones are brightly colored polypoid creatures of the order Actiniaria and were named after the flower.

anesthesia comes directly from the Greek *an-,* "without," + *aisthēsis,* "feeling or sensation." In medicine, anesthesia (the British, more faithful to the Greek, spell it "anaesthesia") has come to have two meanings: (*a*) the symptom wherein a part of the body has lost perception of pain or touch; and (*b*) the procedure whereby a patient has been rendered incapable of sensation, either by inducing a state of total unconsciousness or by blocking the neural pathway of sensation in a part of the body. Both meanings were known and used in ancient times. Herodotus referred to the effect of inhaling the vapor from burning hemp, now known to be the result of liberated cannabis. A diminished but not absent perception is **hypesthesia** (*hypo-,* "below"), while an enhanced perception is **hyperesthesia** (*hyper-,* "above").

aneurysm is a near borrowing of the Greek *aneurysma,* "a widening," which is derived from a combination of *ana-,* "up, through," + *eurynein,* "to widen." In pathology the term designates a localized dilatation of an artery. There are berry aneurysms (the allusion is obvious), dissecting aneurysms (wherein the vessel wall is disrupted and split), fusiform aneurysms (shaped like a spindle), miliary aneurysms (tiny, like a mil-

let seed), and racemose aneurysms (clustered like a bunch of grapes), among other types.

angi- is a combining form derived from the Greek *a*[*n*]*ggeion,* "a vessel." The reference, in medicine, is to a conduit for any of the body fluids, notably blood, lymph, or bile. From "angi-" have come such present-day words as angiology, angiogram, lymphangioma, and cholangitis.

angina is a Latin word meaning "sore throat" and comes from the Latin verb *angere,* "to choke or throttle." In former years, submandibular infection was known as Ludwig's angina, after the German surgeon Wilhelm von Ludwig (1790–1865), and "trench mouth" or necrotizing gingivitis was called Vincent's angina, after the Parisian physician Henri Vincent (1862–1950). Today, "angina" is usually associated with angina pectoris (Latin *pectus,* "the chest"), a crushing retrosternal pain resulting from myocardial ischemia. The relation to ischemia has led "angina" far afield, and one may hear of "abdominal angina" as a reference to severe pain in the abdomen resulting from constriction of the mesenteric arteries. The etymologist might regard this as "abominable angina."

ankylo- is a combining form that means "bent", as in the form of a loop or noose, and is derived from the Greek *a*[*n*]*kylē,* "the bend in the arm" and also the looped thong by which a javelin is hurled. The Greek *a*[*n*]*kylos* means "bent or crooked." **Ankylosis** refers to a fixation of joints, either by disease or design, usually in a bent position. **Ancylostoma** (*ankylo-* + Greek *stoma,* "mouth") is a genus of nematode parasites, including the hookworms. This worm finds its way to the intestine, where it hooks onto the mucosa by means of its crooked mouth. The Latin equivalent of the Greek term is *angulus,* from which we get "angle." We borrow directly from the Latin to obtain **angulus** when referring to the bend in the stomach at the junction of its body and antrum. **Ankle** comes from the Anglo-Saxon *ancleow,* which may be a distantly related word.

anlage is a German word meaning "a plan or arrangement." The noun is derived from the verb *anlegen,* literally "to lay on," particularly in the sense of "to prepare or set up." Biologically, an anlage is whatever precedes, or "sets the stage," for something else. In embryology, an anlage is a forerunner or precursor of a more mature structure.

annulus means "a ring" but appears to be a misspelling of the Latin *anulus,* "ring," as that which encircles, such as a signet ring. By the same token, **annular,** "shaped like a ring," should be spelled "anular," but it isn't and probably never will be.

anodyne is a word seldom heard today, but formerly it was commonly used for any pain-killer. It comes from the Greek *an-,* "without," + *odyne,* "pain." Opium and its derivatives, for example, were and are anodynes.

anomaly is a deviation from the normal and comes from the Greek *an-,* "not," + *omalos,* "even or level" and, metaphorically, "average or ordinary." In biology, an anomaly is usually a structure or organ that is congenitally abnormal, but the word can be used to refer to anything that is out of the ordinary.

Anopheles is the name of a genus of mosquitoes that is notorious for transmitting the malarial parasite and, thus, is directly implicated in perpetuating what is probably the commonest disease of man worldwide. The name comes from the Greek *an-,* "not," + *ophelos,* "of advantage or use," and was bestowed on this pesky creature long before it was identified as the vector of malaria by Sir Donald Ross in 1898. Incidentally, knowing the origin of the mosquito's name also tells us the meaning of the feminine name Ophelia—"useful."

anorexia comes from the Greek *an-,* "lack of," + *orexis,* "appetite," and it still means just that. Incidentally, "Orexin®" is the trade name of a vitamin-B supplement purveyed presumably as a stimulant to appetite. The Greek *orexis* could also mean any other sort of "yearning," and perhaps that might account for a form of the male hormone, testosterone, being named "Oreton®."

anosmia comes from the Greek *an-,* "lack of," + *osme,* "smell," and refers to the condition wherein the sense of smell is lost. The element **osmium** is said to have been so named because of the distinctive odor of its vaporous oxide (OsO_4). The Greek *osme* is not to be confused with *osmos,* "impulse," from which is derived the word **osmosis.**

anoxia means "a deficiency of oxygen in tissues" and is derived from the Greek *an-,* "lack of," + *oxys,* "sharp," in the sense of "acid." This sounds farfetched unless one is acquainted with the origin of "oxygen."

ansa is the Latin word for "handle" but could also mean "a loop, as used to fasten a sandal." In anatomy, the word is used for various looplike structures, particularly small loops of nerves.

antagonist is used in anatomy to designate a muscle that opposes the action of another muscle, and in pharmacology to designate a substance having a blocking or opposing effect. The Greek *antagōnixomai* means "to struggle against," and *antagōnistes* means "an adversary or rival." These words, in turn, come from *anti-*, "against," + *agōn*, "struggle."

anthracosis is a lung disease caused by inhaling coal dust and, therefore, often occurs in coal miners. The condition also is called "black lung disease." The name was taken from the Greek *anthrax*, "coal," which by direct borrowing had, much earlier, been used as the name for quite a different disease, as noted below.

anthrax is an infectious disease of wild and domesticated animals that can be transmitted to man. Its principal feature is a carbuncle that can become necrotic and ulcerated. Such a lesion can have a hard, black center surrounded by red inflammation, thus resembling a burning coal and accounting for its name, taken directly from the Greek *anthrax*, "coal." The causative organism, *Bacillus anthracis*, can lurk in the hides or wool from infected animals, and human anthrax has been known as "woolsorters' disease," among other names. The development of a vaccine effective against anthrax

in sheep went far to advance the career of Louis Pasteur, the celebrated 19th-century French bacteriologist.

anthropo- is a combining form taken from the Greek *anthrōpos*, "a man." This has given us numerous words, such as **anthropocentric** (a perspective that places man at the center of the universe), **anthropoid** ("like a man," in reference to certain subhuman primates), **anthropology** (the study or science of man), and **anthropomorphism** (the attribution of human form or character to nonhuman objects).

antibiotic derives from the Greek *anti-*, "against," + *biotos*, "the means of life." The word has had differing meanings through the centuries. The ancients may have used a similar word to mean resistance, presumably to the vicissitudes of life. In the 19th century, "antibiotic" referred to a belief opposed to the possibility of life, as on other planets. The modern medical use of the word was introduced in 1941 by Selman A. Waksman, who reported finding a strain of actinomyces, an extract of which inhibited the growth of some bacteria. In 1929 Alexander Fleming (1881–1955) first reported an antagonism between certain microorganisms, but it was Selman Waksman (1888–1973) who adapted "antibiotic" to describe the process.

antibody is a word contrived in the late 19th century to include a variety of substances that had been discovered to combat infection and its adverse effects. Among these substances were antitoxins, agglutinins, and preciptins. All of these substances or "bodies" seemed to be "anti" something, so they were called, simply, antibodies. Therefore, the original idea was not that these substances were "against the body" but rather that they were "bodies" (for want of a better term) "against" something else. Only later was the word **antigen** contrived as a name for whatever might induce the formation or activity of these antibodies. Today, "antibody" is restricted to the immunoglobulins of the E-type that are elaborated by immunoreactive B lymphocytes.

antidote is an almost direct borrowing of the Greek *antidotos,* which means "an exchange" and comes from a combination of *anti-,* "against," + *dotos,* "what is given." An antidote is administered "against," or in opposition to, a poison.

antigen is a word contrived to name a substance that induces an immune reaction. As noted above, the word "antibody" came first as a collective term for a variety of newly discovered substances that seemed to have a combative or nullifying effect in infection and its concomitants. "Antigen" was devised as a name for whatever stimulated or activated antibodies. The word "antigen" was suggested by the Greek *anti-,* "against," and *gennaō, "I produce."* The sense, of course, is not that antigens are "against production." Quite the opposite: antigens are conceived to produce or generate "antis." If this sounds confusing, it may be because immunologists seldom are as devoted to semantics as to science. But then, could a semanticist have done any better?

antihelix is the name given to the prominent ridge at the meatus of the outer ear. This is situated opposite the twisted part of the outer ear and accounts for the name, being derived from the Greek *anti-,* "opposite," + *helix,* "that which is twisted."

antipyretic is derived from the Greek *anti-,* "against," + *pyretos,* "fever," and refers to whatever has the effect of reducing or suppressing fever. The root word is the Greek *pyr,* "fire."

antisepsis was contrived from a combination of the Greek *anti-,* "against," + *sēpsis,* "putrefaction." Today we think of antisepsis as any treatment that renders an object unlikely to be a source of infection by pathogenic microorganisms. But the word "antisepsis" actually antedates the promulgation of the germ theory of disease. It was first used in the early 18th century to refer to the elimination of anything thought to be putrefactive as a means of combating the plague. Joseph Lister (1827–1912), the celebrated English surgeon, promoted the modern use of antisepsis as a means of reducing infection in wounds.

antitoxin was made up from the Greek *anti-,* "against," + *toxikos,* "poison." The word was first used to describe the substance that could be induced in the blood of animals to antagonize the toxin of diphtheria.

antrum is a Latin word that means "cave or cavity." Its Greek counterpart is *antron,* also "a cave." In anatomy, "antrum" can refer to any cavity or chamber. The maxillary sinus often is called the antrum, and the lower portion of the stomach is referred to as the gastric or prepyloric antrum.

anus is the nether opening of the alimentary tract through which feces are expelled. The

19

Latin *anus* meant the same thing to the Romans. It also meant "ring," in the sense of encirclement. This would seem appropriate inasmuch as the anus encircles the outlet of the bowel.

anxiety is an ancient complaint for which the Romans had almost the same word in the Latin *anxietas,* "trouble, worry." The patient who, as he is being prepared for examination, is found to be wearing both a sturdy belt and suspenders probably is beset by anxiety.

aorta is almost a direct borrowing from the Greek *aortē,* the name by which Aristotle referred to the main arterial channel issuing from the heart. But where did the Greeks get *aortē*? Authorities are divided in their explanations. Professor H. A. Skinner cites the Greek verbs *aeirō,* "I lift up," or *aortemai,* "I am suspended," as possibilities. However, there is a Greek noun, *aorter,* which meant "a strap over the shoulder to hang anything on." When viewing an anteriorly opened cadaver, it is easy to see how the aorta might look like a curved strap from which hang the heart, the kidneys, and the abdominal viscera. Thus the Greeks, who had no knowledge of circulating blood but thought that arteries contained air, may have likened the aorta to a sturdy strap.

aperture comes from the Latin *aperire,* "to uncover or to reveal." An aperture, then, is an opening through which something can be seen. In years past, what we now call laxatives were known as **aperients,** the allusion being obvious.

apex is a direct borrowing from the Latin word and means the topmost point of anything. It is said to have originally referred to the peak of a high priest's cap. The plural is **apices.** Thus we refer to the apex of one lung and to the apices of both lungs.

aphasia is made up of the Greek *a-,* "without," + *phasis,* "speech," and is used to describe a defect or loss of expression or comprehension of language. It is a symptom of various destructive brain lesions.

aphonia is from the Greek *a-,* "without," + *phōnē,* "voice," and means an inability to speak. *Aphonia* refers to a loss of the voice of any cause, from laryngitis to cerebrovascular disease.

aphrodisiac describes a substance said to enhance libido. Aphrodite was the daughter of Zeus and Dione, the goddess of moisture, and was so named because she sprang from the foam of the sea. Aphrodite was the goddess of beauty and sexual love. Her counterpart in Latin mythology is Venus, from whose name we get **venereal,** which means whatever pertains to the act of love.

aphthous refers to ulcers in the mucous membrane of the mouth. The Greek *aphtha* was used as a name for thrush, an exudative inflammation of the oral mucosa. This, in turn, came from the Greek verb *aptō,* "I set afire or inflame." The Greeks had a great fear of *aphthai,* because for them the term also included diphtheria, which they recognized as often fatal to children.

apnea means a suspension of breathing, either voluntarily as in "holding one's breath," or involuntarily as when breathing is impaired by disease. This is just what *apnoos* meant to the Greeks, who derived their word from *a-*, "not," + *pneō*, "I breathe."

aponeurosis is a thin, wide tendon where the dense connective tissue is broadly splayed into the muscle for which it serves as an attachment. That being so, why does the name sound as if it has something to do with nerves? The answer is that the ancient Greeks could not and did not distinguish between tendons and nerves. Dense, white strands looked all the same to them and were called by the collective term *neuros.* "Aponeurosis" is a combination of *apo-*, "from," + *neuros,* in this case "a tendon."

apophysis as the Greek word means "an off-shoot" and was derived from *apo-*, "from," + *physis,* "growth." "Apophysis" now means a projection from a bone other than an **epiphysis** (which has a different meaning).

apoplexy is from the Greek *apoplēxia,* which meant "a seizure" in the sense of being "struck down." The word came from a combination of *apo-*, "from," + *plēxē,* "a stroke." The common belief was that anyone seized by sudden disability was "struck down" by the gods. This idea persists in our use of the word "stroke" to refer to the consequence of an abrupt, severe, cerebrovascular disturbance. It is curious, too, that we habitually refer to "cerebrovascular accidents," as if these tragic events were the result of a "falling out" among the heavenly bodies that guide our courses. Incidentally, by knowing the origin and meaning of "apoplexy," one can avoid the fatuous redundancy of speaking of an apoplectic stroke or a stroke of apoplexy.

apothecary comes closer than one might guess, in its original meaning, to the modern American drugstore with its many departments dealing in everything from animal crackers to zippers. "Apothecary" is derived from the Greek *apothēkē,* which means "a storehouse." It was not until the 17th century that England's "chemists" and grocers formally agreed that henceforth apothecaries would sell only drugs, while grocers would limit their trade to foodstuffs. Now, it would seem we've come full circle: modern supermarkets have long shelves laden with over-the-counter medicaments, while drugstores offer almost anything under the sun. By a strange quirk, an apothecary shop today is one that deals exclusively in prescription drugs, eschewing even a soda fountain.

appall is not strictly a medical term but it has a kind of physiologic origin. It comes from the Latin *ad* "toward," + *pallere,* "to turn pale." Related is our word **pallor,** a deficiency of color, usually in the face, caused by stimulation of the sympathetic nervous system that results in constriction of the cutaneous arterioles. Anything that appalls may be so dismaying as to make one turn pale.

apparatus comes from the Latin *apparare,* "to prepare," and is a combination of *a- (ad),* "to," + *paratus,* "ready." This brings to mind the motto of the U. S. Coast Guard, *Semper paratus,* "Always ready." From its derivation, then, "apparatus" carries the implication of some arrangement or device "made ready" or prepared for a special purpose. A meaningless device could not properly be called an apparatus.

appetite is an almost direct borrowing of the Latin *appetitio,* "grasping or craving," which, in turn, is a combination of *ap-,* "toward," + *petitus,* "desire" (*petitus* being the past participle of *petere,* "to seek, attack, or fall upon"). Petulant, impetuous, impetus, complete, and repeat are all similarly derived. (However, the English noun "pet" and the verb "to pet" are not related; their origin is obscure.) Appetite can be a craving for almost anything, although usually we think of appetite in terms of a hearty desire for nourishment. But when a Frenchman, with a twinkle in his eye, wishes us "Bon appétit!" who knows what he may have in mind?

aqua is the Latin word for "water." Some have said that *aqua* is related to the Latin *aequa,* meaning "smooth or level," the idea being that the surface of water in a bucket or a pond, when not unduly disturbed, is level. But most scholars attribute *aqua* to the postulated Indo-European form *akwā.* Surely the earliest speaking man had a word for water. (The English **water,** incidentally, comes from the Anglo-Saxon *waeter,* presumed to have been derived from the Indo-European form *awer,* "wet, or to flow.") Medieval alchemists combined "aqua" with all sorts of romantic terms to describe various liquids: aqua fortis, "strong water," was nitric acid; aqua regis, "royal water," was a mixture of nitric and hydrochloric acids, so called because it alone could dissolve gold (which would seem a royally extravagant, even if remarkable, feat); aqua vitae, "water of life," became a collective term for spiritous liquors. This suggests that prevailing attitudes haven't really changed through the years. The Celtic *uisge-beatha* became "whiskey," and the Slavic *voda* (water) became "vodka." The Scandinavians hardly bothered to change the Latin when they named "akvavit."

aqueduct is borrowed from the Latin *aquaeductus,* which, in turn, is a combination of *aqua,* "water," + *ductus,* "a conduit" (from *ducere,* "to lead"). In anatomy, the name "aqueduct" is given to several channels through various structures, usually for the passage of fluid. For example, the "aqueduct of Sylvius" is the canal connecting the third and fourth ventricles of the brain and serving as a passage for the cerebrospinal fluid. Note that despite its relation to *aqua,* "aqueduct" in English contains an "e" and not a second "a." The classical spelling would be "aquaeduct," but usage has worn away the second "a."

arachnoid comes from the Greek *arachnē,* "spider," + *eidos,* "like," and refers to whatever may resemble a spider. The patient with advanced cirrhosis can have a large belly swollen by ascites and spindly arms and legs shrunken by wasting of the flesh. Such a patient is said to have an "arachnoid" habitus. Also, the arachnoid membrane is a delicate, weblike covering of the brain and spinal cord. The Greek word comes from Arachne, the name of a mythological Lydian maiden who was so adept at weaving that she challenged the goddess

Athene to a contest of skill. Athene tried to warn her of the consequence of her presumption, but Arachne would not yield. The contest proceeded, and both the maiden and the goddess were incredibly deft in their weaving. From this point, there are two versions of the story. In one, Arachne finally recognizes her folly and is so stricken with remorse that she hangs herself; Athene brings her to life, but as a spider. In the other version, Athene feels threatened and uses her supernatural power to imbue Arachne with such guilt that the maiden hangs herself, whereupon Athene turns Arachne into a spider hanging from its web so as to forever serve a warning to mortals who might fall into Arachne's error of challenging the gods.

arcus is the Latin word for "bow," and from it came our words such as "arch" and "archery." **Arcuate** describes whatever is bow-shaped. Arcus senilis is a bow-shaped or circular cloudy opacity at the periphery of the cornea and is often seen in the eyes of elderly persons.

areola is the diminutive of the Latin *area,* "an open space, courtyard, or park." An areola, then, is "a little space." In anatomic description, an areola is usually a small area set apart by being of different color or texture, particularly around a central point. Hence, the areola surrounding the nipple or the zone of erythema around a pustule qualifies by this definition. **Areolar** tissue presumably was so named because of the little spaces between the fibers of loose connective tissue.

argentum is the Latin word for "silver," coming from the Greek *argyros,* "silver," and *argos,* "white or shining." With a bit of license, these words were abbreviated as the chemical symbol "Ag." According to Professor H. A. Skinner, the Greek and Latin words probably originated in the Sanskrit root *radj,* "to shine." **Argyria** and **argyrosis** are terms for the deposition of silver salts in the tissues. This condition is evident as a peculiar, slate-gray cast of the skin and as a dark line of silver pigment at the gingival margin. Years ago this was seen in patients who had consumed large quantities of "Argyrol," a proprietary, silver-protein medicament formerly prescribed for sore throats and nervous disorders. An eccentric Philadelphia doctor, Albert C. Barnes, amassed a fortune from the sale of this concoction. Thereby he acquired a world-renowned collection of French paintings that for many years were jealously guarded from public view in his own private museum.

arm has its analogues in Old Frisian and other Teutonic languages. The Old Norse *armr* referred to that portion of the upper extremity between the shoulder and the elbow, probably more specifically to the shoulder. The Aryan form *ar* meant "to fit or join." The Latin *armus* refers to the shoulder and upper arm. But the word usually used by the Romans was *bracchium,* from which we take the anatomic adjective **brachial,** "of the arm," as in the brachial plexus (of nerves) and the brachial artery and vein. (This is not to be confused with the prefix **brachy-,** derived from the Greek *brachys,* "short.")

armamentarium is a direct borrowing of the Latin word meaning "arsenal or armory" and, thus, a collection of weapons. In medicine, a "therapeutic armamentarium" refers to the assortment of remedies available to combat disease or injury.

arse is a time-honored, if somewhat archaic, word descended from the Teutonic and meaning "the fundament, posterior, or rump" of any animal, including man. Commonly the word is corrupted, through ignorance, by deleting the "r" and "e," then adding an extra "s." This results in a wholly unrelated word that properly designates the long-eared, slow, patient, surefooted, domesticated mammal *Equus asinus.* To the Romans, the Latin *asinus* meant both "a donkey" and "a fool," which seems a shameful degradation of the faithful beast of burden. The Greek word for donkey was *onos,* and the Latin *onus* means "burden." To avoid mistaking "ass" for "arse," remember the limerick:

> There once was a maid from Madras
> Who had a magnificent ass.
>   Not rounded and pink
>   As you probably think—
> It was gray, had long ears, and ate grass.

arsenic comes through the Old French from the Latin *arsenicum (arrenicum)* and the Greek *arsenikon (arrenikon),* "a yellow ointment." Because ointments containing arsenic were thought to be "strong," some writers relate the term to the Greek adjective *arrenikos,* "masculine or male." Another connection may be with the Persian *zarnika,* wherein *zar* means "gold."

arteriosclerosis is a word introduced by Johann Lobstein (1777–1835), a Strasbourg surgeon, in 1833. It is a combination of the Greek *artēria,* "vessel," + *sklēros,* "hard," + *-osis,* "a condition," thus "a hardening of the arteries."

artery has been handed down through the ages as a word for efferent vessels leading from the heart, but it all began with a misconception. The term is derived from the Greek *artēria,* which, in turn, came from *aēr-,* "air," + *tēreō,* "I keep," thus "an air duct." The ancients used *artēria* to refer to the windpipe, but because the efferent vessels from the heart usually were empty when cadavers were dissected, the term *artēria* was applied to these, too. *Phlebos,* from *phleō,* "I flow," was applied to veins and sometimes to blood vessels generally. Although it soon became apparent, even to the ancients, that efferent vessels also carried blood, the term stuck as *artēria leiai,* "smooth artery," in distinction to *arteria tracheia,* "rough artery," which we know simply as the **trachea.**

arthritis comes from the Greek *arthros,* "a joint," with the suffix denoting "inflammation." **Arthralgia** (+ the Greek *algos,* "pain") refers to sore joints. **Arthrodesis** (+ the Greek *desmeō,* "to bind") means a procedure designed to immobilize or stiffen a joint. **Arthroplasty** (+ the Greek *plassein,* "to form or to fashion") means to reconstruct a joint. Remarkably, the first report of an operative attempt to fashion an artificial joint was recorded in 1826 by John Rhea Barton (1794–1871), an American surgeon (*N Amer Med Surg J* 3:279). Only recently, with the development of new materials and innovative techniques, has arthroplasty become widely applied.

articulation refers to the joining or juncture of two structures, usually bones, and comes from the Latin *articulus,* "a joint." This, in turn, is a diminutive of the Latin *artus,* meaning "fitted, close, or narrow." "Articulated" is an adjective applied to any jointed structure. When applied to the act of speech, "to articulate" means to properly join the tongue, palate, teeth, and lips so as to produce intelligible sound.

arytenoid is the descriptive name given to the two opposing cartilages of the larynx. Their pyramidal shape suggested a ladle or cup; hence, their name was derived from the Greek *arytaina,* "a pitcher," + *eidos,* "like."

asafetida is nowadays seldom seen (or smelled), but in years past it was not unusual to find children or adults with a little bag containing this substance tied about their necks for the purpose of warding off infectious diseases. Asafetida is obtained from the roots of certain plants, originally from Persia, of the order *Umbelliferae,* which also includes celery and parsnip. The name "asafetida" is from the Persian *aza,* "gum or mastic," + the Latin *foetidus,* "stinking." The name is well deserved. The presumed protective effect, if any, was because persons wearing asafetida bags usually were kept at a distance by others.

asbestosis denotes a condition caused by exposure to asbestos. Presently, asbestos is recognized as a carcinogen, giving rise to mesothelioma in pleural or peritoneal surfaces. The mineral substance got its name from the Greek *a-,* "not," + *sbennumi,* "to quench," i.e., "unquenchable." The name is said to have been originally that of a mythical substance which, once ignited, could not be extinguished. In some strange way the reference was reversed when the name was given to a substance that would not burn. In a manner of speaking, one might suppose, whatever could not burn would also be unquenchable. In any event, asbestos was known as a mineral fiber to the ancients, who used it as wicks for lamps and as cremation cloths.

ascaris is a direct borrowing from the Greek *askaris,* the name given to intestinal worms. The origin of this term is obscure, but it might relate to the Greek *asketos,* "fidgety, irrepressible," which would aptly describe a person sorely infected by intestinal worms. The common nematode or roundworm was named *Ascaris lumbricoides* by Linnaeus. This would seem a redundancy, because *lumbricus* is the Latin word for "worm." Professor H. A. Skinner has suggested that *lumbricus* and *lubricus* may have been unintended variants due to an error by an ancient scribe, so that the original reference might have been to "slippery."

ascites comes from the Greek *askos,* "a pouch or sack," such as that made of leather and used to carry oil, wine, or water. That the fluid-filled abdomen was thought to resemble a wine sack is ironic in that we now recognize alcoholic liver disease as the commonest cause of ascites.

ascorbic acid (also known as vitamin C) is a sovereign remedy for scurvy, as its name implies, being from the Latin *a-,* "not," + *scorbutus,* "scurvy." The disease was known to the ancients, but not its cause or cure. A dietary relationship had been long suspected. Jacques Cartier, the 16th-century French explorer, is said to have learned from the Indians of Canada how to cure scurvy by making a decoction of spruce needles. But it remained for James Lind (1716–1794), surgeon in His Britannic Majesty's Royal Navy, to prove the ascorbutic properties of certain foods. In 1747, while serving aboard HMS *Salisbury,* Lind gave sailors stricken with scurvy either cider, vinegar, elixir of vitriol, seawater, nutmeg, various cathartics, oranges, or lemons. After six days, those given citrus fruits miraculously recovered; the others languished. This probably was the first "controlled," even though not "double-blinded" or strictly "randomized," clinical trial in medical history.

-ase is a suffix used to designate an enzyme. It is a contraction of **diastase,** a neologism contrived as a name for the first recognized enzyme. This happened to be a substance obtained from malt that was found to be capable of hydrolyzing starch. The word "diastase" appears to have been coined about 1833 and was borrowed from the Greek *diastasis,* which meant "a separation." This, in turn, was a compound of *dia-,* "through or apart," + *histemi,* "to stand." Thus, the substance found to make the components of starch "stand apart" was called "diastase," and this was later recognized to be an enzyme (a word coined later). With the discovery of a multitude of enzymes, "-ase" was conceived of being a handy suffix to append to the name of any number of substrates, thereby designating an enzymatic action.

asepsis comes from the Greek *a-,* "without," + *sēpsis,* "putrefaction." Thus, asepsis pertains when no putrifying agent, such as bacteria, is present. The origin of the term denotes the distinction between asepsis and antisepsis.

Aspergillus is a genus of fungi whose structure was thought to resemble an *aspergillum,* the Latin name for a small brush used by priests to sprinkle holy water. This, in turn, comes from the Latin verb *aspergere,* "to sprinkle."

asphyxia has become a somewhat misplaced term. The word is from the Greek *a-,* "without," + *sphyxis,* "pulse," and should mean "pulseless." Originally the term was applied by the ancients to any condition marked by a diminished or absent pulse. Commonly, in such instances, breathing had ceased also, and the term came to be associated mainly with impaired respiration. In actual fact, when breathing has been impeded, the heart continues to beat, and the pulse persists for a remarkably long time. Nevertheless, the use of the term "asphyxia" has persisted much longer.

aspirate is a term that, in reference to its use in medical parlance, has been turned around from its original meaning. The Latin *aspirare* means "to breathe or blow upon" (from *ad-,* "toward," + *spiro,* "I breathe"). An "aspirate," as a noun in phonetics, is the slightly coughed "h" sound and thus preserves the original sense. But in medicine, "aspirate" is used as a verb with two meanings: to remove gas or fluid by suction, and to inhale foreign substances into the respiratory passages. To suck or to inhale are just about the opposite of "to blow upon," but at least we seem to know what we mean when we talk of "aspirating" joint fluid or when we say the patient "aspirated" gastric contents.

aspirin was originally a trademark that has passed into the general language. "Aspirin," originally with a capital "A," is the name given by the Bayer company of Germany to its preparation of acetylsalicylic acid. Salicylic acid was first extracted from the plant *Spiraea ulmaria,* and the principal component of this extract was known by the German term *spiroylige Säure,* later shortened to *Spirsäure.* An "A," to designate "acetyl," was added to "spir," with "-in" as a suffix, and "Aspirin" was concocted.

astereognosis is the loss of ability to identify familiar objects by feeling their shape. A patient so afflicted, for example, cannot recognize, with his eyes closed, a key that is placed in his hand. The term is from the Greek *a-,* "without," + *stereos,* "solid, three-dimensional," + *gnōsis,* "knowledge, recognition."

asterixis describes the clonic movements, especially of the hands, by patients afflicted with various encephalopathies, but particularly that associated with advanced liver disease. The term comes from the Greek *a-,* "without," + *sterixis,* "a fixed position." The patient with hepatic encephalopathy cannot hold his hands in a fixed position. Sometimes this alternating motion is called a "liver flap."

asthenia means "weak" and is the opposite of "strong." Thus, the word was derived from the Greek *a-,* "without or lacking," + *sthe-*

nos, "strength." The asthenic habitus is that of the thin, frail person. Rather than being content with "sthenic," we describe the husky, muscular person as **hypersthenic.**

asthma is a direct borrowing of the Greek word for "gasping or panting," which, in turn, came from *aō,* "I blow." Asthma was defined as "sonorous wheezing" by Celsus in the 1st century A.D.

astigmatism comes from the Greek *a-,* "without," + *stigma,* "a point"; hence "no point." In ophthalmology, this means "no point of convergence" as a cause of impaired vision. The condition was recognized in the early 19th century and soon after was shown to be corrected by the use of slightly cylindrical lenses.

astringent is the property of a substance, when applied to a moist or weeping surface, to dry up discharges. An example is the use of aluminum chloride in antiperspirants or deodorants. The source of the term is the Latin verb *astringere,* "to tighten, bind, or compress."

astrocyte is from the Greek *astēr,* "star," + *kytos,* "a cell," and is the name given to a star-shaped cell found in the supporting tissues of the central nervous system. An **astrocytoma** is a neoplasm arising from these cells.

asylum is a direct borrowing of the Latin word for "refuge or sanctuary." This, in turn, came from the Greek *asylon,* "refuge," which came from a combination of *a-,* "without," + *sylē,* "violence or right of seizure." In ancient Greece, certain temples or sacred places had the privilege of protecting from seizure slaves or persons accused of criminal acts. From this, the meaning of "asylum" was extended to any place that offered refuge for persons needing protection or shelter. In years past, in our own country, reference commonly was made to "an orphan asylum" or to "an insane asylum."

atavism refers to "the apparent inheritance of a characteristic from remote rather than immediate ancestors due to a chance recombination of genes or to unusual environmental conditions favorable to their expression" (Dorland). The word is derived from the Latin *at-*, "beyond," + *avus,* "grandfather." Hence, an atavistic expression cannot be blamed on Grandfather, but relates to someone farther up on the family tree.

ataxia comes from the Greek *a-*, "without," + *taxis,* "order or arrangement." The term refers to a lack of motor coordination, particularly that disturbing the gait, which is a sign of a neurologic disorder.

atelectasis comes from the Greek *a-*, "without," + *telos,* "complete," + *ectasis,* "extension or expansion." The term usually is applied to the lungs and refers either to a failure of expansion at birth or to a collapse of previously expanded lung tissue.

atheroma is from the Greek *athērē,* "gruel or porridge," + *ōma,* "tumor," thereby having the sense of a swelling with the consistency of mush. In ancient times the term was used to describe any mushy swelling, such as a sebaceous cyst. Now it refers to the fatty excrescences that accumulate in the endothelium of arteries.

athetosis is a condition marked by involuntary, writhing movements, especially of the hands and arms. Such a sign is seen in patients with various forms of chorea. The Greek *athetos* means "lacking a fixed position" and represents a combination of *a-*, "without," + *tithēnai,* "to bring into position." This last part suggests our word "tether," which comes from the Old Norse *tjōthr* but probably shares a common Indo-European root with the Greek word.

atlas is the name of the first cervical vertebra and is also used to designate a collection of pictorial illustrations. What is the connection? The original Atlas was the name of one of the mythical Titans, descendants of the primordial deities. After a falling out with Perseus, son of Jupiter, Atlas was turned into stone and condemned to carry on his shoulders the weight of the earth and its heavens. A depiction of Atlas bearing the globe became a common adornment of maps, and soon a compilation of maps and other illustrations became known as "an atlas." Meanwhile, the bone bearing the globe of the head, i.e., the uppermost cervical vertebra, also came to be known as the atlas.

atom is from the Greek *atomos,* meaning "uncut or indivisible," being derived from *a-*, "without," + *temnein,* "to cut." The idea that all matter is composed of particles was accepted by the ancient philosophers. The ultimate particle that could not be further divided or cut was the *atomos.* Only in relatively recent times did it become apparent that even the atom was made up of constituent parts, the nature of which remains an active field of investigation.

atresia is derived from the Greek *a*-, "without," + *trēsis,* "a hole." Thus, atresia refers to a condition wherein there is "no hole." The term was first used in the 17th century. By "atresia" we now refer to a failure of a structure to become tubular, as in a congenital defect, or to the collapse of a ductular structure. Atresia, either congenital or acquired, can result, for example, in obstruction of the biliary ducts.

atrium was the Latin word for the open area in the center of a classic Roman house. The same word is used anatomically to describe the two smaller chambers of the heart, which consist of open spaces with recessed walls.

atrophy is a close approximation of the Greek *atrophia,* "a want or lack of nourishment," being a combination of *a*-, "without," + *trophē,* "nourishment." The ancient term was used to describe a condition or circumstance wherein nourishment was lacking for any reason. The modern medical use is to designate the consequence of that condition, as when we refer to atrophy of a muscle. Moreover, the sense of the term has been broadened to include the consequence of causes other than nutritional deficiency, as when we speak of muscular atrophy due to disuse.

atropine is named after Atropos, one of the trio of Fates, all daughters of Themis, who served as counsel to Zeus. According to Greek mythology, these three ladies spun the web of destiny for all mankind. Of the three, Atropos made the final and immutable decision. This explains the derivation of her name from *a*-, "no," + *tropos,* "turn-

ing." Atropos usually was depicted as holding shears with which she cut the threads that all human lives hang by. The alkaloid atropine was obtained from a genus of plants well known to be poisonous. Therefore, the drug, too, could sever the thread of life, and so it was named "atropine."

attenuate comes from the Latin verb *attenuare,* "to weaken or diminish." The double "t" is important because it indicates an additive rather than a negative prefix. The Latin verb was derived from *ad*-, "toward," + the adjective *tenuis,* "being thin, delicate, or puny." An attenuated virus is one made weak or nonvirulent by various means.

auditory is from the Latin *audire,* "to hear or to give attention to." This in turn is derived from the postulated Indo-European form *awēi,* "to become aware or to notice." The same form, through Anglo-French, gives the bailiff's cry "Oyez! Oyez!" as he calls for attention in the courtroom.

aura is the Latin word meaning "a breeze, a wind, or the atmosphere." This, in turn, is related to the Greek *aō,* "I blow." Now, the word is used both in the sense of a premonitory sign (as a quickening breeze might signal a change in weather) and in the sense of a surrounding evidence (as an atmosphere).

auricle is from the Latin *auricula,* the diminutive of *auris,* "the ear." The external portion of the ear or pinna is called the "auricle" because it is only a small part of the ear, the main structure for hearing being inside the head. The atrial chambers of the heart were formerly called auricles, presumably because their floppy appendages suggested the ears of a dog.

auscultation comes from the Latin *auscultare,* "to listen keenly." The Latin word also carried the connotation of obedience to what was heard. Therefore, when we perform auscultation in the course of physical examination, we should both listen intently and heed what we hear.

autochthonous comes from the Greek *autochthōn,* meaning "of the land itself," being derived from *auto,* "self," + *chthōn,* "the earth." Thus, to the Greeks an *autochthōn* was an aboriginal inhabitant. In pathology, whatever is autochthonous is found in that part of the body where it originates, as, for example, an autochthonous neoplasm.

autoclave is a hydrid word contrived from the Greek *auto,* "self," + the Latin *clavis,* "key." The original device was a pressure cooker so constructed that the generated steam tightened the lid. In other words, the autoclave was "self-locking." The term now is used for the chamber in which instruments are sterilized by heat.

autogenous comes from the Greek *auto,* "self," + *gennaō,* "I produce." The term, then, means "self-produced." An autogenous vaccine is produced by using bacteria obtained from the patient for whom the vaccine is being specifically prepared.

autonomic is a combination of the Greek *auto,* "self," + *nōmos,* "law." Accordingly, whatever is autonomic is "a law unto itself." When the concept of the autonomic nervous system was introduced in the early 19th century, it was thought the system was self-controlled and not under the governance of higher centers in the brain. This is no longer held to be true.

autopsy is a misapplied term when used to refer to a postmortem examination. The Greek *autopsia* (derived from *auto,* "self," + *opsis,* "seeing") meant, in fact, "seeing for oneself." According to Professor Alexander Gode (*JAMA* 191:121, 1965), for the Greeks this had an even more mystical meaning in the sense of "a contemplative state preceding the vision of God." Professor H. A. Skinner noted that Galen used *autopsia* to mean "personal inspection." Possibly from this sense came the application of "autopsy", in the early 19th century, to designate a dissection of the body after death. Nevertheless, "autopsy" has little but currency to recommend its use and, if "postmortem examination" is too cumbersome, **necropsy** (Greek *nekros,* "corpse") is the preferred term.

avulsion comes from the Latin *avulsus,* the past participle of *avellere,* "to pluck, to pull away, or to tear off." This, in turn, is a combination of *ab-,* "away," + *vellere,* "to pull." An avulsed nerve is one that is torn away from its supporting structures, as by injury.

axilla is borrowed directly from the Latin. To the Romans, as to us, the *axilla* was the armpit. Its more remote derivation is uncertain. *Axilla* may be an abbreviated combination of *axis alae,* "the axle or pole of the wing."

axis is the name of the second cervical vertebra, presumably because the uppermost cervical vertebra (the atlas) rotates around the odontoid process of the one below it. The Latin *axis* means "axle or pole" and is related to the Greek *axōn,* "axle," coming, in turn, from *agō,* "I carry."

axone is an almost direct borrowing of the Greek *axōn,* "axle." The conducting core of a nerve fiber, encased in a tubular sheath, is the axis of the structure.

azo- is a prefix denoting the presence of nitrogen. Thus, azotemia is "nitrogen in the blood." The prefix comes from *azote,* the name given by Antoine Laurent Lavoisier (1743–1794), the pioneering French chemist, to nitrogen. The story is that Lavoisier placed a lighted candle and a live mouse in a sealed jar. When the candle was extinguished, its flame having consumed all the oxygen, the mouse, too, soon expired. Lavoisier knew that gas remained in the jar and observed that this gas was incapable of supporting life. Hence, he called the gas *azote,* contriving the name from the Greek *a-,* "without," + *zōn,* "life." Lavoisier was a little off the mark. Scholars have pointed out that the Greek *azōtus* actually meant "ungirt." In this instance, it appears that Lavoisier was caught with his pants down.

azygous is the name given by Galen (131–201) to the unpaired vein traversing the right thorax. The Greek *azygos* means "unyoked" or "not a pair," and comes from *a-,* "without," + *zygon,* "a yoke."

31

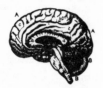

B

bacillus is from the Latin *bacillum,* "a small staff or wand," this being a diminutive of *baculum,* "a rod or scepter." The allusion, of course, is to the rodlike shape of certain bacteria. When first introduced in microbiology, the term was restricted to straight "little rods," in distinction to **vibrio,** which are wavy forms.

bacitracin is an antibiotic substance produced by the Tracy I strain of *Bacillus subtilis,* an aerobic, gram-positive, sporulating bacillus isolated in 1943 from the contaminated wound at the site of a compound fracture sustained by a young girl named Margaret Tracy (B. A. Johnson et al., *Science* 102:-376, 1945).

bacteria is the plural of the Latin *bacterium,* "a small staff," which comes from the Greek *bakterion,* the diminutive of *baktron,* "a cane." In 1853, Ferdinand Cohn (1828–1898), a German botanist, categorized microorganisms as bacteria (short rods), bacilli (longer rods), and spirilla (spiral forms).

balanitis is derived from the Greek *balanos,* "acorn." The Greek word was early used also to describe various things that were thought to be shaped like an acorn, such as small pegs, suppositories, pessaries, and the glans penis. The last reference has persisted in balanitis, an inflammation of the glans penis.

ballotte comes through the French from the Greek *ballō,* "I throw." This led to the sense of tossing an object back and forth. In physical diagnosis, "ballottement" refers to the maneuver whereby a solid mass immersed in fluid, such as the liver in an ascitic abdomen, tends to bounce back when quickly tapped.

balm comes through the French *baume* as a contraction of the Latin *balsamum,* the name of a tree that yielded an aromatic resin that was made into a healing ointment. The

Greek *balsamon* meant "a fragrant gum." Anything that soothes or mitigates pain can be used to excess (perhaps *balsamum* was sniffed), hence the word "balmy" when used to mean "silly or mildly eccentric." **Canada balsam** is a resin obtained from the balsam fir and is used to mount tissue sections on slides for microscopic examination.

bandage originated with the Indo-European *bhendh,* "to bind," and this led to the Anglo-Saxon *banda.* Through the French this became *bandage,* meaning "that which binds." A bandage to the Greeks was *desmos,* and to the Romans *fascia.*

barber comes from the Latin *barba,* "beard." To the Romans, a barber or shearer was a *tonsor.* From this comes "tonsorial parlor," a highfalutin name for a barbershop. The original barbers also were authorized to use their knife blades for the purpose of therapeutic bleeding and were known as "barber surgeons." Their symbol was a white staff, grasped by the patient during the ordeal; around this was draped the red, blood-stained bandage used to dress the wound. The staff was topped by a basin in which blood was collected. This became the familiar barber pole that used to adorn every barbershop.

barbiturate refers to a derivative of barbituric acid. This name was given in 1863 by Adolf von Baeyer (1835–1917), a German chemist. According to a report communicated to Professor H. A. Skinner, Baeyer's synthesis of the substance, from a combination of malonic acid and urea, was aided by the contribution of urine specimens from a Munich waitress named Barbara. Later, "Veronal" was a name given to the hypnotic barbital, presumably in honor of the city of Verona, in Italy. Did those who bestowed the name remember that Verona was the setting for Shakespeare's *Romeo and Juliet* and the place where the hapless maiden quaffed her fatal sleeping potion?

barbotage refers to the technique in spinal anesthesia wherein a small volume of cerebrospinal fluid is withdrawn by needle from the subarachnoid space, mixed with an anesthetic agent, then re-injected. Occasionally, "barbotage" is used more generally to describe any aspiration and re-injection or flushing procedure, as in gastric lavage. The word is French and comes from *barboter,* "to dabble, as a duck in the mud."

barium comes from the Greek *baros,* "heavy." The ore was originally referred to as "heavy earth," and the element was discovered and named in 1808 by Sir Humphrey Davy (1778–1829). The density or "heaviness" of barium is attested to by its widespread use, as barium sulfate, in contrast radiography of the gastrointestinal tract.

basophil is the name of a cell that stains with a basic or alkaline dye because its contents have an affinity for basic substances. The word is a combination of "bas(e)" + the Greek *philo,* "fond of."

bedlam is a word describing a scene of confusion and uproar. It is a slurred contraction of Bethlehem, as in the name of the Hospital of Saint Mary of Bethlehem, formerly an asylum in southeast London for persons then called lunatics. The hospital was popularly known by a name pronounced "Bedlam" and is said to have been frequented by onlookers in search of macabre entertainment.

belladonna is an extract of the leaves and roots of the plant called "the deadly nightshade" *(Atropa belladonna)*. The extract is capable of producing a potent anticholinergic effect, including dilatation of the pupils. *Belladonna* is Italian for "beautiful lady," and the story is that the drug was taken by ladies of Italy to induce a limpid look that was presumably deemed attractive. **Atropine,** the name given to a principal alkaloid of belladonna, also has a feminine connection in its derivation from Atropos, one of the trio of mythological Fates.

belly is descended from an Old Norse word meaning "bag or sack." The Oxford English Dictionary hints that its origin may also have been related to the notion that the belly was the container of the soul. "Bellyache" is used colloquially as both a noun and a verb. When used as a verb, it refers derisively to a common complaint of alleged malingerers.

benign is from the Latin adjective *benignus,* meaning "kind, affable, friendly, or favorable." This, in turn, was derived from a combination of the Latin *bene,* "well," + [g]*natus,* "to be born." A benign person, then, is kind and gentle, presumably because he is "well born." A benign neoplasm came to be thought of as relatively harmless because it was presumed to arise from "well" tissue. Of course, a benign tumor is not always of a favorable disposition.

beri-beri is the Singhalese word for "weak," the duplication being commonly used in Eastern languages for intensification or emphasis. The affliction, now recognized as a polyneuropathy, was endemic in the Far East and resulted from a diet too severely limited to polished rice. Now we know the deficiency to be mainly that of thiamine (vitamin B$_1$).

bezoar is derived from the medieval Arabic *badizhar,* which, in turn, comes from the ancient Persian *podzahr,* the name given to the hair ball extracted from the rectum of a wild Asiatic mountain goat. The hair ball was said to have been prized for its magical efficacy as a universal antidote. Indigestible agglomerations of hair that accumulate in the digestive tract, usually in demented persons who pluck and swallow their own hair, are known specifically as **trichobezoars,** the prefix being the Greek for "hair." Those concretions composed of indigestible plant fibers are **phytobezoars,** the prefix being the Greek for "plant."

biceps is a Latin word meaning "two-headed" and is derived from *bis-,* "double," + *caput,* "head." Anatomically, the biceps is a muscle with two "heads" of origin. The biceps brachii is in the upper arm; the biceps femoris is in the thigh. There is no such thing as a bicep.

bifurcate is from the Latin adjective *bifurcus,* "double pronged," being derived from a combination of *bis-,* "double," + *furca,* "fork." Incidentally, the fork as an eating tool is a relatively recent utensil. The Romans used "forks" more often to support vines or as yokes applied to the necks of slaves.

bigeminal refers to a cardiac rhythm wherein heartbeats occur in series of two. The word comes from the Latin *bis-*, "double," + *geminare*, "to repeat." Also, in Latin a *geminus* is a twin and, in the plural, *gemini* are twins. The Gemini are among the signs of the zodiac (from the Greek *zōdiakos*, "of or pertaining to animals"). Formerly, it was common to swear by the Gemini, hence the old expletive "By jiminy!" (though another possible source is *Jesu Domine*, O Lord Jesus).

bile comes from the Latin *bilis*, which means "gall or bile" and also "wrath or anger." To the Romans, *bilis* accounted for two of the four "humors" of the body: yellow bile, black bile, blood, and phlegm. *Bilis* is said to have been derived from a combination of *bis-*, "double," + *lis*, "contention," the idea presumably being that there are two forms of bile that are responsible for two types of temperament. The reason for this may have been the observation of thin, yellow bile emanating directly from the liver, while a more viscid, darker bile was found to be stored in the gallbladder. This had its modern counterpart in the "A" and "B" bile described by B. B. Vincent Lyon, a Philadelphia gastroenterologist, who analyzed bile obtained by duodenal intubation for evidence of biliary tract disease. Lyon's "A" bile was thin and yellow; "B" bile, obtained after the gallbladder had been stimulated to contract, appeared darker and more viscid.

bilirubin is derived from the Latin *bili-*, "bile," + *ruber*, "red." The purpose of the term, apparently, was to distinguish bilirubin from what were thought to be other forms, namely, "biliflavin" (Latin *flavus*, "yellow") and "biliverdin" (French *verd*, from Latin *viridis*, "green"). When the chemistry of bile was later adduced, there was no need for two words to describe the principal pigment of bile, which, although yellow, was called bilirubin. "Biliflavin" was abandoned. "Biliverdin" remained as the designation of dehydrobilirubin or oxidized bilirubin.

biopsy is derived from the Greek *bios*, "life," + *opsis*, "vision," and thus literally is the "viewing of live tissue," as in the examination of a tissue specimen obtained from a living organism. This is in distinction to **necropsy**, a "viewing of the dead." In common parlance, "biopsy" is used to refer both to the procedure and to the specimen thus obtained and examined. Only the former is correct, but the incorrect use probably will gain legitimacy by currency.

bladder is said to have originated with the postulated Indo-European root *bhel*, "blade, bloom, or sprout." This led to the Anglo-Saxon *blaedre*, "blister," meaning a watery swelling that sprouts from the skin. Thus, **blister, bleb,** and bladder seem to have a common source.

blast- as a combining form also seems to have originated with the postulated Indo-European root *bhel*, "blade, bloom, or sprout." This led to the Greek *blastos*, "germ or offspring." In embryology, the **blastoderm** is the initial mass of cells produced by cleavage of a fertilized ovum. When used as a suffix, "-blast" refers to a primitive cell type from which more highly differentiated cells emerge, as in "myeloblast." A **blastoma** is a tumor resulting from the "sprouting" of primitive cells.

blephar- is a combining form from the Greek *blepharon,* "eyelid." Thus, **blepharitis** is an inflammation of the eyelid, and **blepharoplasty** is a repair or refashioning of the eyelid.

blood is still another word said to have originated with the postulated Indo-European root *bhel,* "bloom or sprout," though the connection is less than certain. The Old English word was *blōd,* pronounced to rhyme with "food." In the early 16th century the vowel sound was shortened to rhyme with "good," and only later did the spelling change to "blood," the pronunciation coming to rhyme with "flood."

boil as a term for a focal suppurative swelling in the skin is said to have originated with the Gothic *uf-bauljan,* "to blow up." The Old English word was *byl,* and in some archaic dialects "boil" is still pronounced as "bile."

borborygmus is an almost direct borrowing of the word that meant to the Greeks what it means to us, "gut rumbling or growling bowels." The inference that it is a classic example of onomatopoeia is inescapable.

botulism comes from the Latin *botulus,* "sausage." The word refers to a toxic condition first observed in 19th-century Germany and immediately attributed to the eating of contaminated sausage. The poisonous substance was called "botuline," that is, "a derivative of sausage." Not until the end of the century was a bacterial source identified and named *Bacillus botulinus.*

bougie is a direct borrowing of the French word for "taper or candle." The idea is not that candles were used to dilate orifices (although this is possible) but rather that dilators were shaped like candles, being smaller at the tip than at the base. Our adjective "tapered" seems to convey this sense. A taper in Old English was "tapur," said to be a dissimilated form of "papur" and derived from the Latin *papyrus,* a sort of paper. The wicks of candles were made from a paper-like substance.

bowel originated with the Latin *botulus,* "sausage," which in Vulgar Latin became *botellus.* This was shortened in French to *boel,* and became *bouele* in Middle English. It would seem that the external appearance of the intestine suggested a sausage. The fact that sausages were originally encased in segments of animal bowel, usually that of sheep, is merely incidental. The Romans had a perfectly proper name for the bowel, *intestina.*

bradycardia is made up of a combination of the Greek *bradys,* "slow," + *kardia,* "heart." The reference is to a heartbeat slower than normal.

bradykinin was discovered as a substance resulting from the action of snake venom on plasma globulin. When injected into experimental animals, the substance caused lowering of blood pressure and slowly developing contraction of the gut. Because of this slow response by the gut, Rocha e Silva and his associates (*Am J Physiol* 156:261, 1949) named the substance "bradykinin," from the Greek *bradys,* "slow," + *kinein,* "to move."

brain is said to have its origin in the Old Teutonic root *bragno*[*m*], Old English *braeg*[*e*]*n.* While this may have a tenuous relation to the Greek *bregma,* "the top of the head," it should not be surprising that there is no classical term, handed down through the ages, for the brain as an organ. The ancients had only a vague and uncertain concept of the brain's function.

breast is a distant relative of the Middle High German *bruistern,* which meant "to swell up." Similarly, **bosom** is attributed to the Sanskrit *bhasman,* "blowing, as of a bellows." **Buxom,** on the other hand, was once spelled *bughsom* and was derived from the Old English *būgan,* which meant "to bow or bend." Hence, in the old days, a "buxom bride" was much admired as one who gave promise of being pliant and obedient. Later, the meaning changed to approach that of "blithe" and, still later, to "full of health and vigor." To have arrived at its present meaning, "buxom" must have suggested to someone that generously proportioned female breasts connoted vim and vitality.

bronchus is a dissimilated borrowing of the Greek *bro[n]gchos,* by which the ancient Greeks referred to the conduits of the lung. This may, in turn, have been derived from the Greek *brechein,* "to be moistened," in the sense that the bronchial lining is always moist.

brucellosis is named after Sir David Bruce (1855–1931), an English army surgeon who identified the cause of undulant, or Malta, fever in 1887. Bruce found the infecting bacteria, *Bacillus melitensis,* in the spleens of British soldiers who died of undulant fever on the Mediterranean island of Malta. The infection came from contaminated goat's milk. *Melitensis* is the Latin form that means "of or pertaining to Malta."

bruise comes from the Old French *bruiser,* "to break, smash, or shatter." When we refer to a hefty bulk of a fellow capable of "taking the place apart" as a "bruiser," we are using the term in the original sense.

bruit comes through the French from the Latin *brugitus,* "to rumble." This, in turn, may have been derived from the Latin *rugire,* "to roar." The Oxford English Dictionary suggests that the initial "b" may have been added for an onomatopoeic effect.

bubo comes from the Greek *boubon,* which was variously used to refer to the groin or to swelling in the groin. An association between pestilential fever and glandular swelling in the groins was recognized as early as the 1st century A.D. Reaching an epidemic scale and more than decimating the population of Europe in the Middle Ages, the disease became known as the **bubonic plague.** The infection is now known to be caused by *Pasteurella pestis.*

buccal in reference to the inside of the cheek is said to have originated in the Hebrew *bukkah,* "empty, hollow." The Latin *bucca* means "cheek" and also "a loudmouthed person." Professor H. A. Skinner recalls that "in Roman comedy Bucco was a clown who kept his cheeks distended in order to receive a sounding smack." The Latin *buccina* (from the Greek *bukanē*) means "trumpet." The buccinator muscle gives tonus to the wall of the cheek and is essential to blowing a horn. However, a buccaneer, while he may be a bold fellow with "cheek," takes his name from the French *boucanier,* originally "one who hunts wild oxen" (the popular meaning of the French *boucan* is "rowdy").

buffer as a term for any substance in solution that serves to maintain a given pH when an acid or an alkali is introduced is said to have originated indirectly from the writings of Søren P. L. Sorensen, a Danish chemist, about the turn of the century. Actually, Sorensen wrote in French and used the word **tampon,** a nasalized variant of the Old French *tapon,* "a wad of cloth used to plug a hole." This was translated into German as "buffer" and so into English, in the sense of "warding off a blow."

bulimia means "excessive hunger." The word comes from the Greek *bous,* "ox," + *limos,* "hunger." The Greeks often used an allusion to the ox to describe whatever was huge or monstrous. In this same sense, we allude to the horse in our use of "horseradish" or "horselaugh."

bulla in Latin was "a bubble, stud, or knob," hence, any rounded protrusion, particularly that which was hollow or cystic. The ethmoid bulla is a rounded projection of the ethmoid bone into the lateral wall of the nasal cavity, enclosing an air cell or sinus. Also, blisters of the skin or blebs on the pleura are called bullae.

bunion comes from the Italian *bugnone,* "a lump." This, in turn, probably is derived from the Greek *bounos,* "hill or mound," which may be of Cyreniac origin.

burking is an eponymic addition to the English language, seldom used today but of interest to medical students. As the study of human anatomy became widespread and essential to the instruction of doctors-to-be, cadavers became increasingly difficult to procure. With no legal provision for dissectable subjects, the practice of body-snatching and grave-robbing flourished. Two proficient procurers in Edinburgh were named Burke and Hare. When corpses were in short supply, Burke undertook to ignore the distinction between the quick and the dead by murdering those poor persons whom they judged to be worth more dead than alive. Robert Knox, then professor of anatomy at Edinburgh, made insufficient inquiry into the source of the specimens delivered to him and became an innocent victim of these nefarious acts, which, when discovered, ended the careers of Burke, Hare, and Knox. Meanwhile, the practice had become a cause for concern throughout Britain and came to be called "burking." The wicked business ended when the sale of legitimately dead bodies for dissection was legalized by Warburton's Anatomy Act of 1832.

bursa is a direct borrowing of the Medieval Latin word for "bag or purse." This came from the Greek *bursa,* "a hide or wineskin." The English word "bursar" is similarly derived and designates "the one who holds the purse." In medical parlance, a bursa is a sack-like structure containing a viscid fluid that serves as a shock absorber and lubricant in bony joints.

buttock refers to one of the two gluteal prominences of man or animals and is a diminutive of *butt,* meaning the thick stump or end of anything. In Old English, -*ock* was a diminutive suffix, as in "bullock," meaning "a small bull," or "hillock," meaning "a small hill."

butyric is from the Greek *bouturos,* "butter," which in turn was derived from *bous,* "ox," + *turos,* "cheese." According to Professor H. A. Skinner, cheese was known before butter, and the Romans considered butter useful as a salve or source of oil for lamps but not as food. Butyric acid was originally discovered in rancid butter.

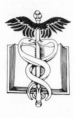

C

cachexia is from the Greek *kakos,* "bad," + *hexis,* "condition or state." Cachexia describes the grossly debilitated condition of a patient with advanced disease or malnutrition. Such a patient is, indeed, in a bad state.

cadaver is derived from the Latin *cadere,* "to fall, perish, to be slain, or to be sacrificed." A cadaver, obviously, is the body of a person who has perished. But why, then, are not all dead bodies so called? Why are only the bodies used for anatomic dissection called cadavers? And only human bodies? Perhaps the answers lie in the Latin sense of "to fall, to be sacrificed." Often, though not always, the body laid on the dissecting table is that of an unfortunate person who has "fallen" in life's struggle and at whose death the mortal remains are unclaimed and unburied, and hence deemed suited for "sacrifice" to the learning of medical students.

caduceus is a winged rod entwined by two serpents. As such it became the symbol of Mercury, the swift messenger of the gods and, in his own right, the god of science and commerce. Also, Mercury was the patron of travelers, rogues, vagabonds, and thieves. By some misconception, the caduceus became the insignia of the U.S. Army Medical Corps. The proper symbol of medicine is the staff of Aesculapius, which is a coarse rod or staff entwined by a single serpent. Why a serpent? To the ancients, the serpent embodies renewal of youth and health, probably because it periodically shed its skin and emerged to all appearances as a freshly transformed creature.

Caesarean section is the procedure whereby an infant is removed from the pregnant uterus by incising the anterior abdominal wall of the mother. In ancient times this was regularly undertaken on the death of a child-bearing woman near term. Julius Caesar, or perhaps one of his antecedents, was said to have been born in this manner, hence the eponym.

caffeine is an alkaloid present in coffee, tea, cola, cocoa, and other beverages. The term is from the French *café,* "coffee," to which the suffix "-ine" was added to indicate a derivative. Coffee, in turn, is said to have originated in the Arabic *qahwah,* pronounced in Turkish as "kahveh." It has been suggested further that the root word was the Arabic *qahiya,* "to have no appetite," the inference being that the beverage was thought to be a stimulus to appetite.

calcaneus is a name for the heel bone (also called the **os calcis**) and comes from the Latin *calx,* "limestone." This, in turn, is related to the Greek *chalix,* "gravel or cement," and to the Arabic *kalah,* "to burn." Lime (calcium oxide) is formed by heating limestone (calcium carbonate). Actually, *calcaneus* came not from the classical Latin but from the Late Latin of monkish scribes. Apparently, something about the heel bone suggested a lump of chalk, which word comes from the same source as does **calcium** and its derivatives.

calculus in Latin means "a pebble," presumably being the diminutive of *calx,* "limestone." Because pebbles were used in counting at one time, we now have our verb "calculate" and its various derivatives, including the name for that branch of mathematics employing highly systematized algebraic notations.

calf as a term referring to the rounded, muscular back of the lower leg comes from the Anglo-Saxon *cwealf,* which meant

the same and is postulated to have originated in the Indo-European *gelbh,* "to bunch up." When the muscles extending the foot contract, they appear to "bunch up." Incidentally, a quite distinct root word, *guelbh,* "womb" (and later, "cub"), is said to have led to the Anglo-Saxon *cealf,* meaning the offspring of an animal, especially a cow.

calorie is said to have had its origin in the Indo-European root *kāl,* "gray, brown, or warm," whence the Latin *calere,* "to be warm." From this came the French *chaleur,* "heat," and then the English "nonchalant," meaning cool or not hot. Incidentally, the Latin *caldarius,* "warm water," led to the French *chaudière,* "boiler," and to our "chowder." A French *chauffeur* was originally "a stoker" and only later a driver of a motorcar. A calorie (spelled with a small "c") is the French unit of heat and is defined as the amount of heat required to raise one gram of water through one degree Celsius. The biomedical unit now generally used is the Calorie (with a capital "C"), also known as the **kilocalorie,** which is a thousand times greater, i.e., the amount of heat required to raise one kilogram of water through one degree Celsius.

calvarium comes directly from the Latin word for a bald scalp or the dome of the skull. More familiar to lay persons is the name "Calvary," given to "the place of the skull" in the outskirts of Jerusalem where Jesus was crucified in the year that came to be A.D. 33. Another name for the same place is "Golgotha," which is Aramaic and also means "skull."

calyx is a direct borrowing of the Greek word for "the covering of a bud or flower," this in turn being derived from the Greek *kalyptō,* "I cover or conceal." This is the sense in which "calyx" is used in botany. The Latin *calix,* "cup or beaker," came from the Greek *kulix* of the same meaning. Whether the calyces of the renal pelvis were fancied as buds of a flower or represent a variant spelling of the Latin *calices* is uncertain.

campto-, campylo- are combining forms taken from the Greek *kamptēr,* "a bend, an angle," and *kampylos,* "bent, curved." **Camptodactyly** (+ Greek *daktylos,* "finger") is a fixed flexion of one or more fingers. **Campylobacter** (+ Greek *baktē-rion,* "a little rod") is a genus of small, curved, gram-negative bacteria that have been only recently recognized to cause dysentery in man. The species so implicated is *Campylobacter fetus,* formerly known as *Vibrio fetus.* The species designation is explained by the fact that the organism was earlier identified as a cause of abortion in cattle, sheep, and goats.

canal comes from the Latin *canalis,* "a pipe, conduit, or gutter." A **canaliculus,** as the diminutive, is "a little conduit."

cancellous refers to a lattice-like configuration of bone and comes from the Latin *cancellus,* meaning "a grating or latticework." Incidentally, a cancelled check or ticket is rendered unusable by inscribing scratch marks or making perforations, as a lattice.

cancer is a direct borrowing of the Latin word for "crab." The ancients also used the word in reference to malignant tumors.

The allusion, doubtless, was to the manner in which invasive neoplasms firmly grasped the tissues in which they grew. Also, Galen (A.D. 131–201) observed, probably of a breast cancer, "Just as a crab's feet extend from every part of the body, so in this disease the veins are distended, forming a similar figure." In Old English, any chronically inflamed induration, particularly about the mouth, was commonly called "a canker sore," probably because the Latin word was pronounced "kanker." *Chancre,* as the French term for the lesion of primary syphilis, also was derived from the Latin *cancer.*

Candida albicans is a species of yeastlike fungus that can infect human tissues. The disease it produces in the mouth or throat is known as **thrush** (a term of obscure origin). An older term for the infecting organism is **monilia,** from the Latin *monile,* "necklace," perhaps because of its strand-like growth pattern. *Candida albicans* would seem to be a redundancy, inasmuch as *Candida* comes from the Latin adjective *candidus,* "gleaming white," and *albicans* is from the Latin verb *albicare,* "to make white." An explanation might be that the growth of the fungus itself is white, and the infection produces a characteristically white exudate on mucosal surfaces.

cannabis is both the Greek and the Latin word for "hemp." The word is related to *canna,* "a reed." Hemp *(Cannabis sativa),* a member of the mulberry family of plants, often grows in marshy areas and this, presumably, is its association with reeds. The tough fibers of the hemp stalk can be fashioned into rope or twine. A coarse fabric woven from this material was referred to as "cannabaceous," hence our word "canvas."

cannula is the diminutive of the Latin *canna,* "a reed," and came to mean any slender, tubular instrument. The double "n" distinguishes this from "canal," though a cannula could be inserted in a canaliculus.

canthus is the Latin derivation of the Greek *kanthos,* "the corner of the eye." Because the Greek word also meant the iron binding of a cartwheel, it is probable that the ancients thereby applied *kanthos* to the entire margin of the eyelid.

capillary comes from the Latin *capillus,* "a hair of the head," being derived from *caput,* "head," + *pilus,* "a hair." The use of "capillary" to designate an exceedingly fine, tubular vessel has been attributed to Leonardo da Vinci in his 15th-century writings.

capsule is from the diminutive of the Latin *capsa,* "box," hence "a little box." In this sense, "capsule" can refer to any encompassing structure or to the small container used for a dose of medicament.

caput is the Latin word for "head, top, or summit." This, in turn, is related to the Greek *kara* and *kephalē,* having the same meaning. In anatomy the term is applied to anything having the shape of a head. **Caput Medusae** refers to a collection of dilated veins around the umbilicus, consequent to portal-vein hypertension. The mythical Medusa was once a voluptuous maiden whose crowning glory was her blonde tresses. By captivating Neptune, Medusa incurred the wrath of Minerva, who, in a rage, turned Medusa's hair into writhing serpents

and transfigured the poor girl into a hideous Gorgon. So frightful was the sight of the transformed Medusa that whoever looked on her was turned to stone. It was the heroic Perseus who succeeded in beheading Medusa, whereupon he presented the trophy to Minerva, who emblazoned the figure of Medusa's head on her breastplate.

carbohydrate is a hybrid term combining the Latin *carbo,* "charcoal," and the Greek *hydōr,* "water," thus designating substances composed of carbon, hydrogen, and oxygen (the last two in the proportions found in water).

carbuncle is the diminutive of the Latin *carbo,* "coal or charcoal." The allusion is to "a little, live coal." To the Romans, *carbunculus* also referred to the garnet, a red gemstone. For a focal, inflamed swelling in the skin and subcutaneous tissues to be called a "carbuncle" seems natural. Interestingly, **anthrax,** producing a similar lesion, is so called from the Greek word for coal.

carcinoid tumors, found usually in the gastrointestinal tract but occasionally elsewhere, are so called because, when first described in the early 19th century, they appeared to resemble cancerous neoplasms but were thought benign in their limited growth and lack of adverse effects in their hosts. Hence, the name was contrived by combining "carcin-" (from "carcinoma") + "-oid" (from the Greek *eidos,* "like"). However, in 1954 Jan Waldenström and his Swedish associates, among others, demonstrated a peculiar syndrome of cutaneous flushing and endocardial lesions occurring in patients whose carcinoid tumors had metastasized from the small intestine to the liver. Such tumors were found to secrete toxic amounts of serotonin and various vasoactive peptides.

carcinoma is supposed to have originated with the Indo-European root *kar, karkar,* "hard." From this came the Greek *karkinos,* "crab," presumably because of the crustacean's hard shell. In Hippocratic writings, *karkinos* is used to refer to any firmly indurated, nonhealing ulcer, whereas *karkinōma* (the suffix designating "a swelling") indicated a malignant tumor. Not until the 19th century was "carcinoma" restricted to malignant neoplasms of epithelial origin.

cardiac is said to have been traced to the Indo-European root *kered,* which meant "heart," as does the Greek *kardia* in Hippocratic treatises. The term also has been applied to structures near the heart, especially the most proximal portion of the stomach at the entrance of the esophagus. Probably in such usage the adjective "cardial" rather than "cardiac" would help to avoid confusion.

caries is the Latin word for "decay or rot" and has been applied to such foci in teeth and bones.

carina is the Latin word for "keel of a boat" and has been borrowed by both plant and animal anatomists to refer to any projecting ridge. For example, the carina of the trachea is the semilunar ridge marking the bifurcation leading into the mainstem bronchi.

carminative refers to any medication given to allay indigestion, particularly that to relieve gas, belching, and flatulence. The newer physiology has validated the old empiric use of certain carminatives. For example, peppermint was long included in prescriptions for its carminative effect. Now it is known that peppermint tends to relax the lower esophageal sphincter, thus allowing the eructation of troublesome stomach gas. The mints provided at the exit of a restaurant, therefore, serve a rational function, although it is unlikely that the proprietor ever heard of the lower esophageal sphincter. The origin of "carminative" is uncertain. Some say it may have been derived from the Latin *carmen,* "a song, lyric poem, or ritual formula." Others contend that it is more likely to have come from the Latin *carminare,* "to card wool," the allusion being to the effect of clearing out the adventitious substances causing dyspepsia.

carotid is taken from the Greek *karotides,* an ancient term for the principal arteries in the neck leading to the head. The Greek *karotikos* meant "stupefying," as apparently it was known that sustained pressure on the arteries of the neck caused insensibility. "To garrote," originally a Spanish technique for inflicting capital punishment by tightening an iron collar around the neck of the condemned, can be similarly traced to the Greek *karotikos.* On the other hand, "karate," a term for one of the martial arts, cannot. This comes from a Japanese word meaning "empty hands," thus signifying that in karate no weapon is used other than the bare hands.

carpal is from the Greek *carpos,* "wrist." The Indo-European root has been postulated as *k[w]erp,* "to twist." For centuries, the eight carpal bones were only numbered, and it was not until the early 18th century that they were given individual names.

cartilage is from the Latin *cartilago,* "gristle." The Greek word for cartilage is *chondros,* and this provides **chondro-,** the usual combining form applied in anatomic terms.

caruncle is from the Latin *caruncula,* the diminutive form of *caro,* "flesh"; hence *caruncula* means, literally, "a little bit of flesh." The term was applied to various fleshy projections from mucous membranes. An example is the lacrimal caruncle, the small, red body at the inner canthus of the eye.

cáscara sagrada is Spanish and means "sacred bark." In the usual English pronunciation, the accent is on the second syllable of "cascara." The source of the substance is *Rhamnus purshiana,* better known as "the buckthorn tree." The tree was held sacred by the ancient Greeks for reasons that are not now clear. Not until the 13th century is there a record of an extract from the bark having been used as a cathartic in Europe. The cathartic property owes to its content of anthroquinones.

casein comes from the Latin *caseus,* "cheese." Casein now refers to the protein of milk, a particularly valuable source of nourishment inasmuch as it contains all the essential amino acids.

castor oil formerly was called *oleum ricini,* and its active cathartic ingredient is now known as ricinoleic acid. The oil is expressed from the seeds of *Ricinus communis,* also known as "the castor bean" or "palma Christi," probably because the appearance of the bean was likened to the scarred palm of Christ. The Latin *ricinus*

referred to "the sheep tick," and apparently the castor bean was thought to resemble this small creature. An explanation of "castor" is uncertain. It is not related to the Latin word for "beaver," and castor oil is not to be confused with "castoreum," a substance obtained from certain glands of the beaver and used as a base for perfume. Rather, it has been suggested that "castor oil" was a confused expression of "Christi oil."

castrate comes from the Latin *castrare,* "to prune, to cut off" and specifically "to remove the testicles." Women are said to be castrated when the ovaries are removed. The Indo-European root word is said to have been *kes,* "to cut, or a knife."

catabolism is a borrowing of the Greek *katabolē,* "a throwing down." This, in turn, is a combination of *kata,* "down," + *ballein,* "to throw." Thus, catabolism is a throwing or tearing down of body tissue.

catalepsy is an almost direct borrowing of the Greek *katalēpsis,* which was used by Hippocrates to designate any abrupt seizure or sudden incapacitating sickness. The Greek word is derived from *kata,* "down," + *lambanein,* "to get hold of." The term is used now to indicate a state of unresponsive rigidity.

cataract is probably from the Greek *katarraktes,* "something that rushes down." This could apply to the rapid descent of water in a stream or to the dropping of a gate or grating of a window. In reference to an opacity in the ocular lens, the allusion presumably is to the closure of a window. An alternative explanation is that the term for the ocular lesion comes rather from the

Greek *katarraptes,* "to cover over by stitching or patching," and that "catarapt" was mistakenly converted to "cataract."

catarrh is from the Greek *katarroia,* "a running down." The Greek *katarrein,* "to flow down," came from *kata,* "down," + *rhein,* "to run or flow." The Greeks used *katarroia* to refer to any supposed humor that had formed in excess and was discharged by the body. Ordinary nasal catarrh or "a runny nose" was attributed to a running down of fluid from the brain into the nose. "Catarrh" also was once used loosely to refer to any inflammation, especially that implying congestion. Infectious hepatitis was formerly called "catarrhal jaundice."

catatonia is a nearly direct borrowing of the Greek *katatonos,* "a stretching down." Hippocrates is said to have used the verb *katateinein* in the sense of "to stretch for the purpose of setting a bone." The word now refers to a manifestation of schizophrenia wherein the patient exhibits a stubborn negativism, often with a stuporous rigidity alternating with impulsive excitement.

catgut is a suture material that was never made from the gut of a cat. Rather, it was fabricated from the intestine of sheep. Why, then, the cat? Probably this was a transliteration of "kit," an old word for a fiddle, the strings of which were made from gut. Kit, in turn, probably came to be used as a contraction of the Greek *kithara,* "a lyre, harp, or lute." From this also came the name of the familiar guitar.

catharsis is a direct borrowing of the Greek *katharsis,* "a cleansing." Originally the term "cathartic" was applied to all medi-

cines supposed to cleanse or purify, thus ridding the body of disease. Later it was restricted to purgative agents. Willard Espy observes that the given name Catharine is taken from the same Greek source, meaning "pure." His arch comment: "Whether you trace cathartic to Catharine or back to the original Greek depends, I suppose, on how, if a woman, you feel about yourself, or how, if a man, you feel about women."

catheter was used by the Greeks, as *katheter,* to refer to any instrument that was inserted for a purpose, such as a plug or pessary. The word came from the Greek *kathiemai,* "to send down or to sound," as a probe. The ancients used a hollow metal tube as a means of emptying the urinary bladder, and this they called a *katheter.*

Caucasian as sometimes used to designate a person whose skin is white, or nearly so, has a curious origin. According to Professor Alexander Gode (*JAMA* 185:574, 1963), the association of "Caucasian" and "white" goes back to 1781, when a German anthropologist, Johann Friedrich Blumenbach (1752–1840), proposed on the basis of his craniometric researches a fivefold division of mankind into whites (Caucasians), blacks (Negroes), yellows (Mongols), browns (Malaysians), and reds (Americans). Blumenbach called the whites "Caucasians" because what he regarded as the ideal whiteman's skull was most nearly represented by a specimen from the southern Caucasus, a mountain range between the Caspian and Black seas in what is now the southwest corner of the Soviet Union. Even today in case reports one occasionally finds a "white man" called a "Caucasian male." This is a pseudoscientific pomposity.

cauda is the Latin word for "tail." The **cauda equina,** the array of sacral and coccygeal nerves emanating from the tapered end of the spinal cord, is so called because it resembles "a horse's tail." The **caudate** lobe of the liver extends downward along the posterior surface as a sort of tail of the liver.

causalgia is a combination of the Greek *kausis,* "burning," + *algos,* "pain." The term refers to a burning pain, especially in an extremity, associated with atrophic skin changes owing to peripheral nerve injury.

caustic comes from the Greek *kausteira,* "burning," in the sense of whatever is capable of inducing a corrosive burn.

cautery comes from the Greek *kautērion,* "a branding iron." In the past, a distinction was made between "actual cautery" and "potential cautery." In actual cautery, searing heat was delivered to an area by an instrument made hot in a flame. A potential cautery was effected by a caustic substance that, when applied to a surface, produced coagulation by a chemical reaction, usually attended by a burning sensation.

cecum is spelled *caecum* by purists and is taken from the Latin *caecus,* "blind." It refers to the *cul de sac* (French, "bottom of the sack") of the proximal colon just below the entrance of the ileum. The cecal sac is "blind" in that its lumen leads nowhere. An earlier term for this appendage of the colon was the Greek *typhlos* "blind," from *typhos,* "smoke," from the sense in which smoke obscures vision or shuts out light. An old term for inflammation of the cecum was

typhlitis; inflammation of the vermiform appendix was **perityphlitis.**

-cel- is a combining form that can be attributed to either of two Greek words which, while distinct, have somewhat related meanings: *kēlē,* "a rupture or hernia," and *koilos,* "hollow, as a cavity." In the Anglicized forms, the "k" is made "c" (except in "keloid"), and the Greek *koil-* is usually spelled "coel-." Here is where the confusion begins. **Hydrocele** is sometimes misspelled "hydrocoele." **Celiac,** as it is usually spelled in the U.S., actually comes from *koilos,* which is why purists insist on spelling it "coeliac," and they are right. Some people think it a pedantic affectation to use "coel-" for "cel-," but there is more to it than that; these are different derivatives. **Celom,** the primitive body cavity of the embryo, really should be spelled "coelom." The "celiac" artery and plexus are so named because they serve the contents of the abdominal cavity; thus, the spelling should be "coeliac." *Coeliaca* was used by the ancients to describe any condition marked by swelling of the belly. Coeliac (often spelled "celiac" by Americans) disease, a feature of which is abdominal distention, now refers specifically to primary intestinal malabsorption as it occurs in children or adults (and is otherwise known as "nontropical sprue").

cell is from the Latin *cella,* its earliest meaning being "a place to hide and store grain, fruits, oil, or wine." The origin of our common word "cellar" is thus evident, as is the use of "jail cell." Later, *cella* came to refer to any relatively small, confined space, and it is in this sense that it was applied to the basic organic unit of life that we recognize now as a cell. **Cellulose** is derived from the Latin *cellula,* "a little cell." This is the substance which forms the exoskeleton of plant cells.

centigrade is a French word derived from the Latin *centum,* "one hundred," + *gradus,* "a step or degree." In 1742 the Swedish scientist Anders Celsius (1701–1744) proposed an eminently sensible scheme of dividing the span in temperature from the freezing to boiling points of water into one hundred degrees (0° to 100°), thus providing a centigrade scale. It is only a coincidence that the initial "C," used to designate temperature readings from such a scale, stands for both "centigrade" and **Celsius** (who, of course, is not to be confused with Celsus, the renowned 1st century A.D. Roman encyclopedist). Thus, on the centigrade scale, the normal human body temperature is 37° C., this having now supplanted the formerly familiar 98.6° F. The "F," as everyone knows, is the initial of the surname of Gabriel Daniel Fahrenheit, a German physicist who was born and lived (from 1686 to 1736) in the Baltic seaport of Gdańsk, then under Prussian domination and known as Danzig. The **Fahrenheit** scale, now used popularly only in the U.S., makes very little sense (with 32° F. being the freezing point of water and 212° F. its boiling point) and seems almost arbitrary. The probably apocryphal story goes that on one bitterly cold winter day in Danzig, Fahrenheit decided the outdoor temperature could hardly go lower, so he set that reading for his scale at 0°; also he had a cold, felt feverish, took his own body tem-

perature, and called that 100°. Ever since, most of us have gauged temperatures according to this seemingly whimsical scale. Fortunately, the centigrade, or Celsius, scale is now coming into almost universal use.

cephalic comes from the Greek *kephalē,* "head." An exception in usage, however, is the "cephalic" vein, which courses along the outer aspect of the upper arm. In Arabic, according to Professor H.A. Skinner, this vein was called *al-kifal,* "the outer," and by mistaken translation this became *"cephalic."* This may have led to the erroneous notion that bleeding from the cephalic vein would draw blood from the head. Note that there is no corresponding cephalic artery (excepting, perhaps, the brachiocephalic, or innominate, artery, a trunk serving both the right arm and the head).

cerebellum is so called as the diminutive of the Latin *cerebrum,* "the brain." Hence, the cerebellum is "the little brain." The distinctive function of the cerebellum in coordinating muscular action was not recognized until the early 19th century.

cerebrum is the Latin word for "brain." The Romans used the same word variously to refer to the head, the skull, understanding, and a hot temper.

ceruloplasmin is an alpha-2 globulin in serum that transports copper. The name is a hybrid concoction of the Latin *caerulus,* "azure," + the Greek *plasma,* "anything molded, as a pervading substance." The reference to a blue color relates to the reaction for copper in qualitative analysis. In another usage, the **locus ceruleus** is a pigmented eminence ("blue spot") in the superior angle of the floor of the fourth ventricle.

cerumen is from the Latin *cera* and the Greek *keros,* both meaning "wax." But the Romans used no such word for the waxy accumulation in the external auditory canal. To them it was *sordes aurium,* "the dirt of the ear."

cervix is Latin for "neck," particularly the nape or back of the neck. In anatomy, "cervix" is used to describe the narrow or neck-like portion of a structure, as in the uterine cervix. From the Latin noun comes the adjective **cervical,** which can describe anything pertaining to any sort of neck.

cestode is from the Latin *cestus,* "girdle or belt." This, in turn, is said to have been derived from the Greek *kestos,* "stitched or embroidered," especially as a girdle might be so fabricated or decorated. In medicine, "cestode" refers to any tapeworm of the phylum Platyhelminthes. Such a long, flat worm made up of segmented proglottids might be thought to resemble an embroidered belt.

chalazion is the diminutive of the Greek *chalaza,* which meant both "hail," referring to pellets of ice, and "a small pimple or tubercle." The relation between the two meanings is somewhat obscure. In any case, "chalazion" is now used as the term for an inflamed swelling of a Meibomian gland in the margin of the eyelid. The gland was so named after Heinrich Meibom (1638–1700), a German anatomist.

chancre is a French word meaning "ulcer," coming from the Latin *cancer,* "crab," probably because chronic ulcers often are hard and indurated like a crab's shell. In modern times, "chancre," both in French and in English, has come to refer to the venereal sore of primary syphilis. **Chancroid,** the lesion caused by infection with *Hemophilus ducreyi,* somewhat resembled a chancre but was recognized as a different disease.

charlatan is a derogatory term applied to a physician or quasi-medical practitioner held in disrepute because he makes claims for remedies that lack efficacy. The word is borrowed from the French, where it was adapted, in turn, from the Italian *ciarlare,* meaning "to babble, to prattle, or to chatter." Thus, a charlatan is one who talks a good game but can't produce. The allusion is similar to that which gave rise to **quack.**

charley horse is a term commonly used to describe intense pain and stiffness, usually in thigh muscles and especially consequent to athletic stress. The explanation is said to be that Charley was the name given customarily to an elderly, often partially lame horse that was retired from more strenuous service and reserved for family use.

cheek is said to go back to the Anglo-Saxon *cē[a]ce,* "the jaw." Later, the Middle English *cheke* referred to the fleshy part of the jaw or the jowl. Sometimes the fleshy roundness of the fundament is called "the cheek of the buttocks," but this is a long way from the jaw.

chemo- is a combining form taken from the Late Greek *chēmeia,* which had a meaning similar to "chemistry," albeit consonant with the primitive science then known to the ancients. The origin of the Greek word is obscure. Some authorities have contended that it relates to a similar word that was an arcane name for Egypt and also meant "black." It seems that conjuring the chemical substances was early referred to as "the Egyptian or the black art." Passing into Arabic, the prefix *al-* was added, and the word became **alchemy.** Much of the medieval preoccupation with seeking a transmutation of base metals into gold was known by this term. After the 16th century, the *al-* was dropped, and modern **chemistry** is said to date from 1661, when Robert Boyle (1627–1691), an English natural philosopher, established a distinction between chemical elements and compounds. **Chemotaxis** (+ Greek *taxis,* "an orderly arrangement") is the movement of an organism or a cell in response to a chemical concentration gradient. **Chemotherapy** (+ Greek *therapeia,* "treatment") is a term first used by Paul Ehrlich (1854–1915), the German bacteriologist (who shared with Elie Metchnikoff the Nobel prize for medicine and physiology in 1908), in reference to the effects of chemical agents on living cells, including microorganisms. Ehrlich's concept of selective chemical destruction of infecting organisms led to his discovery of arsphenamine, an arsenical compound then better known as "Salvarsan," as a treatment for syphilis and other treponemal infections. Salvarsan was designated by Ehrlich as "606" because it was the product of his 606th experiment in his search for such a compound. Today, "chemotherapy" is thought of principally in regard to the use of chemical agents to combat cancer.

cheno- is a combining form taken from the Greek *chē,* "goose." Chenodeoxycholic acid is a bile acid first obtained from goose gall and is currently being investigated as a medication for the dissolution of gallstones. Ursodeoxycholic acid, first obtained from the bile of bears (Latin *ursus,* "bear"), is being similarly studied.

Cheshire cat syndrome refers more to the physician than to the patient and was the term used by Dr. E. G. L. Bywaters (*Postgrad Med J* 44:19, 1968) to describe his plight at being confronted by a trio of patients exhibiting all the signs of polyarteritis nodosa but not, in fact, having the disease. The allusion is to the befuddlement of Alice in Wonderland at seeing the grin without the cat. Should one address oneself to the grin, thought Alice, or wait until the features of the cat were more clearly discernible? Should one treat the patient who appears to have a suggestive sign of disease, mused Bywaters, or withhold treatment until unmistakable evidence of the disease is in full array?

chest comes from the Greek *kiste,* "a box." In Old English, the word was variously spelled cist, ciest, cest, and finally chest.

chiasma is a Greek word meaning "crossed like the letter 'X.'" Hence, the optic chiasma, a decussation of the optic nerve tracts, has an X-configuration.

chicken pox is said to be so called not because the disease was thought to come from the familiar fowl but to distinguish its typically mild course from that of the more grave smallpox. The distinction between the two diseases was first established by William Heberden (1710–1801), an English physician. "Chicken" has been used otherwise to connote weakness or pettiness, as in "chicken-hearted" and "chicken feed."

chimera is an almost direct borrowing of the Greek name for a mythologic monster having a lion's head, a goat's body, and a dragon's tail. The fire-breathing *chimaira,* as it was spelled by the Greeks, was among the unpleasant creatures that inhabited the infernal regions of Pluto's domain. In medicine, a chimera is "an individual organism whose body contains cells derived from different zygotes, of the same or different species, occurring spontaneously as in twins (blood-group chimeras) or produced artifically, as an organism that develops from combined portions of different embryos or one in which tissue or cells of another organism have been introduced" (Dorland).

chiropractic is a system of therapeutics based on the contention that disease results from neural dysfunction, and that this can be corrected by manipulation of the spinal column and adjacent structures. The word is a concoction of the Greek *cheir,* "hand," + *praktikos,* "fit for doing." The term thus emphasizes the manipulative aspect of treatment.

chloroform is so called because it is a compound of chlorine (named from the Greek *chloros,* "green," because of its color as a gas) and formyl ($CHCl_3$). Its use as a surgical anesthetic agent was first demonstrated in 1847 by Sir James Simpson (1811–1870), an obstetrician of Edinburgh. This was the year following the initial public demonstration of ether in Boston. Chloroform became popular, especially in Britain during the en-

suing century, in part because it was administered successfully to Queen Victoria during childbirth. With increasing recognition of its hepatotoxic and cardiodepressant effects, and because better agents became available, its use in anesthesia eventually was abandoned.

cholecyst- in its various combinations comes from the Greek *cholē,* "bile," + *kystis,* "bladder." Thus, **cholecystectomy** is "a cutting out of the gallbladder"; **cholecystography** is "a recording of the gallbladder"; and **cholecystokinin** is "a substance that 'moves' the gallbladder," i.e., causes it to contract.

choledochus is a Latinized name for the common bile duct which is, by itself, seldom heard. It is derived from the Greek *cholē,* "bile," + *dochē,* "a receptacle." "Choledocho-," however, is a more familiar combining form used to indicate whatever may pertain to the common bile duct.

cholera is a direct borrowing of the Greek name for a disease characterized by intense vomiting and diarrhea. Whether such cases so called by the ancients included those that would be identified as cholera today is uncertain. Several possible derivations of the Greek *cholera* have been proposed. One is that the word combined *cholē,* "bile," + *rhein,* "to flow," the allusion being that acute vomiting and diarrhea reflected a profuse discharge of body "humors," including bile. Another holds that "cholera" relates to the Greek *cholos* or *cholades,* "the intestines," to which *rhein,* "to flow," was added. In its epidemic form, the disease often was called "Asiatic cholera," at least by Europeans. It was Robert Koch (1843–

1910), the German bacteriologist, who discovered in 1883 the *Vibrio cholerae* as the infectious cause of the disease.

cholesterol or as it was formerly known "cholesterin," is a complex alcohol often occurring as a fatlike, pearly substance. Because it was first recognized as a constituent of gallstones and thought to represent solidified bile, its name was made up of the Greek *cholē*, "bile," + *stereos*, "solid." The ending "-ol" was later added to indicate its chemical structure as an alcohol.

chondro- is a combining form signifying cartilage and is taken from the Greek *chondros,* which, as an anatomic term, meant "cartilage or gristle." Actually, the Greek *chondros* generally referred to cereal grains which, when cooked, form gruel. Apparently, to the Greeks, cartilage resembled a thick gruel. A **chondroblast** (from the Greek *blastos,* "germ or seed") is a precursor of the **chondrocyte,** the cell producing cartilage. **Chondrodystrophy** is a disturbed growth of cartilage resulting in **achondroplasia,** literally a lack of proper form in cartilage and a cause of dwarfism.

chord is an almost direct borrowing of the Greek *chordē,* "a string of gut used in musical instruments or as a bowstring." The Greek word also refers to "sausage." The "ch" from the initial Greek letter chi is preserved in musical and most anatomic terms, such as *chorda tympani* (the latter word from the Greek *tympanon,* "a drum") and *chordae tendinae* (the latter word from the Greek *teinein,* "to stretch"). The "h" is dropped in the spelling of "cord" as a kind of string.

chorea is manifested by convulsive twitchings or movements that suggest a grotesque dance. The word is derived from the Greek *choreia,* "dancing, especially group or choral dancing." The symptom, in older days, was known as "Saint Vitus's dance."

chorion is a direct borrowing of the Greek word for "skin or leather." In Hippocratic writings, the word was used to refer to membranes, particularly those that enclose the intrauterine fetus. The **choroid plexus** is so called because of its resemblance to the vascular chorion. The **choroidea** (or simply "the choroid," as it is usually called) is the thin, vascular coat investing the eyeball between the retina and the sclera.

chrom- is a combining form taken from the Greek *chrōma,* which means "the surface of the body, particularly the color or complexion of the skin," and hence has a relation to "color" generally. **Chromium** is so called because its compounds are highly colored. **Chromatin** and **chromosome** were so named because they appeared as particles deeply stained by dye applied to sections examined microscopically. **Chromaffin** (the latter portion coming from the Latin *affinis,* "a relationship, especially by marriage") is a term applied to cells that stain readily with various chromium salts.

chronic comes from the Greek *chronos,* "time." A distinction between illnesses that are abrupt, sharp, and brief ("acute") and those that are protracted over a long time ("chronic") was made in early Hippocratic writings.

chrysotherapy is derived from the Greek *chrysos,* "gold," + *therapeia,* "treatment," and means just that: the use of gold salts as medicaments. Such therapy is prescribed, for example, in selected patients with rheumatoid arthritis.

chyle is from the Greek *chylos,* "juice or fluid." Professor H. A. Skinner points out that in ancient Greek, *chylos* and *chymos* had almost identical meanings, Both meant "juice," but *chymos* referred more to natural juice, while *chylos* referred to a processed juice, as in decoctions wherein a juice was formed by boiling. In reference to the contents or products of the digestive tract, the two Greek words often were confused. However, their respective derivatives, **chyle** and **chyme,** are clearly distinguished in modern physiology. Since the discovery of the lymphatic channels, chyle has been recognized as a product of digestion represented by the fat-laden lymph transported from the small intestine. Chyme is the semifluid content of the alimentary lumen, representing a mixture of ingested food and various digestive juices.

cicatrix is the Latin word for "scar." This is an example of a classical, polysyllabic word having no advantage when compared to a simple, well-known word. To call the mark of a healed wound "a cicatrix" is pompous.

cilium is the Latin term that refers to the edge of the eyelid. The word may have come from the Greek *kylix,* "a cup," the allusion being to the eyelid forming a cup for the eyeball. An alternative origin is the Greek *kylisma,* "a place to roll in." In any case, only much later was "cilia," as the neuter plural, used to refer to eyelashes. It is in this same sense that the term was then applied to the fine, hairlike processes emanating from the surfaces of certain cells, such as those of the respiratory epithelium. The **ciliary** body and muscle of the eye were so called because their plicated appearance suggested that of the eyelashes. The Latin word for eyebrow is *supercilium,* and from this we have our adjective "supercilious," meaning haughty or disdainful, as expressed by raising the eyebrows.

cinchona is the name given to the bark of a tree indigenous to South America. The chief alkaloid in an extract of cinchona is quinine, and thereby hangs a tale. The early Spanish invaders of Peru learned of a "fever tree" whose bark, when pulverized and brewed as a beverage, effected miraculous cures of "the fevers and the tertians," by which was meant malaria. A persistent legend is that the brew was given to the acutely ill Countess Anna del Chinchón, wife of the Spanish viceroy in Peru. On her prompt recovery, her husband introduced the wonder drug to Europe, where it confirmed its reputation by curing the **ague.** The drug was then variously known as "the Countess' powder," "the Peruvian bark," "the Jesuits' bark" (because members of that religious order were the principal importers), and "the cardinal's bark" (because the eminent Cardinal de Lugo in Rome was among its promoters). Carl von Linné (1717–1783), also known as Linnaeus, the famous Swedish botanist and taxonomist, named the genus of rubiaceous trees bearing the bark *Cinchona* in honor of the countess, though in so doing he misspelled her name.

circadian is a neologism presumably concocted from the Latin *circa,* "around," + *diem,* "a day." It is used to refer to events occurring within a 24-hour period, as in a circadian rhythm exhibited by certain phenomena in living organisms.

circulation is from the Latin *circulare,* "to make a circle." Galen (131–201), the celebrated Greek physician, came close to comprehending the circulation of blood but was confused by lacking knowledge of the capillary connection between arteries and veins. It remained for William Harvey (1578–1657), the English physician, to establish the physiologic concept of the circulation. Harvey described his convincing experiments and reasoning therefrom in his monumental *De Motu Cordis,* published in 1628.

circum is the Latin preposition meaning "around or about." From this as a combining form, we get a host of words, including **circumcision,** "to cut around," usually used in specific reference to the prepuce; **circumflex,** "to bend around"; **circumscribe,** literally "to write around" or figuratively "to delimit"; and **circumvallate,** "walled around."

cirrhosis was so named by René Théophile Hyacinthe Laënnec (1781–1826), the distinguished French physician. In describing the scarred livers of alcoholics, Laënnec was impressed by their abnormal color and related this to the Greek *kirrhos,* "tawny," a dull, yellowish-brown. Thus "cirrhosis" as a name has nothing to do with fibrosis, even though fibrosis is a feature of the disease. Unfortunately, "cirrhosis" is commonly confused with other words of a similar sound, such as "sclerosis" or "scirrhous," which are quite unrelated. Also, it should be kept in mind that there is only one cirrhosis, and that relates to the liver. To say "cirrhosis of the liver" or "hepatic cirrhosis" is redundant. There is no such thing as "cirrhosis of the heart" or any other structure.

cisterna is the Latin word for "reservoir" and is related to *cista,* "a box or chest." Thus, the cisterna chyli is a dilated segment in the lumbar region of the lymph channel that becomes the great thoracic duct. Incidentally, this name was disputed as inaccurate because the Roman cistern actually had no incoming or outgoing channels, but the use of "cisterna chyli" was so well established that it defied change. The cisterna magna is an enlargement of the subarachnoid space between the cerebellum and medulla oblongata where cerespinal fluid collects.

clap is a vulgar but venerable term for gonorrhea, appearing in English literature as early as the 16th century. A popular and probable explanation is that the word comes from *Le Clapier,* the medieval name for a red-light district of Paris. The French name means "rabbit warren," the allusion being obvious. A common French term for brothel was *clapise,* a shortened form of which became attached to the disease often acquired therein.

claudication is a symptom of arterial insufficiency in the legs and is commonly misunderstood to refer to pain. The term comes from the Latin *claudicare,* "to be lame or to limp." Ischemia in an exercising muscle causes pain but also impairs contraction, thus causing lameness. "Intermittent claudication" was originally described in horses going lame with exercise and then recovering with rest.

clavicle comes not from the diminutive of the Latin *clavis,* "key," as is frequently suggested, but rather from the Latin *clavicula,* meaning "tendril," the shoot from the stem of a vine by which the plant gains support. The thin, curved bone connecting the sternum and the scapula suggests the tendril of a vine.

climacteric now refers to that time in life when procreative powers cease. The Greek *klimakterikos* was "the step in a stair or the rung of a ladder," hence a point of change at which one went either up or down. The ancient Greeks considered that five climacteric periods marked changes in one's life, the critical years being usually calculated as multiples of seven, viz., at the 7th year, the 21st year, the 49th year, the 63rd year, and the 77th year. The decline in procreative power was thought to be marked by the 49th year.

clinic comes through the French *clinique,* "at the bedside," from the Greek *klinē,* "a couch or a bed." Late Latin writers used *clinicus* to refer to medical instruction given at the bedside as contrasted to abstract lectures and disputations. Nowadays, "clinic" is used to mean *(a)* a gathering of students for instruction in the practical aspects of any endeavor (there are even clinics devoted to baton-twirling, of all things); and *(b)* a place for the assembly of patients, particularly (and contradictorily) those who are ambulatory and not confined to bed, in contrast with those in a hospital. **Clinical** refers to those aspects of a medical problem determined directly from patients rather than from laboratory testing, and a **clinician** is a practitioner primarily concerned with the care of patients, in distinction to an academician or a laboratory worker. The **clinoid** processes are the bony projections that demarcate the pituitary fossa and resemble the four posts of a bed.

clitoris is an almost direct borrowing of the Greek *kleitoris* and is said to be related to *kleis,* "a door latch," the clitoris being likened to a "latch" on the vagina.

cloaca is the Latin word for "sewer or drain." In biology, a cloaca is, aptly, a common ampullary terminus of both the alimentary and urinary tracts, such as normally characteristic of birds, reptiles, amphibians, many fishes, and a few mammals. In human pathology, a cloaca is an anomaly.

Clonorchis designates a genus of Asian liver flukes. The name is composed of the Greek *klon,* "branch," + *orchis,* "testicle." The organism is featured by branched testes. The most common species is *Clonorchis sinensis,* the latter term referring to its Chinese origin.

clonus is from the Greek *klonos,* "any violent motion or tumult." The ancients used this term to describe epileptic convulsions. Now, in medicine, clonus refers to rapidly alternating rigidity and relaxation, such as may occur at the ankle joint. This is in contrast to a tonic, or sustained, contraction of a muscle.

Clostridium designates a genus of anaerobic, spore-forming bacteria commonly infecting ischemic or necrotic tissue. The name comes from the Greek *klōstēr,* "a thread or yarn." The microorganism most frequently found in gas gangrene, *Clostridium perfringens,* is so called from the Latin *perfringere,* "to break up," presumably because it elaborates necrotizing enzymes. *Clostridium difficile,* an opportunistic invader in ischemic bowel disease, is so called simply because it is so extremely difficult to culture.

coarctation is from the Latin *coartare,* "to press together," hence its application to a stricture, particularly in a major blood vessel such as the aorta.

coca is said to be the Spanish spelling of the Peruvian Indian name *cuca,* given to a shrub growing on the eastern slopes of the Andes mountains, but the word may have been derived from the Aymara *kkoka,* which has the same meaning. In pre-Columbian times, it was known that the leaves of this plant, when chewed, yielded a euphoric sensation, thus inuring the user to a harsh life. When the active principle of coca leaves was isolated in the mid-19th century, the alkaloid was called **cocaine,** the "-ine" suffix indicating "a derivative." This name should be pronounced in three syllables, as "koh-kah-een." Alas, it proved too easy to say "koh-kane." When synthetic analogs were developed, it was imagined that "-caine" was a suffix denoting a local anesthetic property, and there followed a host of misnomers, to wit, "procaine," "lidocaine," "benzocaine," "hexylcaine," ad erratum. It is said that the original recipe for the Coca-Cola beverage, concocted in 1886 by John Styth Pemberton, an enterprising Atlanta,

Georgia, druggist, included a pinch of coca leaves. If so, this could have accounted for the drink's early popularity. The Coca-Cola company de-cocainized its coca leaves in 1906, the year of the Pure Food and Drug Act. "Coca" is, of course, not to be confused with "coco" or "cocoa"; all are quite different. The coconut (often misspelled "cocoanut") is the fruit of the coconut palm; its hollow center contains a milky substance, its meat often is shredded for use in flavoring or decorating various baked foods, and its outer covering is used to make mats. "Coco" is from the Portuguese word for "grimace"; three depressions at the nut's base give the appearance of a scowling face. Cocoa, as the familiar breakfast beverage, is a transliteration of *cacao,* derived from the Nahautl Indian name for a small evergreen tree, *Theobromo cacao,* that grows in Central and South America and yields seeds which, when dried and pulverized, provide cocoa and chocolate. The brew contains the xanthine alkaloids theobromine and caffeine. *Theobroma,* as the name for the genus of plants bearing cacao beans, was contrived by Linnaeus in 1737 from the Greek *theos,* "god," + *broma,* "food," thus "a food for the gods"; alternatively, the "theo-" may be a Latinized form of "tea."

coccus is from the Greek *kokkos,* "a kernel or berry." Giving this name for the small, round forms of bacteria is said to have been suggested in 1874 by Theodor Billroth (1829–1894), the celebrated Viennese surgeon. The **gonococcus** is the microorganism of the species *Neisseria gonorrhoeae* and is so called from the Greek *gonē,* "seed, as in semen," because of the mistaken belief that the urethral discharge resulting from infection by this organism was an abnormal flow of semen. The **staphylococcus** is so named from the Greek *staphylē,* "a bunch of grapes," because that is the way the microorganisms tend to cluster. The **streptococcus** occurs in short chains, hence its name from the Greek *streptos,* "twisted, as in a chain or necklace."

coccyx is from the Greek *kokkyx,* "the cuckoo bird." Professor H. A. Skinner points out that the ancients gave this name to the rudimentary tail vertebrae of man because of their resemblance to the bill of a cuckoo. The coccyx was at one time called "the whistle bone," because of its anatomic relation to the source of flatus.

cochlea is the Latin word for "snail," coming from the Greek *kochlias,* "a small spiral shell." The structure of the inner ear closely resembles that of a snail's shell.

codeine is from the Greek *kodeia,* "the head of a poppy," thus alluding to the source of the alkaloid. The name was conferred by Pierre-Jean Robiquet (1780–1840), a French physician, in 1832.

colchicine is an alkaloid useful in the treatment of gout, and the name is obtained from *kolchikon,* the Greek term for the meadow saffron or autumn crocus, the original herbal source of the alkaloid. The Greek name came from Colchis, the district south of the Caucasus mountains where the plant grew.

cold turkey is a vernacular way of referring to the total, abrupt cessation of a drug. The expression alludes to the "gooseflesh" or "duck bumps" that appear in the skin of persons withdrawing from addiction to opiates. The nodular appearance is that of the skin of a plucked, uncooked, cold turkey.

collagen is a combination of the Greek *kolla,* "glue," + *gennaō,* "I produce." The name, contrived in the 19th century, refers not to any phenomenon that occurs in living tissue but rather to the early observation that dense connective tissue, when boiled, yields a gluey gelatin. **Colloid** (+ Greek *eidos,* "like") is, literally, "a glue-like substance." The term was proposed in the 19th century to distinguish the two main classes of soluble substances, the first being the crystalloids. Glue or gelatin was cited as an example of the second type, to which the name "colloid" was given.

colon as a term for the large intestine is from the Greek. But from which Greek word? There are three candidates. *Kolon* meant "the large intestine" to the Greeks and may have come from *kolos,* "curtailed or stunted," thus alluding to the observation that the large intestine is only about one-third the length of the small intestine ("large" and "small" referring, of course, to the caliber of the two segments rather than to their length). A different Greek word, *kōlon,* meant "a limb" in the sense of a member of the body. Perhaps the jointed configuration of the large intestine, as in its ascending, transverse, and descending segments, suggested a limb, such as an arm or a leg. Finally, *koilia* meant "the hollow of the abdomen." The reader can take his choice and be as right (or wrong) as any expert. As a combining term, **colo-** yields **colostomy,** literally "a mouth of the colon"; **colotomy,** "a cut in the colon"; and **colectomy,** "the removal of the colon." **Colic** is a cramping abdominal pain caused by spasmodic contraction of the smooth musculature of the abdominal viscera, commonly observed in infants. Presumably, colic was originally thought to arise in the colon.

colors often are included in biomedical terms of classical origin. Among the root forms so used are:

> **alb-**, "white" (L)
> **anthrac-**, "black (as coal)" (Gr)
> **argent-**, "silver" (L)
> **argyr-**, "silver" (L)
> **ater-**, "dull black" (L)
> **auro-**, "golden" (L)
> **azul-**, "blue" (Sp)
> **beryl-**, "pale- or sea-green" (Gr)
> **caerul-**, "blue" (L)
> **candid-**, "bright white" (L)
> **chlor-**, "green" (Gr)
> **chrom-**, "colorful or tinted" (Gr)
> **chrys-**, "golden" (Gr)
> **cirrho-**, "tawny yellow" (Gr)
> **cneco-**, "pale yellow" (Gr)
> **coccin-**, "scarlet" (L)
> **croce-**, "saffron, yellow" (L)
> **cyan-**, "dark blue, blue-green" (Gr)
> **erythro-**, "red" (Gr)
> **flav-**, "yellow" (L)
> **fulv-**, "light brown" (L)
> **fusc-**, "dark brown" (L)
> **iodo-**, "violet" (Gr)
> **leuko-**, "white" (Gr)
> **luteo-**, "yellow (as mud)" (L)
> **mela-**, "black" (Gr)

> **niger-**, "glossy black" (L)
> **pelio-**, "livid, dull gray-blue" (Gr)
> **phaeo-**, "dusky, gray, or brown" (Gr)
> **purpur-**, "purple" (L)
> **rhodo-**, "red" (Gr)
> **rubeo-**, "red" (L)
> **spadix-**, "chestnut brown" (L)
> **violo-**, "violet" (L)
> **virido-**, "green" (L)
> **xantho-**, "yellow" (Gr)

colpo- is a combining form usually referring to the vagina. It comes from the Greek *kolpos,* "any fold, cleft, or hollow." Thus, **colporrhaphy** (+ Greek *rhaphē,* "suture") is "a repair of the vagina"; **colposcopy** (+ Greek *skopein,* "to observe") is "an inspection of the vagina"; and **colpotomy** (+ Greek *tomē,* "cutting") is "an incision of the vagina."

coma is directly borrowed from the Greek *kōma,* "a deep sleep." In Hippocratic writings the word was used also for lethargy, but its modern medical meaning is restricted to a state of profound unconsciousness.

comedo is the Latin word for "glutton," being derived from the verb *comedere,* "to eat up." How does this relate to the use of the word in reference to a "blackhead," which is a plugged sebaceous gland in the skin? According to one explanation, the plugged sebaceous gland, when squeezed, exudes a wormlike fragment of waxy material, and apparently the ancients thought this was the remains of a small worm that had burrowed into the skin to devour the flesh. The plural of "comedo" is "comedones."

complaint is that which the patient presents to his doctor. The word is derived from a combination of "com-," as an intensive, + *plangere,* "to wail or to lament." Originally, the Latin verb *plangere* meant "to beat the breast or head as a sign of grief." So the patient who, in anguish, puts his hand to his head and wails, "Oh, doctor, what a pain!" is literally complaining.

complement is a contraction of the Latin *complementum,* "that which fills a void." This, in turn, comes from the verb *compere,* "to fill up." The term was given its biomedical sense by Paul Ehrlich (1854–1915), the famed German immunologist and bacteriologist, to designate the substance necessary to complete certain hemolytic reactions. At the turn of the century, Jules Jean Baptiste Vincent Bordet (1870–1961), a Belgian, and Octave Gengou (1875–1957), a Frenchman, showed that other substances could "fix" complement, thus preventing an otherwise expected hemolytic reaction in sensitized red blood cells. This became the basis for a variety of diagnostic "complement fixation tests."

complexion is derived from the Latin *com-,* "together," + *plectere,* "to plait or to braid." Ancient philosophers thought in terms of four elements or basic attributes: "fire" being hot and dry, "air" being warm and moist, "earth" being cold and dry, and "water" being cold and moist. How these attributes were "woven together" would determine a person's visage, or appearance, or "complexion."

concha is the Latin word for almost any crustacean, particularly its shell. The word is related to the Greek *ko[n]gche,* "a cockleshell." The ancients used these terms to describe various shell-like cavities in anatomy. In modern nomenclature, the conchae are the small bones of the inner nasal passages and, also, the hollows of the external ears.

condom is attributed alternatively *(a)* to the Latin verb *condere,* among its meanings being "to conceal, hide, or suppress"; or *(b)* as an eponym immortalizing an 18th-century English physician whose name may have been Condon, or something similar, and who is said to have prepared a prototype of the device using an inverted cecum of a sheep.

condyle is derived from the Greek *kondylos,* "a knuckle or knob." Its later use, in anatomy, was restricted to the rounded articular surfaces of various bones. The term **condyloma** has the same origin but came to be used to describe the warty cutaneous excrescences around the anus or genitals, usually associated with venereal diseases.

conjunctiva is the feminine of the Latin adjective meaning "connecting or joining together." In anatomy, the modified noun "membrane" is implied but not used when referring to the covering membrane that connects the globe of the eye with the lid.

constipation is derived from the Latin *constipare,* "to crowd together," being a combination of *con-,* "against," + *stipare,* "to cram or stuff." To the Romans, *constipare* meant to pack anything tightly. It was not until the 16th century that the derived word was applied to the state of a dilatory bowel stuffed with inspissated feces.

consumption is an archaic term for any wasting disease, notably tuberculosis. It comes from the Latin *consumere,* "to use up." The acute, fulminant form of disseminated, military tuberculosis was known, of yore, as "galloping consumption."

contagion is from the Latin *contingere,* "to touch closely." The Indo-European root is said to have been *tag,* "to seize," a word we still use in a similar context. A contagious disease is one that might be transmitted by close touch with someone who has the disease.

contre coup is French for "counterblow." The reference is to traumatic lesions, especially of the cranium, that occur on the side opposite where a blow was struck.

control is derived from a combination of the Latin *contra,* "opposite to or facing against," + *rotula,* "a little wheel," in the sense that the little wheel is a roll or a ledger. Thus, a "counter roll" would be a ledger for checking or verifying accounts. In biomedical investigation, a control is a subject or procedure against which an experimental counterpart is compared. Charles Darwin (1809–1882) spoke of "control experiments" in 1875, although James Lind (1716–1794), the British naval surgeon, was probably the first clinical investigator to undertake a controlled experiment in 1747 when he proved the efficacy of ascorbic acid in preventing scurvy.

contusion is from the Latin *contudere,* "to crush, pound, or bruise." About A.D. 1400 reference was made in Middle English to a *counteschown,* the lesion that results from being smitten with a staff or by falling.

convalescence is from the Latin *convalescere,* "to grow strong or to regain strength." This, in turn, was derived from a combination of *con-,* "with," + *valere,* "to be strong." Convalescence, then, is a period during which strength, lost by injury or illness, is regained.

copro- is a combining form denoting a relationship to feces. It comes from the Greek *kopros,* "dung." **Coprolalia** (*copro-* + the Greek *lalia,* "babble") is a term for scatologic raving. "Scato-" is derived from the genitive of the Greek *skōr,* which also means "dung or excrement."

copulate comes from the Latin *copulare,* "to couple or to join, as with a bond."

cor is the Latin word for "heart" but also means "the seat of feelings." *Cor* is used as a component of numerous medical terms, such as "cor biloculare" and "cor pulmonale." Moreover, the Latin word has a host of English offspring, such as core, cordial, accord, concord, record, courage, encourage, and discourage.

coracoid is from the Greek *kōrax,* "a crow or raven." "Coracoid" has been used to describe whatever may resemble a crow's beak.

corium is the Latin word for "skin or hide" and refers specifically to the zone of dense connective tissue underlying the epidermis. The corresponding Greek word is *chorion.*

cornea is the feminine form of the Latin adjective meaning "horny." The cornea is the thin, transparent structure forming the anterior part of the fibrous tunic of the eye. *Cornu* is the Latin word for "horn or hoof," referring especially to the dense material of which these structures are composed. The cornu Ammonis is another name for the hippocampus major, given because it resembles a ram's horn, the symbol of Jupiter of Ammon. In English, "a corn" came to refer to any horny, knotty excrescence of the skin, hence the name for the common lesion of the toes and feet.

coronary is from the Latin *corona,* "crown." The corresponding Greek word appears to be *chorōnos.* "Coronary," then, refers to anything resembling a crown, or that which surrounds or encompasses, as a garland. Some confusion has arisen because the Greek *korōne* meant "a sea crow." The same word was used to refer to the heel of a bow where a notch secured the bowstring. It seems to be an allusion to such a notch that the **coronoid** processes of the ulna and mandible were so named.

coroner comes from the Latin *corona,* "a crown." In olden days, a coroner was an officer of the English crown. Among the duties of this officer were looking into and recording the deaths of the king's subjects. In many American jurisdictions, the title "coroner" has been superseded by "medical examiner." Whatever the name, the principal charge of this officer is to investigate sudden, unnatural, or suspicious deaths.

corpus is the Latin word for "body, matter, or substance"; hence it has had a wide application in anatomy. The plural is **corpora.** The corpora Arantii, the nodules of cartilage in the semilunar valves of the heart, were described by Giulio Aranzi (1530–1589), an Italian anatomist. The corpora mammillaria, two small rounded protuberances at the base of the brain, were so named because of their fancied resemblance to the female breasts. The corpus callosum is so called

from the Latin *callosus,* "hard or thick-skinned." From this same Latin origin come **callus** and **callous,** the noun and adjective, respectively. The corpus luteum is, literally, "a yellow body," from the Latin *luteus,* "mud-colored."

corpuscle is an almost direct borrowing of the Latin *corpusculum,* the diminutive of *corpus,* hence "a little body."

cortex is the Latin word for "bark, shell, hull, or rind," all in the sense of an outer covering. In anatomy, the cerebral cortex is the outer layer of the principal part of the brain; the renal cortex is the outer portion of the kidney; and **cortical** bone is the dense outer part, in contrast to the inner marrow. **Corticosteroid** describes a substance found in the adrenal cortex.

coryza is an ancient and now somewhat pompous word for "a cold in the head." It is said that the Greek word *koryza* was derived, paradoxically, from *kara,* "head," + *zeō,* "I boil." The allusion was to the runny nose, which suggested an effluent of a nasty humor.

cosmetic comes from the Greek *kosmein,* "to arrange or adorn." Thus, cosmetic surgery can be thought of as a rearrangement of certain anatomic features for the purpose of adornment. As such, its cost is excluded from coverage by most health-insurance schemes.

costa is the Latin word for "rib." The combining form **costo-** and the adjective **costal** refer to whatever may pertain to the rib or ribs.

cough is a word of uncertain origin, but almost surely it must have begun as an onomatopoeic expression of just what it represents, that is, a forceful expulsion of air from the lungs and bronchial tree.

coxa is the Latin word for "hip," which, in turn, is said to have come from the Sanskrit *kaksha* of the same meaning. The Latin *coxa* led to the French *coussin* and, thence, to our word "cushion."

cranium is the Latin word for "skull" and is related to the Greek *kranion.* Generally, the word refers to the skull minus the mandible, that is, to the major portion which serves principally as the brain case. **Craniotomy** is an ancient and venerable operation for cutting an opening into the skull. The old belief was that this provided a sure means of allowing the escape of bad spirits.

crazy has no medical significance but still is often heard and used. Its origin has been traced to Old Norse, whence came the Middle English *crasen,* "to crack or break." Words that may be related are "crackle" (full of cracks) and "crash." Whatever is "crazy," then, is cracked, broken, or defective.

cream as a vehicle for dermatologic medicaments is said to have had its origin in the Indo-European *ghrei,* "to smear or rub." The Greek *chrisma* means "anything smeared on, such as a scented unguent." The Greek *christos* means "anointed"; hence "the Christos" or "Christ" was "the anointed one." The Anglo-Saxon *crisma,* through French, became "cream."

creatinine is the anhydride of **creatine,** both words derived from the Greek *kreas,* "flesh or meat." The two nitrogenous substances were first discovered in meat extracts.

cremaster is an almost direct borrowing of the Greek *kremastēr,* "a suspender." The ancient anatomists gave this term to the muscles that suspend the testicles in the scrotum. The cremasteric fascia invests the spermatic cord.

crena is the Latin word for "notch or cleft" and is so used in certain anatomic terms, such as "crena ani" for the cleft between the buttocks. **Crenated** erythrocytes are red blood cells with notched or burrlike surfaces.

crepitus meaning the peculiar sound or tactile sensation of gas, usually air, that has infiltrated soft tissues, as in subcutaneous emphysema, is a direct borrowing of the Latin *crepitus,* "a rattle or a crackling sound." The noun, in turn, was derived from the Latin verb *crepare,* "to make rattle or to chatter noisily about."

cretin is from the Old French *chrêtien,* which literally meant "a Christian," but became a somewhat contemptuous term applied to certain benighted human beings who were looked upon as hardly more than brutes. As a consequence of persecution in France, a group of adherents to Arianism, judged to be a heretical sect, sought refuge in remote valleys of the Pyrenees. Because of a chronically deficient diet, notably lacking in iodine, children of these people often were born with stunted bodies and minds. Philippus Aureolus Theophrastus Bombastus von Hohenheim (1493–1541), better known as Paracelsus, a celebrated Swiss physician, was the first to recognize the relation between goitrous parents and cretinous children. A cretin is the victim of the congenital, juvenile form of hypothyroidism, **myx-edema** being the condition in adults.

cribriform is a combination of the Latin *cribrum,* "a sieve," + *forma,* "likeness." The cribriform plate of the ethmoid bone and the cribriform fascia of the thigh are so called because of their numerous perforations.

cricoid comes from the Greek *krikos,* "a ring," being a variant of *kirkos,* "a circle." The cricoid cartilage was so named because it resembled a signet ring. The **cricopharyn-geus** muscle encircles the lowermost portion of the hypopharynx.

crisis is derived from the Greek *krinō,* "I decide or judge," particularly in the sense of choosing or separating. Thus, a crisis occurs when an acutely ill patient appears to be on the verge of either survival or death. In effect, it can be said that a judgment is thus made between the quick and the dead. The ancients observed that there were critical days in the course of various acute diseases, especially those marked by fever. Fevers are said "to break" either by crisis, i.e., rapidly, as though a prompt decision had been rendered; or by lysis, i.e., gradually resolving. A related word is "criterion," a direct borrowing of the Greek *kritērion,* "a standard or means by which a judgment is made."

crotch is a vernacular term for the region where the legs come together. It is so used in the sense of a fork or a point of division. The crotch of a tree is where its limbs divide. The origin of the word is obscure. It may have come from the Middle English *croche,* which meant "a shepherd's crook or crosier." This, in turn, probably came from the Old Scandinavian *krokr,* "hook." From

this also was derived our word "crouch," meaning to assume a "hooked" position. A probably related word is **crutch,** the stick used to aid the lame and taken originally from the crotch of a tree.

crus is the Latin word for the leg, more specifically the shin. The term also is associated with the Latin *crux,* "cross," perhaps because *crus* was considered the perpendicular leg of a cross. In any event "crus" is used in anatomy to describe various formations in the shape of V or X. The crus of the diaphragm is the crossing of muscles at the esophageal hiatus. **Crural** refers to the leg or whatever appears shaped like a leg.

crux is the Latin word for "cross." **Cruciate** ligaments, as in the knee, are so named because they cross each other. A related word is "crucial," in the sense of decisive, the reference being to the choice one must make when arriving at a "crossroad."

crypt is from the Latin *crypta,* "an underground passage or gallery." In turn, this came from the Greek *kryptō,* "I hide." The crypts of Lieberkühn are the lumens of glands in the intestinal mucosa. **Cryptorchidism** refers to an undescended testicle that remains "hidden" in the abdomen. **Cryptogenic** means, literally, "of hidden origin" but often is used as a pseudosophisticated way of saying "I don't know where it comes from."

culture comes from the Latin *cultura,* "a tilling of the soil for the purpose of raising crops." This is closely related to the Latin *cultus,* which had a variety of meanings, all having to do with "raising up, training, refinement" and the like. In referring to a bacterial culture, one adheres closely to the original Latin meaning.

curare is the toxic essence of a plant described as *Strychnos toxifera* and found in limited areas of Guiana. The poison applied to the tips of arrows was concocted by Indians of the Macusi tribe, who called the plant source *urari-yé* and the poison *urari*.

cure comes from the Latin *cura,* "care, concern, or attention." The current use of the word seemingly sprang from the belief that proper and sufficient "care" was tantamount to "cure." Would that this were so! The familiar admonition to "Cure occasionally, relieve often, console always" comes from the ancient French aphorism "Guérir quelquefois, soulager souvent, consoler toujours."

curette is the French word for "scraper" and comes from the verb *curer,* "to clean out." **Curettage** or **curettement** are French words and refer to the operation of scraping a wound or other lesion for the purpose of cleansing.

cusp comes from the Latin *cuspis,* "a pointed end, as of a spear." The term is used in anatomy to refer to the pointed extremity of anything, such as the cusp of a tooth or the cusp of a valve. **Bicuspid** means "two-pointed ends" and may refer to a tooth or to a heart valve. **Tricuspid** refers to the heart valve with three points.

cutis is the Latin word for "skin." The diminutive **cuticle** means "the little skin," as that emanating from the perionychium. The Greek *kutos* referred to any hollow vessel. Indeed, the skin can be considered as the vessel containing the body.

cyanosis comes from the Greek *cyanos,* "dark blue." This is the color assumed by the skin and mucous membranes when deprived of oxygenated blood.

cyclops is borrowed from the Greek *Kyklōpes,* the name given to a mythical race of lawless, giant shepherds who inhabited Sicily. Their most striking feature was a single, large, rounded eye situated in the middle of the forehead. The name came, literally, from *kyklos,* "a rounded ring," + *ōps,* "eye." Medically, a cyclops is a monster born with a single, centrally placed eye.

cyst is derived from the Greek *kystis,* "a bladder, bag, or pouch." In turn, this comes from *kyō,* "I hold." In anatomy, "cystic" refers to any sort of bladder. A **cystocele** (from the Greek *kēlē,* "hernia") is a protrusion of the urinary bladder into the vagina. **Cystine** is an amino acid first discovered as a hydrolytic product of protein in urine, where it crystallized as a concrement in the bladder.

cyto- is a combining form, also appearing as **-cyte,** indicating whatever pertains to a cell. It is derived from the Greek *kytos,* "hollow, as a cell or container." In combination, "-cyto-" can describe all sorts of cells. **Anisocytosis** (Greek *an,* "not," + *iso,* "the same") describes a group of cells, normally regular, that vary markedly in size. **Poikilocytosis** (Greek *poikilos,* "varied") describes a condition wherein cells are of markedly abnormal shape. A **karyocyte** (Greek *karyon,* "a nut or kernel") is a nucleated cell, particularly an early normoblast or an erythrocyte that normally would not harbor a nucleus.

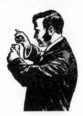

D

dactyl- is a combining form referring to a finger, or sometimes a toe, and is derived from the Greek *daktylos*, "finger." Thus, **syndactyly** (the Greek *syn-*, "together") means that adjacent digits are joined by a congenital web.

data is the plural (a point not always remembered by American speakers and writers) of the Latin *datum*, "a thing given," the neuter past participle of *dare*, "to give." In science, data are assembled as facts, statistics, or the like; one rarely encounters *datum* in reference to a single fact or statistic, but such use would be entirely proper.

deaf in Middle English was spelled (and pronounced) "deef." So the old-timer who pronounces the word to rhyme with "reef" is not being comical; he is being archaic. The word was so said in many parts of England until the 18th century. The original Indo-European root probably was *dheubh*, "dull to perception." Our adjective "absurd" is

taken from the Latin *absurdus*, "senseless or silly," being a combination of *ab-*, "from," + *surdus*, "deaf, unheeding."

debridement is a French word that combines *de-*, "not," + *brider*, "to bridle," thus, literally, "an unbridling." Originally, the term was used for the process of cutting constrictive bands but later, in surgery, came to refer to the cutting away of injured or necrotic tissue.

deceased is a delicate way of saying "dead." Not only is it delicate, it is used almost invariably as a passive verb. No one with a civil tongue speaks of "deceasing" himself, or anyone else for that matter. "Deceased" comes from the Latin *decedere*, "to go away." This is akin to referring to death as a "passing away." **Demise** is a delicate noun for "death." Its origin is somewhat tortuous but probably goes back to the Latin *mittere*, "to send away." "Demise" and "dismiss" would seem to be related in origin but are quite distinct in meaning. A worthy suggestion might be to leave "deceased" and "demise" to persons given to unctuous speech, such as morticians. "Dead," even though a four-letter word, is perfectly respectable.

decidua is from the Latin verb *decidere,* "to cut away or to fall away." Deciduous trees are those from which the leaves fall away at the chill of autumn, and deciduous teeth are those that are shed by the youngster in the course of normal development. Decidua commonly refers to the mucosa of the uterus that "falls away" after parturition. The "menstrual decidua" is the hyperemic endometrium that is shed in the normal menstrual cycle.

decrepit is a term to describe a person or thing that has become infirm or broken down by age. The word is an almost direct borrowing of the Latin *decrepitus,* "broken down," which in turn is a combination of *de,* "from," + *crepare,* "to make rattle or creak."

decubitus is from the Latin verb *decumbere,* "to lie down," and is related to the Latin *cubitum,* "the elbow." The Romans habitually rested on their elbows when reclining. Decubitus describes a reclining position and usually is further specified as, for example, "the left lateral decubitus." A "decubital ulcer" is a bedsore, the consequence of pressure necrosis on a dependent part from lying in one position too long. The **antecubital** fossa is the hollow in front of the elbow. Some related words are "cubicle" (a small chamber in which to lie down), "incumbent" (a state of lying in or occupying), and "concubine" (one who lies with another).

decussation is from the Latin verb *decussare,* "to divide crosswise," i.e., in the form of an X. The decussation of the anterior pyramids of the medulla oblongata is the crossing of fibers from one side to another so as to form the lateral spinothalamic tracts.

defecate comes from the Latin *defecatio,* "a cleansing," this being, in turn, derived from *de,* "out of," + *faex,* "dregs or sediments." The allusion is to feces being the "dregs" of the bowel.

degenerate comes from the Latin *degenerare,* "to disgrace, to fall short of, or to be inferior to one's ancestors." The derivation is from *de,* "down from," + *genus,* "the race." In biology, a degenerated cell is one that has deteriorated in structure or function when compared with its normal counterparts of the "race."

deglutition is a combination of the Latin *de,* "down," + *glutire,* "to gulp." Now the term is used in the gentler sense of simply swallowing. A related word is "glutton."

delirium is said to have been first used by Aurelius Cornelius, better known as Celsus, the celebrated Roman medical encyclopedist of the 1st century A.D. The term is from the Latin *de,* "away from," + *lira,* "a furrow." Whoever is mentally confused or incoherent cannot plow a straight furrow and may be said to be out of his groove.

deltoid refers to the shape of Δ (delta), the fourth letter of the Greek alphabet. Hence, it describes anything triangular in configuration.

delusion comes from the Latin *deludere,* "to dupe or deceive." The Latin *ludere* means "to play or to amuse oneself," and a *ludio* was an actor. One who suffers delusions is being misled by imaginary circumstances.

dementia is the Latin word for "madness" and comes from a combination of *de,* "out of," + *mens,* "mind." Whoever is demented is out of his mind. In a now outmoded classification, one form of mental derangement was referred to as "dementia praecox," the second word being the Latin for "premature" (and the source of our word "precocious"). **Praecox,** in turn, comes from the Latin *prae-,* "before," + *coquere,* "to cook," thus, literally, "uncooked" or "half-baked."

demulcent comes from the Latin *demulcere,* "to stroke lovingly or to caress," this being a combination of *de,* "down," + *mulcere,* "to stroke or to pet; to caress or soften." The Romans used *demulcere* particularly for the soothing stroking of horses. In medicine, a demulcent is a soothing drug, especially one topically applied to allay the irritation of inflamed surfaces.

dendrite means "treelike" and is derived from the Greek *dendron,* "a tree." The term, in anatomy, refers particularly to the branching protoplasmic processes of nerve cells. In botany, a "rhododendron" is a "red tree," and a "philodendron" is a climbing plant with evergreen foliage that clings to trees, so called because it has an affinity for or "loves" trees.

dengue is the name of an acutely painful, febrile illness endemic in the West Indies, the Middle East, India, and the South Pacific. It is also known as "breakbone fever." Its victims often exhibit contortions because of intense muscle and joint pains. One explana-tion is that the name originated in the Swahili word *dinga,* "a sudden cramp or seizure." Another explanation relates the name to the Spanish *denguero,* which means "affected or finicky." Slaves in the West Indies were said to have called the disease "dandy fever," presumably because of the affected gait or postures of persons so afflicted.

dermis comes from the Greek *derma,* "the skin." A related Sanskrit word was *dartis,* "leather or hide." When used alone, dermis refers to the corium or dense layer of connective tissue underneath the stratified squamous epithelium. More often, "derm-" is a combining form making up a host of words pertaining to the skin, such as **dermatology** (the science of the skin), **dermatitis** (an inflammation of the skin), **dermatome** (an instrument for slicing the skin), **dermatographia** (a condition wherein gentle stroking induces a localized swelling, or "writing," on the skin), and many others.

desiccate comes from the Latin *desiccare,* "to dry up or to drain," this being derived from a combination of *de,* "away," + *siccus,* "dry." The **sicca** syndrome is characterized by excessive dryness of the normally moist membranes of the eye and mouth. The French *sec,* "dry," particularly as it refers to wines lacking sweetness, is a related word.

desmo- is a combining form derived from the Greek *desmos,* "a band or fetter." Consequently, "desmo-" has come to refer to dense fibrous or connective tissue. **Desmoplasia** is a growth of fibrous tissue, particularly that investing certain neoplasms. A

desmoid tumor is a hard, fibrous neoplasm, such as can occur in persons afflicted with Gardner's syndrome.

desquamate is from the Latin *de,* "away," + *squama,* "scale." The Latin verb *desquamare* means "to take the scales off a fish." In medicine, "desquamate" refers to the scaling and shedding of the outer layers of the skin.

detritus is the past participle of the Latin *deterere,* "to rub off or to rub away." Detritus, then, is that which is rubbed away and refers, as a medical term, to debris collected in or around degenerating or necrotic tissue.

detrusor comes from the Latin *detrudere,* "to push down or to dislodge." The detrusor muscle of the urinary bladder serves to aid in the expulsion of urine.

dexter is the Latin word for "right," as opposed to "left." Because a majority of persons are right-handed, **dexterity** has come to mean skill and facility. This may be true for the right hand of such persons, but for anyone acquainted with elementary physiology, a disturbing question arises: if the left side of the brain controls the right side of the body, then are left-handed persons the only ones in their right mind?

dextrin is an intermediate product of the hydrolysis of starch and is so called because of its dextrorotary ("turning to the right") effect on polarized light. **Dextrose** is a colorless, crystalline hexose that has a similar dextrorotary property. Actually, it is d-glucose, the "d" standing for "dextro-."

dia- is a busy combining form taken from the Greek preposition *dia,* which has many meanings, including "through, throughout, thoroughly, completely, across, and opposed to." It has been used to concoct new words, and it appears as a prefix in many truly Greek words. **Diabetes** is a direct borrowing of the Greek *diabētēs,* which means both "a siphon" (*dia-* + *bainō,* "to pass or to run") and "a pair of compasses" (that is, the sort used to inscribe circles). Areteus the Cappadocian, a famous Greek physician of the 2nd century A.D., explained that *diabētēs* as a disease was so called because its victims "passed water like a siphon." The common sort of diabetic urine is laden with sugar, and hence the second part of "diabetes **mellitus**" is the Latin word for "sweetened with honey." The urine of patients with "diabetes **insipidus,**" on the other hand, while voluminous, is lacking in sugar, and therefore tasteless or insipid. To the Romans, *insipiens* meant "foolish," as derived from *in-,* "lacking," + *sapientia,* "taste or sense." The Latin *sapor* means "taste" in the concept both of flavor and of refinement. **Diagnosis** is a direct borrowing of the Greek *diagnōsis,* but to the Greeks this meant specifically "a discrimination, a distinguishing, or a discerning between two possibilities," in the sense of resolving or deciding. The word combines *dia-* in any or almost all of its meanings + *gnōsis,* "knowledge" when applied to the discernment of disease as it affects a given patient. **Dialysis** is a direct borrowing of the Greek word for "a loosening of one thing from another." It is almost exactly in that sense that "dialysis" is used in medicine as "a process of separating crystalloids and colloids in solution by the difference in their rates of diffusion through a semipermeable membrane" (Dorland). **Dia-pedesis** (+ Greek *pedesis,* "a leap") was used by ancient writers to refer to serous oozing from small blood vessels. In modern physiology, "diapedesis" refers to the escape of blood corpuscles through the discontinuous endothelium of intact vessels, particularly as this occurs in response to inflammation. **Diaper** refers not to the shape or function of the familiar "three-cornered pants" but to the fabric and its color. The word combines *dia-,* "thoroughly," + the Greek *aspros,* "white." In ancient times the fabric was a pure linen of fine texture that was pristinely white. **Diaphoresis** is a Greek word used by ancient writers for "sweating." It includes the Greek *phoreō,* "I carry." "Diaphoresis" is still used as a rather pompous medical synonym for sweating. **Diaphragm** is a near borrowing of the Greek *diaphragma,* "a partition," this being a combination of *dia-,* "across," + *phragma,* "a fence or wall." Certain ancient writers ascribed great significance to the muscular diaphragm separating the chest from the abdomen, some even attributing to it powers of the mind. This explains the naming of the **phrenic** (Greek *phrēn,* "the mind") nerve that supplies the diaphragm. **Diaphysis** incorporates the Greek *physis,* "growth." Originally the term referred to "the bursting of a bud" or "the point where a branch grew from a stalk." Later, in anatomy, "diaphysis" came to be applied to the shaft of a long bone, particularly as a growth center, in distinction to the epiphysis. **Diarrhea** is an almost direct borrowing of the Greek *diarrhoia,* "a flowing

through," which incorporates the Greek verb *rheō,* "I flow." The ancients used the term, as we do, in reference to an excessive, watery evacuation from the bowel. **Diastase** is a word coined in the 19th century as the name for a substance (later identified as an enzyme) capable of breaking down or separating starch into its component sugars. It was derived from the Greek *diastasis,* "a standing apart." Because diastase was thought of as the prototype of an enzyme, the last three letters, **"-ase,"** came to be a suffix designating an enzymatic property. The Greek *diastasis* is still used in its original meaning when applied to a separation of the abdominal muscles, as in "**diastasis recti.**" **Diastole** is a direct borrowing of the Greek word meaning "a distinction or difference" and is related to the Greek verb *diastellō,* "I separate or distinguish." With separation there is the idea of introducing or expanding a pause between two circumstances or events. It is in this sense that "diastole" came to be, in physiology, the name for the period of relaxation and dilatation of the heart muscle between systolic contractions. **Diathermy** is a contrived term incorporating the Greek *therma,* "heat," thus referring to "penetrating heat." **Diathesis** is a Greek word meaning "an order of arrangement," particularly in the sense of "a disposition." Ancient writers conceived that certain persons, because of their make-up or temperament, were particularly disposed to certain diseases. We use the term in much the same way when we refer, for example, to "a hemorrhagic diathesis."

diet comes from the Greek *diaita,* "a way of living or a mode of life." Originally the term was used for a hygienic regimen generally, but later it was restricted to a mode of eating considered conducive to good health.

digestion is derived from the Latin *digerere,* "to arrange, sort out, or distribute." Medieval chemists used the term in the sense of "dissolving." In the 17th century a device was introduced wherein bones could be softened by cooking under pressure, and this was called "a digester." The early physiologists borrowed the term in the belief that ingested food was treated in the stomach in a manner similar to digestion as carried out in the chemist's laboratory. As it turned out, they may have been closer to the mark than they might have guessed.

digit is a contraction of the Latin *digitus,* "a finger or a toe." A "digitation" is a finger-like process, and "to interdigitate" means to appear as interlocking fingers. "Digit" as a term for a number came from the custom of counting on the fingers. This also accounts for the metric system of numbering on a base of ten.

digitalis comes from the Latin *digitus,* "finger." The allusion is to the tubular blossoms of the plant whose dried leaves, when pulverized, provide the drug. The shape of the flower suggests the empty finger of a glove. In part, this explains the plant's common name, "the foxglove." But why the "fox"? No one really knows. By curious coincidence, "digitalis" was proposed as the Latinized name of the plant in the 16th century by a German botanist, Leonhard Fuchs (1501–1566). *Fuchs* is German for "fox."

Apparently he chose "digitalis," a Latin way of saying "pertaining to the finger," because the common German name for the plant is *Fingerhut,* which means, literally, "a finger hat" or a thimble. But we are still left wondering why the foxglove was so called as early as the 11th century.

diopter comes from the Greek *diopteuō,* "I watch closely and accurately." The Greek *dioptra* referred to an optical instrument used for measuring angles. "Diopter" was adopted as a name for the unit of the refracting power of lenses, the standard of one diopter being a focal distance of one meter.

diphtheria got its name from the Greek *diphthera,* "a prepared hide or leather." The allusion is to the parchment-like membrane in the throat characteristic of the disease. Diphtheria was known to the ancient Greeks, but they did not call it by that name. To them it was "the Egyptian disease" or "the Syrian ulcer," another example of blaming a malady on someone else.

diplopia is contrived as a combination of the Greek *diploos,* "double," + *opsis,* "vision." The term first appeared in print in the early 19th century.

dipsomania is the result of combining the Greek *dipsa,* "thirst," + *mania,* "madness." The term first appeared in English in the mid-19th century to describe "a frenzy to drink," specifically referring to alcoholic beverages, and was considered a form of insanity.

disease comes from the Old French *desaise,* a combination of *des-,* "away from," + *aise,* "ease." In its early use, the term referred to any tribulation that disturbed one's ease.

Only later did disease acquire its restricted medical sense.

disk is a near borrowing of the Greek *diskos,* "a circular, flat stone," which the Greeks were much given to hurl. Sometimes the *diskos* had a hole in the center, either for a strap by which to swing it or so it could be used as a quoit (a doughnut-shaped object to toss at a peg). "Disk" now refers to any circular, plate-like structure as, for example, the "intervertebral disk."

dispensary comes from the Latin *dispensere,* "to weigh out." Originally, the term referred to a place where medicinal agents were measured and distributed. Later, it came to mean a place where the sick or injured were treated but not kept as inpatients. In the past, outpatient departments often were called "dispensaries."

dissect is from the Latin verb *dissecare,* "to cut apart," this being a simple combination of *dis-,* "apart," + *secare,* "to cut." An anatomic dissection, then, is "a cutting apart." The Latin verb *resecare* meant "to cut back, trim, or curtail." Thus, a surgical **resection** is an operation wherein an organ is "cut back" or removed in whole or in part.

distill is derived from the manner in which a liquid is heated so that its vapor can be condensed and collected, drop by drop. Hence, the word is a combination of the Latin *de-,* "from," + *stilla,* "a drop." To **instill** originally meant to introduce something drop by drop.

diuresis is made up of a combination of the Greek *dia-,* "thoroughly," + *oureseiō,* "I want to make water," thus "to promote uri-

nation." Of course, there is a distinction between stimulating the excretion and flow of urine from the kidney and stimulating contraction of the smooth musculature of the urinary bladder so as to cause its evacuation. By common acceptance, a diuretic agent is understood to be that which promotes the formation of urine. An example, among many, would be chlorothiazide. On the other hand, bethanechol, which stimulates smooth muscle contraction, is a bladder evacuant, not a diuretic.

diverticulum is a direct borrowing of the Latin word for "a bypath or a wayside shelter," coming from the verb *divertere,* "to turn aside." The "-culum" implies the diminutive and indicates that a diverticulum is subsidiary to the main channel. It is important to remember that "diverticulum" is the neuter singular and that "diverticula" (not "diverticuli") is the neuter plural, a point that many careless or unknowing speakers and writers seem to ignore.

doctor comes from the Latin verb *docere,* "to teach." In years past, "doctor" was a title of courtesy and respect bestowed on any learned man. Later, it became associated with the title of the highest academic degree. Meanwhile, "doctor" acquired a specifically medical connotation. Probably this was because, of all learned scholars, only members of the medical faculty became familiar to the public at large.

dolicho- is a combining form derived from the Greek *dolichos,* "long." Thus, **dolichocephalic** refers to a long head, and **dolichocolon** to an unusually long and redundant large intestine.

dope comes from the Dutch *doop,* meaning "a sauce or viscous fluid." It became applied to narcotics because as raw opium is being processed, it becomes a thick liquid when heated. Later, any substance having a numbing or stupefying effect became known as "dope." By extension, the person who was the victim of a narcotic effect was called, in slang, "a dopehead" or simply "a dope." But there is more to the vagaries of this little word. Unscrupulous racehorse promoters found they could oftentimes ensure the outcome of a race by giving dope to the mount preselected for winning. Anyone privy to this illicit information was said to have "the inside dope." Soon, any worthwhile intelligence came to be called "the dope."

dorsum is Latin for "back." Thus, the dorsum of the hand or foot is the "back" of that part. Seldom, if ever, is "dorsum" used to refer to the whole backside of the human body, but the adjective **dorsal** is understood to pertain to the back of the thorax. The dorsal vertebrae are the thoracic vertebrae. "Dorsal" also is used to mean "posterior," as in the dorsal roots of the spinal nerves. Incidentally, to endorse a check means to sign one's name on the back of the slip.

dose is said to have had its origin in the postulated Indo-European root *dō,* "to give." A descendant is the Greek *dosis,* "that which is given." A related word is the Latin *donare,* "to bestow," and from this we derive "donate." A dose, then, is a "giving" of medicine.

dram is an almost forgotten unit of measure. It came originally from the Greek *drachmē,* a coin approximately equivalent in value to a Roman *denarius.* The coin also was used as a weight, and later a "drachm" or dram became one-eighth of an ounce as an apothecary's weight (but one-sixteenth of an avoirdupois ounce). Before adoption of the metric system, a dram of fluid was commonly taken as one teaspoonful, the symbol on a prescription being written as "ℨ."

dropsy is now an archaic term for a condition wherein the body tissues are swollen by an accumulation of excess fluid. Its use in English comes through the French *hydropisie,* from the Greek *hydrops,* which meant the same thing, *hydōr* being the Greek word for water of any kind. In former times, "dropsy" often was used as a diagnosis in itself. Now we refer to edema, ascites, or anasarca as more descriptive signs, and we require a designation of the underlying cause, such as cirrhosis or congestive heart failure, as the diagnosis. This enhanced perception accounts for the disuse of "dropsy."

duct is a contraction of the Latin *ductus,* "a drawing or a leading," which is related, in turn, to the verb *ductare,* "to draw, to lead, or to escort." However, Latin authors never used *ductus* when they referred to a conduit for fluids. Rather, they used *canalis,* "a pipe or gutter."

duodenum began as the Greek *dōdeka-daktulon,* "twelve fingers," the idea being that the proximal, retroperitoneal portion of the small intestine was about twelve fingerbreadths long. This came to be translated, through the Arabic, as the Late Latin *duodenum.* In classical Latin this would have been *duodecim,* "twelve" (from *duo-,* "two," + *decem,* "ten"). In German, the duodenum is *der Zwölffingerdarm,* "the twelve-finger gut."

dura mater is the name for the tough, outer membrane encasing the brain and spinal cord. It is composed of the Latin words *dura,* "hard or tough," and *mater,* "mother." This makes little sense until one knows that the Latin *dura mater* is a literal translation of its precedent, the Arabic term which meant "strong mother [in the sense of "protector"] of the brain."

dys- is an inseparable combining form, originating in the Greek, that confers a bad sense on whatever word it is hooked onto. "Dys-" conveys a meaning of defective, difficult, ill, or painful. There are a host of medical terms beginning with "dys-." Some of them are closely related to Greek words. **Dyscrasia** is an almost direct borrowing of the Greek *dyskrasia,* "a bad mixture of humors, a bad temperament"; the Greek *krasis* means "mixture or make-up." The term originally referred to any diseased condition but now, for some obscure reason, is restricted to hematology, as in "blood dyscrasia." **Dysentery** is the condition of a painful gut, usually attended by diarrhea. The Greek *dysenteria* (+ *enteron,* "intestine") means "a bowel complaint." **Dyspareunia** comes from the Greek *dyspareunos,* "ill-mated," but now means painful sexual intercourse. The Greek *pareunos* (*para-,* "beside," + *eunos,* "bed") means "lying beside." **Dyspnea** relates to the Greek *dyspnoia* (+ *pneō,* "I breathe"), and both mean "difficult breathing." Some "dys-" words have been contrived from the Greek. **Dyspeptic** (+ Greek *pepsis,* "digestion") describes a nondescript digestive malaise. **Dystrophy** (+ Greek *trophē,* "nourishment") is abnormal growth or development. Some "dys-" words are merely (and sometimes painfully) contrived. An example is "dysfunction." Incidentally, "dys-" is not to be confused with "dis-," a prefix borrowed from the Latin and meaning "apart, asunder, or deprived of."

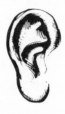

E

ear is from the Old Norse *eyra* and is related to the Latin *auris* and the Greek *ous,* all of which mean "ear." The Greek *oukein,* "to hear," is the forerunner of "acoustic," and the Latin term provides the adjective **aural** and the combining form **auri-,** "pertaining to the ear" (except for the "auricle" of the heart, a sort of nickname for the atrial appendage, thought to look like the floppy ear of a dog). The Latin *auris* is not to be confused with the Latin *aura,* "a breeze or atmosphere," or the Latin *aurum,* "gold."

eburnation comes from the Latin *ebur,* "ivory," and thus means a conversion to the appearance of ivory. In eburnation, bone becomes abnormally hard and as dense as ivory. In dentistry, it refers to a condition wherein exposed dentin assumes an ivory-like look.

ecchymosis is from the Greek *ekchymesthai,* "to pour out," which combines *ek-,* "out," + *chymos,* "juice." The juice, of course, referred to blood, and *ekchymōsis* was used in Hippocratic writings to refer to the escape of blood from the rupture of a small vessel and the consequent infiltration of surrounding tissues. To lay persons, an ecchymosis is a **bruise.** This less sophisticated term comes, as might be expected, from the Anglo-Saxon *brȳsan,* "to break."

echinococcus is derived from a combination of the Greek *echinos,* "a hedgehog or a sea urchin" (the allusion being to the prickly or spiny surface of such animals), and the Greek *kokkus,* "berry." The name was suggested by the numerous, spiny hooklets seen in the minute, berrylike scolex of the larval form of the parasite.

echography is a method of diagnostic imaging, also known as ultrasonography. The image is produced by the "echo" of high-frequency ultrasound waves as they encounter body tissues of varying densities. In Roman mythology, Echo was the name of a lovely nymph whose one failing was that she talked too much. One day Juno, Queen of Olympus, was searching for her errant husband, Jupiter, who she suspected was cavorting with the nymphs. By her prattling, Echo detained Juno, thus allowing the nymphs to escape. Juno was so incensed by this ploy that she cursed Echo by depriving her of the use of her tongue, except in reply. Juno's harsh sentence on poor Echo: "You shall still have the last word, but no power to speak first!" So it is the "reply" to the ultrasound wave that creates the image in echography.

eclampsia is derived from the Greek *eklampsis,* "a shining forth." The allusion is to the scintillating flashes of light in the visual field that may be symptomatic of toxemia of pregnancy.

eclectic is a term that once applied to a certain "school" of medicine. In ancient times, eclectic medicine was that purportedly selecting those methods of treatment deemed best from the variety of cults then extant. In more recent times, eclectic physicians were those who selected single remedies, particularly those of botanical origin, for specific maladies. The term comes from the Greek *eklektikos,* "selective."

ecology is a word introduced in 1869 by Ernst Heinrich Haeckel (1834–1919), the celebrated German zoologist and votary of classical Greek. The word then was half-forgotten but was recently revived to find a place in almost everyone's vocabulary. "Ecology" was derived from the Greek *oikos,* "house or place to live," + *logos,* "word or study," and means the science of the habitat of living things, particularly as that habitat is affected by its environment.

ectoderm is derived from the Greek *ektos,* "outside," + *derma,* "skin." The term refers to the outermost germ layer of the embryo, from which the skin and its appendages originate. The other two layers are the **endoderm** (from the Greek *endon,* "within or inner") and the **mesoderm** (from the Greek *mesos,* "middle"). The triad of germ layers was conceptualized in 1845 by Robert Remak (1815–1865), a German neurologist and embryologist.

-ectomy is a combining form and means "a cutting out." It comes from the Greek *ek,* "out," + *tomē,* "a cutting," Preceded by the name of almost any anatomic structure, it forms a word for the surgical removal of that structure. An example is "appendectomy."

ectopia is from the Greek *ektopia,* "displacement," a combination of *ek-,* "out," + *topos,* "place." The word was not used by the Greeks as a medical term but is said to have been given as a name for an extrauterine pregnancy by Robert Barnes (1817–1907), an English obstetrician.

eczema is a direct borrowing of the Greek word for "anything thrown off or out by heat" and is derived from a combination of *ek-,* "out," + *zeein,* "to boil." To the ancients, a skin eruption was a "boiling over" of the body "humors." Formerly used to refer to almost any vesicular or scaly rash, "eczema" now is usually restricted to immunopathic eruptions. In this sense, the term may be reverting to the original concept of unruly humors.

edema comes from the Greek *oidēma,* "a swelling." The original Greek is more favored in the British spelling of "oedema" than in the American version. In ancient writings, the term was applied to any tumorous condition but later was restricted to swelling in tissues resulting from the accumulation of fluid.

effervescence comes from the Latin *effervescere,* "to boil over," which was derived from a combination of *ex-,* "out," + *fervescere,* "to become boiling hot." Now the term describes any liberation of gaseous bubbles from a solution, hot or cold.

effete means "exhausted or worn out" and comes from the Latin *effeta,* which means "exhausted from bearing young" and is made up of *ef-,* "out of," + *feta,* "breeding." The latter, in the masculine form, is **fetus,** a familiar medical term.

ego is the Latin "I," the first person singular pronoun. In psychiatry, the ego is purported to be "that portion of the psyche which possesses consciousness, maintains its identity, and recognizes and tests reality" (Dorland).

egophony is from the Greek and is spelled *aegophony* by purists. It is a combination of *aix,* "goat," + *phonē,* "voice or sound." The auscultatory sign is a bleating sound heard just above collections of pleural fluid and is best elicited by having the patient voice the letter "a" as in "bake"; the resulting egophonous sound comes through the stethoscope as "e" in "beet" (or "bleat").

elbow is derived from the Anglo-Saxon *elnboga,* literally "the arm-bending." The related Latin word is *ulna,* "elbow or arm."

electron is a direct borrowing of the Greek word for "amber," the yellow-brown, translucent, fossil resin that was found capable of gaining a negative electric charge when rubbed. An interesting analogue comes from Arabic, in which amber is *kahraba* and a closely related form means electricity. The ancient Greeks were aware that rubbed amber exerts an attracting force, but it remained for William Gilbert (1544–1603), an English physician and natural philosopher, to use the term "electrified" to describe this form of magnetism.

element comes from the Latin *elementum,* "a rudiment, beginning, or first principle." The origin of the Latin word is not known, but the suggestion has been made that it might have come from a euphonious recitation in sequence of the three letters "L," "M," "N," as "el" + "em" + "en," just as we refer to our "ABCs."

elephantiasis is the name for a condition marked by thickened, corrugated skin and an obvious allusion to the pachyderm, or elephant (from the Greek *pachys,* "thick," + *derma,* "skin"). The Latin name for the animal is *elephantus,* and the Greek name was *elephas.* Some say there may be a relation to the Hebrew *aleph,* sometimes given as *eleph,* which is the first letter of the Hebrew alphabet and also the symbol for "ox," signifying anything huge.

eliminate is derived from the Latin *e-,* "out or beyond," + *limen,* "threshold." What we eliminate, then, we discard or "throw out beyond the threshold." "Preliminary" as used to describe, for example, a tentative diagnosis means something we consider "before crossing the threshold."

elixir to the pharmacist is a fluid, usually a mixture of alcohol and water, with coloring and flavoring added, to serve as a vehicle for a medicinal agent. An example is "elixir of phenobarbital." Most authorities trace "elixir" to the Arabic *al-iksir,* literally "a dry powder" but more specifically an essence that was sought by alchemists to turn base metals into gold. Therefore, to medieval practitioners of the arcane arts, "elixir" had the connotation of magic. When the goal of alchemy proved too elusive, the search continued for an *elixir vital,* a potion intended to ensure eternal youth. This, too, remains undiscovered. On a more prosaic note, we are reminded that there is a Latin adjective *elixus,* meaning "wet through and through; soaked," and this seems more in keeping with the pharmacologic term "elixir" as we know it. But somehow that faint aura of magic still clings to "elixir."

emaciation is derived from a combination of the Latin *e[x],* "out of," in the sense of "because of," + *macerare,* "to make soft or thin." The emaciated patient is in that condition because of whatever has depleted his tissues of their normal substance.

embolism comes from the Greek *embolos,* "a wedge or plug," which is a combination of *en,* "in," + *ballein,* "to throw or cast." An embolus, then, is something "thrown in." Rudolf Virchow (1821–1902), the famous German pathologist, is said to have suggested the use of "embolus" as the name for a loose blood clot that becomes wedged in a smaller vessel, thus obstructing the flow of blood.

embryo is from the Greek *embryon,* "the fruit of the womb," which in turn was derived from *en-,* "in," + *bryo,* "to cause to burst forth."

emesis comes from the Greek *emein,* "to vomit." To the Greeks, *emetikos* meant "provoking sickness," and from this comes the word **emetic,** referring to an agent that induces vomiting.

emissary describes veins connecting the venous sinuses of the dura mater, through foramina in the skull, with the external veins. The word is derived from the Latin *emissarium,* "drain or outlet." The term was first applied in 1720 by Giovanni Domenico Santorini (1681–1737), the Italian anatomist. The concept was that excessive pressure in the dural vessels could be alleviated by the escape of blood through these "drains."

emollient comes from the Latin *emollire,* "to soften or make mild." In pharmacy, an emollient is a substance that softens or soothes the skin or an irritated mucosal surface.

empathy is derived from a combination of the Greek *en-,* "in," + *pathos,* "feeling." The concept is thought to have originated with the German psychologist Theodor Lipps in the word *Einfühlung.* The concept of "in feeling" connotes the emotional appreciation of another's feeling. But, in comparison with sympathy, empathy implies an awareness of the observer's separateness from the observed. The distinction is nicely made by

Dr. Charles D. Aring (*JAMA* 167:448, 1958), who points out, "Appreciation of another's feelings and problems is quite different from joining in them, and in so doing, complicating them beyond resolving." The good doctor, then, has an empathetic understanding of his patients' feelings.

emphysema is a borrowing of the Greek word meaning "an inflation," this coming from a combination of *en-*, "in," + *physiaō*, "I blow." In the 17th century, emphysema was any swelling of tissues caused by the infiltration of air. "Surgical emphysema" sometimes followed trauma and produced the sign we now call "crepitus." René Théophile Hyacinthe Laënnec, the innovative French physician, described pulmonary emphysema in the early 19th century. The term is now customarily restricted, for the most part, to the disease of the lungs characterized by increased air space.

empirical comes through the Latin *empiricus*, "a self-trained physician," from the Greek *empeiros*, "skilled by experience." This, in turn, was derived from *en-*, "by," + *peira*, "trial." The "empiric school of medicine" arose in the 2nd century B.C., and its adherents were concerned only with what they perceived as the immediate cause of illness and its symptomatic expression. In their search for remedies, they were committed to acting on their own observations and scorned the more traditional and speculative approach of the "dogmatists." The "dogmatists" (or "methodists," as they were sometimes called) in turn looked upon the "empiricists" as charlatans. Fortunately, there is no longer such a heated dis-

pute. All capable physicians recognize and make use of empirical observations and beneficial treatments with the understanding that simply because they cannot yet be wholly or rationally explained does not render them invalid.

empyema is taken from the Greek word for "a suppuration." It is a combination of *en-*, "in," + *pyon*, "pus or corrupt matter." Now the term usually is restricted to a suppurative collection in the pleural space or gallbladder.

encephalo- is a combining form derived from the Greek *enkephalon*, "the brain." This in turn comes from *en-*, "in," + *kephalē*, "the head." Indeed, the Greek word, slightly modified as "encephalon," is still used to designate, collectively, the contents of the cranium, viz., the cerebrum, the cerebellum, the pons, and the medulla oblongata. **Encephalopathy** is a general term referring to almost any disorder of the brain; **encephalitis** is an inflammation of the brain.

endarteritis is an inflammation of the innermost coat, the tunica intima, of an artery. The word has been derived from the Greek *endon*, "within," + *arteria*, "artery." Endarteritis is not to be misconstrued as an inflammation of an "end artery." This term refers to an artery, usually a small terminal branch, that does not anastomose with another arterial channel.

endemic comes from the Greek *endemos*, "native to a place," this being derived from *en-*, "in," + *demos*, "people." The Greek word appears in Hippocratic writings to refer to anything, particularly a disease, peculiar to the people of a given area. In present usage, "endemic" denotes a disease that is not necessarily widely prevalent, but almost always to be found among the inhabitants of a particular place.

endo- is a combining prefix representing the Greek *endon,* "in, inner, or within," and serves a large number of medical terms. The **endocardium** (+ Greek *kardia,* "heart") is the membrane lining the chambers of the heart. **Endocrine** (+ Greek *krinein,* "to separate or put apart") was contrived to describe those glands that "put apart" and secrete substances which are then used within the body in contrast to exocrine glands, which excrete whatever they "put apart" into channels that communicate with the exterior of the body. The endocrine organs sometimes are called the "glands of internal secretion." **Endoderm** (+ Greek *derma,* "skin") is the innermost of the three germ layers of the embryo, the others being the *ecto*derm (outer) and *meso*derm (middle). **Endometrium** (+ Greek *mētra,* "uterus") is the membrane lining the uterus. **Endometriosis** is a condition wherein an endothelial tissue almost identical to that of the uterine mucosa proliferates in ectopic sites, usually in or near the pelvis. **Endorphin** is a generic descriptor of certain opiate peptides recently found to be elaborated in the brain. Dr. Avram Goldstein, among the pioneer investigators in this new field, credits his colleague Dr. E. J. Simon with having coined the term in 1975. Presumably, "endorphin" is a contraction of *endo*genous *morphine*-like substances. Dr. Goldstein explains that this is "analogous to 'corticotropin,'" which denotes the biologic activity rather than a specific chemical structure" (*Science* 193:1081, 1976). **Endoscopy** (+ Greek *skopein,* "to look or inspect") is a technique whereby a diagnostician, using specially designed optical instruments, can peer into the innermost recesses of the body. Hardly any orifice or body cavity has remained virgin by resisting the probes of the endoscopist. **Endothelium** (+ Greek *thēlē,* "nipple") is an oddly derived word. Apparently *epi*thelium was first used to describe the outer covering of the nipple, then later applied to the skin generally, and eventually to any membrane communicating with the exterior of the body. In contrast, *endo*thelium was contrived to denote that type of membrane that lines the cavities of the heart, the blood and lymph vessels, and the serous surfaces of the body.

enema comes from the Greek *enienai,* derived from a combination of *en,* "in," + *ienai,* "to send." The procedure of injecting fluids into the anus was known and practiced by the ancients, probably originating with the Egyptians. The proper medical term, however, in bygone years was **clyster,** coming from the Greek *klyzein,* "to wash out." A Greek *klyster* was "a syringe." The intrarectal administration of fluids, either for cleansing or for the introduction of medicaments, was long held to be solely in the province of the doctor and, as such, was always called "a clyster." When physicians tired of the practice and abandoned it to nurses, the procedure was the same but the name was changed to "enema." The early Dutch were much more straightforward and called it *aarsspuiting.*

ensiform comes from the Latin *ensis,* "a sword," + *forma,* "shape or appearance." Thus, the cartilage at the lower end of the sternum, having the appearance of a small sword, became known as "the ensiform process." Its other name is **xiphoid** and means the same but comes from the Greek *xiphos,* "sword," + *eidos,* "like."

entero- is a combining form derived from the Greek *enteron,* "the gut or intestine," this relating to the Greek *enteros,* "within." The same sense is expressed in the vulgar English term "innards."

entomology comes from the Greek *entoma,* "insects," + *logos,* "a study." The Greek name for insects was derived from *en-,* "in," + *tomē,* "a cutting." The allusion was to the markedly segmented bodies of bugs that gave the appearance of having been "cut into." Of course, the Latin *insectum,* "notched or indented," means the same thing. It goes without saying that "entomology" should never be confused with "etymology" (from the Greek *etymos,* "true or actual," + *logos,* "word or reason"), the subject of this book.

enzyme is contrived from the Greek *en-,* "in," + *zymē,* "a leavening agent or ferment." The term was coined in 1858 by Moritz Traube (1826–1894), working in the laboratory of Ferdinand Cohn (1828–1898) in Breslau, for the substance he could only hypothesize to be responsible for the phenomenon of fermentation. Previously, fermentation of carbohydrates was thought to be dependent on the presence of living yeast cells. It was not until 1897 that the actual enzyme, then called **zymase,** was proven to

exist by Eduard Buchner (1860–1917), a German biochemist.

eosin was given its name from the Greek *ēos,* "dawn." The allusion was to the rosy color of the sky at daybreak and of the dye, tetrabrom fluorescein, commonly used in tissue staining. An **eosinophil** (from the Greek *-philein,* "to love") is a cell that "likes" or has an affinity for eosin and refers specifically to those white blood cells that display prominent red cytoplasmic granules when stained with eosin.

ependyma was given as a name for the lining membrane of the cerebral ventricles and central canal of the spinal cord by Rudolf Virchow (1821–1902), the celebrated German pathologist. How Virchow contrived this name is not clear. The Greek *ependytes* is "an outer tunic," that is, a tunic worn on top of another (from *epi-,* "upon or on top of," + *endyo,* "to put on or clothe"). The idea of "clothing" may be understood, but the allusion to an outer garment for an inner lining is confusing.

ephedrine is the name given to a sympathomimetic alkaloid originally obtained from *Ephedra equisetina,* commonly known as "the horsetail plant." The Greek *ephedraō* means "I sit upon" (from *epi-,* "upon," + *hedra,* "seat or chair"), and a similar term was used in the Hippocratic "Aphorisms" to refer to the buttocks. Apparently there was something about the plant that suggested the tail end of a horse.

epi- is a classical prefix taken from the Greek preposition *epi,* which can mean "on, upon, at, by, near, over, on top of, toward, against, among." **Epidemic** comes from the Greek *epidēmios,* "among the people"; the Greek *dēmos* referred especially to "the common people or citizenry." Hippocrates used *epidēmios* when alluding to diseases rife among the populace. **Epidermis** (+ Greek *derma,* "skin") was also used in Hippocratic writings to refer to the outer layer of the skin. **Epididymis** is a direct borrowing of the Greek word, but to Galen, the famous 2nd-century Greek physician, it meant the outer membrane of the testis. However, Herophilus, the Greek "father of anatomy" who performed his works a century later, used the term as we do, to mean the coiled portion of the spermatic ducts that "sit upon" the testes. The Greek *didymos* actually means "double, twofold, or twins," but also was used to refer to the paired testes and ovaries. "Epididymis" with its three "i"s and one "y" often poses a spelling problem for medical students, young and old. The puzzle of which goes where is solved by remembering the origin of the word, i.e., beginning with *epi-,* followed by the *di-* of "two." **Epigastrium** is an almost direct borrowing of the Greek *epigastrion* (+ Greek *gaster,* "belly"), which referred to the area of the anterior abdominal wall above the umbilicus. The area below the umbilicus was called the *hypogastrion* ("below the belly") or **hypogastrium,** as we know it now. **Epiglottis** is the term for the lid-like cap covering the entrance to the trachea. Apparently the structure was once thought of as an appendage of the tongue, because its name combines *epi-* with the Greek *glōtta,* a variant of *glōssa,* "tongue." **Epilepsy** comes from the Greek *epilēpsis,* "a laying

hold of." To the Greeks the word also meant "a seizure," the notion being that the victim of a seizure was "laid hold of" by some mysterious force or influence, probably instigated by the gods. In fact, the Roman term was *morbus sacer,* "sacred disease." **Epinephrine** was so named from Greek sources in 1898 by J. J. Abel (1857–1938), the physiologist who isolated the sympathomimetic substance from the adrenal gland which happens to be situated above *(epi-)* the kidney (Greek *nephros*). **Adrenalin** also was a logical Latin coinage for the same substance, but this term was taken over as a trade name. **Epiphysis** is a direct borrowing of the Greek word for an outgrowth of bone that is separated in its development by a zone of cartilage from the end of the main portion of a long bone. More particularly, now, the term refers to a secondary center of ossification commonly found at the ends of long bones. The Greek word for "growth" is *physis.* **Epiploic** is from the Greek *epiploon,* the name used for the omentum in Hippocratic writings. This, in turn, came from the Greek *epipleō,* "I sail upon or float upon." The allusion, presumably, is to the omentum "floating upon" the abdominal viscera. The **appendices epiplocae** were so called because they appeared to be small, omentum-like appendages of the colon. The **epiploic foramen** is an opening into the lesser peritoneal space behind the lesser omentum. It is sometimes called "the foramen of Winslow" after Jacob Benignus Winslow (1669–1760), the Danish anatomist who described it. **Episiotomy** is a combination of the Greek *epision,* "the pubes or pudenda," + *tomē,* "a cutting." The term is said to have been proposed in 1857 by Karl von Braun (1822–1891), a Viennese obstetrician, for the procedure of widening the outlet of the birth canal to facilitate delivery. **Epispadias** (+ Greek *spadōn,* "a tear or rent") refers to the congenital defect wherein the urethra opens on the dorsum of the penis. **Epistaxis** is a direct borrowing of the Greek word meaning "a dripping," particularly of blood from the nose. The root verb is the Greek *stazein,* "to let fall, drop by drop." **Epithelium** (+ Greek *thēlē,* "the nipple") originally was used to describe the cellular surface membrane overlying the nipple. Later, Friedrich Gustav Jakob Henle (1809–1885), the celebrated German histologist, applied the term to all surface membranes, including the skin and other surfaces communicating with the exterior of the body. This is in contrast to **endothelium,** which has nothing to do with the nipple, but was somehow contrived from the same origin to refer to membranes lining closed, internal spaces, including blood and lymph vessels. **Epizootic** is a disease rampant among animals (from the Greek *zōion,* "animal"), the bestial counterpart of "epidemic."

eponym is from the Greek *epōnymos,* "named after someone," this being derived from a combination of *epi-,* "upon," + *onoma,* "name." In medicine, a number of anatomic structures, diseases, diagnostic procedures, and methods of treatment have been named after the persons who discovered, described, or promoted them. A modern tendency has been to discourage or even abhor the use of eponyms. In part, this is understandable. "Bright's disease," named for Richard Bright (1789–1858), a notable physician who worked at Guy's Hospital, in London, proved to be too nondescript a term for the various forms of nephritis. On the other hand, "Laënnec's cirrhosis" clearly designates the micronodular consequence of alcoholic injury in the liver, and substitutes are either incomplete or unduly cumbersome. Moreover, eponyms often convey a nice sense of historical tribute.

Epsom salt once was the term for hydrated magnesium sulfate when this was commonly used as a laxative and also as a bath or soak to alleviate inflammation or swelling. An early source for the substance was the mineral springs at Epsom, England. The town now is probably better known as the site of Epsom Downs, a well-known racetrack.

ergot gets its name from the Old French *argot,* "a cock's spur." Rye plants infected by the fungus *Claviceps purpurea* yield grain that is purple and misshapen in a sickle-form that resembles a cock's spur. Such grains are carefully excluded from rye intended for consumption as a cereal, but are deliberately cultivated as a commercial source of various ergot alkaloids (e.g., d-lysergic acid, methysergide, ergotamine, and bromocriptine). The principal actions (but by no means the only effects) of ergot are contraction of uterine muscle and peripheral vasoconstriction. Ergot poisoning, from consumption of rye contaminated by the fungus, was rife in the

Middle Ages. Abortion and gangrene were common consequences of ergot poisoning. The pain suffered by its victims was such that the condition was sometimes referred to as *ignis sacer* ("holy fire"), *ignis infernalis* ("hell's fire"), or Saint Anthony's fire (because it was at shrines dedicated to Saint Anthony that sufferers sought relief).

erosion comes from the Latin *erodere,* "to eat away," which is a combination of *e(x)*-, "out or away," + *rodere,* "to gnaw." An erosion is a lesion wherein the affected skin or mucous membrane appears to have been "eaten away." Incidentally, the Latin term explains why certain gnawing animals are called "rodents," and why mercury bichloride is sometimes called "corrosive sublimate."

eructation is a fussy substitute for "belch" or "burp." It comes from the Latin *eructare,* "to belch or vomit." **Belch** is the present-day spelling of the Old English *bealcian* and may be related to "boil" in the sense of generating gas. The Dutch *balken* means "to bray." **Burp** is an imitative word, that is, it sounds like what it means, and that would seem to be a perfectly sound reason for using it.

erysipelas is a condition marked by redness and swelling of the skin and subcutaneous tissue resulting from infection by group-A streptococci. The name we use is the same as given by the ancient Greeks, although their application of the term may not have been as specific. Professor H. A. Skinner offers two origins of "erysipelas": *(a)* from the Greek *erythros,* "red," + *pella,* "skin";

or *(b)* from the Greek *eraō,* "I draw," + *pelas,* "near" (perhaps because of its tendency to spread to nearby parts). He points out that the sense of the first derivation is better, while the etymology of the second seems more correct.

erythema is a direct borrowing of the Greek word for "redness in the skin, or a blush." The Greek *erythros* means "red." Medically, the use of "erythema" has been extended to describe redness in any surface, external or internal, caused by dilatation and engorgement of the capillary bed.

erythrocyte is so called from a combination of the Greek *erythros,* "red," + *kytos,* "cell." As such, it could refer to any "red cell" but is reserved for those anucleate, disk-shaped cells that circulate in the blood.

eschar comes from the Greek *eschara,* which commonly meant "a hearth or fireplace" but also was used in Hippocratic writings to describe the scab that formed when a wound was sealed by cautery. To call such a seal an "eschar" is a nice usage, but to call every scab an eschar is a turgidity.

esophagus is a name for the gullet and was derived from the Greek *oise,* the future imperative of *pherō-,* "I bear or carry," + *phago-,* a learned combining form taken from the Greek *phagein,* "to eat or devour," and in this sense referring to "that which was eaten." **Gullet** comes through the Old French as a diminutive of the Latin *gula,* "throat," the idea presumably being that the narrower esophagus was sort of "little throat." Until recent times not much attention was paid to what seemed a simple conduit connecting the pharynx with the stomach. Now we know that appearances are deceiving, and that the esophagus is actually a quite sophisticated organ, subject to a variety of disturbances and disorders.

essence has long been used to refer to the active principle of a drug, particularly one of botanical origin. The word comes from the Latin *essentia,* which in turn was derived from *esse,* "to be." Thereby, the "essence" is the "being" or fundamental quality of anything. For example, in a solution of a volatile oil in alcohol, where alcohol is the vehicle, the volatile oil is the "essential oil." Aristotle added a "fifth element" that he called "essence" to his basic categories of matter: fire, air, earth, and water. This came to be called the "quintessence" (from the Latin *quintus,* "fifth"). We now use this term for the most nearly perfect embodiment of something.

ester is a term said to have been coined by Leopold Gmelin (1788–1853), a German physiologist. His purpose was to generally designate compound ethers. The new term was made up of the first and last syllables of *Essigäther,* the German word for "acetic ether."

estrus refers to the regularly recurring periods of maximal sexual receptivity in female mammals, also known as periods of "heat" or "rut." "Estrus" (which is spelled "oestrus" by the proper British) comes from the Greek *oistros,* "the gadfly," an insect whose sting puts cattle in a frenzy. In gynecology, estrus refers to the cycle of changes in the female genital tract consequent to ovarian hormonal activity. **Estrogen** is the generic

term coined for hormonal substances that induce estrus in female mammals. It is a contrived combination of "estro-," denoting *estrus,* + "gen" (from the Greek *gennaō,* "I bring forth").

ether comes through the Latin *aethra* from the Greek *aithēr,* "the upper, purer air" (as opposed to *aēr,* "the lower air or immediately surrounding atmosphere"). This explains why "ether" is used to refer to whatever is conceived to fill the vast upper regions of space and thus serves to transmit waves of the electromagnetic spectrum. The colorless, transparent, and highly volatile diethyl ether was known and named long before its use as an anesthetic agent was demonstrated. It was first called *spiritus aethereus,* "ethereal spirit," presumably because of its clarity and extreme volatility.

ethmoid comes from the Greek *ēthmos,* "a sieve," and *eidos,* "like." The name has been applied to the bone that forms a roof for the nasal fossae and part of the floor of the anterior fossa of the skull. The bone's numerous perforations give it the appearance of a sieve.

etiology is a combination of the Greek *aitia,* "a cause," and *logos,* "a discourse," and means a study or exposition of causes. "Etiology" often is mistakenly used as a synonym for "cause." Doctors of medicine have a penchant for using seemingly learned, polysyllabic terms in the place of simple words. If one chooses the more pretentious of two words that mean the same thing, that is pedantic pomposity. If one uses the more highfalutin of two words that do not mean the same thing, that is ignorance. Other frequently encountered examples are the mistaken use of "methodology" when one means "method," and the almost ludicrous use of "symptomatology" when one means "symptoms." Tacking on an erroneous "-ology" should fool no one.

eu- is a combining prefix that represents the Greek adverb *eu,* "goodly or well," as opposed to the inseparable prefix *dys-,* "hard, bad, or ill." For example, **euthyroid** has been coined to indicate a normal or "good" function of the thyroid gland. **Euphoria** comes from the Greek word *euphorus,* "well or patiently borne," being a combination of *eu-* + *pherein,* "to bear." In present-day usage, "euphoria" has been elevated in sense to mean elation or an abnormally exaggerated feeling of well-being.

ex- is the Latin preposition (sometimes shortened to just *e*) meaning "out of, from" (in the sense of space); "from, after, since" (in the sense of time); "from, by, through, on account of" (in the sense of cause or origin); "after, according to" (in the sense of conformity); or "with, by means of" (in the sense of means). **Exacerbation** is taken from the Latin *exacerbare,* "to provoke or exasperate," this being a combination of *ex-* + *acerbare,* "to embitter, to aggravate." Thus, an acerbic remark is a bitter utterance that may provoke anger. In medicine, an exacerbation is an increase in severity, usually as a repetition, of a disease or its symptoms. **Exanthem** is a near borrowing of the Greek *exanthema,* "a breaking out," as in the blooming of flowers. In this Greek word, the "x" is the letter xi (not chi). *Anthos* is the Greek for "flower," specifically the bloom

or blossom. In medicine, exanthem is used to refer to an outbreak of lesions in the skin, particularly those associated with the familiar childhood diseases, such as measles. Formerly, a companion word, enanthem, was used to refer to lesions appearing in mucous membranes, but this is seldom heard nowadays. **Excoriation** comes from the Latin *excoriare,* "to flay," a combination of *ex-* + *corium,* "the skin." The sense here is that strips of skin are torn away. The violence implicit in the term has been toned down in medicine, where excoriation has come to mean a scratch or the result of scratching. **Excrescence** comes from the Latin *excrescere,* "to grow out, to rise up," being a combination of *ex-* + *crescere,* "to come into being, to arise." In pathology, an excrescence is a lesion of any sort that "grows out" of a surface. **Excretion** is derived from the Latin *excernere,* "to sift out, to separate," a combination of *ex-* + *cernere,* "to distinguish, to decide." Thus the origin of this term makes an interesting and significant point. Whatever is excreted is not merely discarded or "put out" but, rather, has been purposely separated from something else. In physiology, excretion refers to substances separated for external discharge, as from the skin or mucous structures, while secretion refers to substances separated for internal discharge, such as hormones. **Exercise** comes from the Latin verb *exercere,* "to keep someone busy or to keep something in motion, to train, or to drill." *Exercere,* in turn, was derived from *ex-* + *ercere,* the combining form of *arcere,* "to restrain or to keep pent up." Thus exercise is not just moving about but also the release of tension. **Exfoliate** comes from a combination of *ex- + folium,* "leaf," thus "to shed," as leaves. An exfoliative dermatitis is a severe form of inflammation wherein the necrotic skin peels away, as dead leaves fall from a tree. **Exogenous** is contrived from a combination of the Greek *exō-* (where the "x" is xi, not chi) + *gennaō,* "I produce." Whatever is exogenous is produced or arises outside the body, while whatever is endogenous is produced or arises within. **Exophthalmos** describes a protruding eye or the condition of being "bug-eyed," the term being a combination of the Greek *ex- + ophthalmos,* "eye." Exophthalmic goiter is a condition wherein a palpable swelling of the thyroid gland is associated with a hypermetabolic state, a sign of which is protrusion of the eyeballs. Formerly this was called "Graves' disease" in tribute to Robert James Graves (1796–1853), the brilliant Irish physician who lived and taught in Dublin and who published a perceptive account of the disease in 1835. Graves was a reformer of clinical teaching and an innovator who also had a sense of humor. Whereas in his time the dictum was "Feed a cold and starve a fever," Graves requested that his epitaph should read, "He fed fevers." **Exotic** is derived from the Greek *exōtikos,* meaning "foreign or alien." Originally it was used to describe anything strange that came from a foreign land. An exotic disease is one usually observed in a faraway place and rarely, if ever, in one's own habitat. "Exotic" is not to be confused with "esoteric," which means "known only to a select few." **Expectorant** comes from the Latin *expectorare,* "to expel from the chest," being a combination of *ex- + pectus,* "the chest." An expectorant, then, is a medicament that enables the patient to expel phlegm from his bronchial tubes and trachea. To expectorate is not exactly the same as to spit, although often the polysyllabic term is used as a delicate substitute. One spits from the mouth; whatever is spit may or may not come from the chest. "Spit" comes from the Old English *spātl,* "saliva," whence "spittle." **Experiment** is an almost direct borrowing of the Latin *experimentum,* "a test." This, in turn, relates to *experiri,* "to try out." **Extensor** comes from the Latin *extendere,* "to stretch out." An extensor muscle is one that "stretches out" a joint, as opposed to a flexor muscle, which bends a joint. **Extirpate** means to remove completely or "to root out," as a surgeon might wholly resect a tumor. The word comes from the Latin *ex- + stirps,* "stalk, stem, or root."

eye comes through the Anglo-Saxon *ēage,* from the Teutonic *auge,* all of which refer to the organ of vision. Incidentally, the Old Norse *vindauga,* "wind-eye," became our "window." In years past, the upper canine tooth was called the "eyetooth" in the mistaken belief that it was connected to a branch of the same nerve that supplies the eye.

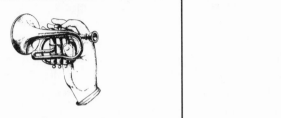

F

facies is the direct borrowing of the Latin word for "face." To the Romans it also meant "visage or appearance," in the sense of what was externally apparent. We also use "face" in the same way when we say "on the face of it. . . ." In medicine, the *facies Hippocratica* is the visage of a moribund patient. In the *Prognostics* of Hippocrates, this was described as a "sharp nose, hollow eyes, collapsed temples; the ears cold, contracted, and their lobes turned out; the skin about the forehead being rough, distended and parched; the color of the whole face being green, black, livid, or lead-colored."

Cassius facies is an expression that comes from Shakespeare's *Julius Caesar* (act I, scene ii), where Caesar observes, "Yon Cassius has a lean and hungry look." Caesar was prescient when he followed this by remarking, "He thinks too much; such men are dangerous."

factitious is taken from the Latin *facticius*, which is related to the verb *facere*, "to make, fashion, or build," and hence refers to whatever is made to occur, as opposed to that which occurs naturally or spontaneously. Thus, a factitious fever is one that is induced, and factitious diarrhea is forced to occur by the deliberate use of cathartics. "Artificial" and "factitial" are nearly synonymous, but, in medicine, "factitious" carries the connotation of surreptitious, with an intent to deceive.

falciform is contrived by a combination of the Latin *falx, falcis,* "scythe or sickle," + *forma,* "shape." The falciform ligament is a sickle-shaped peritoneal fold by which the anterior and superior surface of the liver is attached to the abdominal wall and the diaphragm.

fascia is the singular of the Latin feminine noun meaning "a band or bandage." To the

Romans, the word also meant "a wisp of cloud." Both senses are evident in the anatomic use of the term. In ancient writings, "fascia" meant only a narrow fibrous band, while a broad sheet of connective tissue was called an "aponeurosis." *Fasciculus,* being the diminutive of *fascia,* is "a little bundle." In anatomy the term is applied to various small bundles or clusters of nerve or muscle fibers. **Fasciculation** refers to focal, clonic contractions of a small bundle of muscle fibers resulting from irritability in a single neuromuscular component.

fat comes from the Old English *faētt,* the past participle of *faētan,* "to cram or to adorn." A related word is "vat," which comes from the Old English *faet,* "a vessel." In olden days, for a man or beast to be "well upholstered" was looked upon with favor.

fauces is a direct borrowing of the Latin word for "a small passage," particularly that into the throat or gullet. In anatomy, the "faucial tonsils" (also called "palatine tonsils") are the gland-like aggregates of lymphoid tissue situated in the throat.

favism refers to an acute hemolytic anemia that occurs in persons who have a genetic deficiency of glucose-6-phosphate dehydrogenase in their erythrocytes and who thereby suffer a hemolytic reaction when they eat fava beans. *Fava* is the Italian word for "bean," particularly the "broad bean." The Latin word for bean is *faba,* and this serves as an example of the frequent interchange of "b" and "v" in Romance languages.

favus is a kind of tinea capitis, resulting from infection by the fungus *Trichophyton scho-*

enleini and characterized by the formation of yellow, cup-shaped crusts. *Favus* is the Latin word for "honeycomb," which the crusts resemble.

feces comes from the Latin *faex, faecis,* "dregs or sediment." In the 15th century and for at least two hundred years thereafter, the English used the Latin word, variously spelled, to refer to the dregs of any fermenting substance. Beginning in the 17th century, "faeces" (later Americanized as "feces") became restricted in reference to the "dregs" or excrement of the bowel.

fecund is the contraction of the Latin *fecundus,* "to be fruitful." In the biology of reproduction, "fecundity" denotes the ability to produce offspring.

feldsher as used to describe a physician's assistant comes from the German *Feldscherer.* An old German word for "barber" was *Scherer,* which reminds us of our word "shearer," one who shears sheep or human heads. Taking to the field, as with an army, the Scherer became a *Feldscherer,* among whose duties was also that of pulling teeth and otherwise assisting the military surgeon. Today "feldsher" designates a minimally trained medical practitioner, particularly one who serves in rural Russia. The Chinese counterpart is a "barefoot doctor."

femto is the prefix used in the metric system to denote powers of 15. It is from the Danish *femten,* "fifteen." The units by which the mean corpuscular volume (MCV) of erythrocytes are expressed are femtoliters, i.e., 1×10^{-15} liter, an exceedingly small volume.

femur is the Latin word for "thigh." In anatomy it is used as the name of the thighbone.

fenestra is the Latin word for "window," related to the Greek *phainein,* "show, bring to light, disclose." "Fenestra" is used as an anatomical term to describe certain window-like openings, especially in the ear, such as "fenestra ovalis" (in the middle ear) and "fenestra rotunda" (in the cochlea). A fenestrated structure is featured by openings or apertures. "Fenestration" refers to an operation wherein openings are made. In another context, "to defenestrate" means to throw something (or someone) out of a window.

ferment is a contraction of the Latin *fermentum,* which to the Romans meant "yeast" and was recognized as the ingredient necessary to promote the conversion of sugar or starch-containing substances to alcoholic beverages. The word was derived from the Latin verb *fervere,* "to seethe or to boil," doubtless because gas (carbon dioxide), generated in the process, gives an appearance of boiling. Fermentation occurs normally and abnormally in the human digestive tract.

fettle is a word for "condition or trim" that is now only occasionally heard and then usually in combination as "in fine fettle," meaning physically fit. In Old English, a *fettle* was a girdle of sorts, and to be in fine fettle was to be well girded. This brings to mind a verse composed by German students in 1817 at Wartburg in celebration of the burning of the male corset:

> A corset girds with great élan
> The waist of every proud Uhlan
> So that when he in battle stands
> His heart won't fall into his pants!

fetus is a direct borrowing of the Latin masculine noun, which had numerous meanings, such as "breeding, produce, offspring, fruit," all in the sense of successful reproduction. Probably the term is related to the Latin verb *ferre,* "to carry, to bring forth, to produce." Now the word is restricted to designate the unborn offspring, more mature than an embryo, of any mammal.

fever comes through the Old French *fevre,* from the Latin *febris,* which means "fever." The word is thought to be of Sabine origin. It is related to the Latin verb *fervere,* "to seethe or steam" (from which, incidentally, comes our word "fervent"). In Hippocratic practice, fever was regarded as beneficial in the sense of being a symptom of the body's natural antagonism to disease. The Latin *febris,* then, may also relate to the verb *februare,* "to cleanse or to purify." February is so named as the month for cleansing and purification in anticipation of the coming spring. Only a few generations ago it was customary for people to dose themselves with cathartics, as a "spring tonic." **Febrile,** a Latinized way of saying "with fever," is favored by doctors and nurses. "Feverish" would be a more English way of saying the same thing, but this is a word used by patients and is not quite learned enough for professionals.

fiber is an almost direct borrowing of the Latin *fibra,* which means the same thing, that is, "a tough filament or thread." A **fibril,** as the diminutive, is "a fine thread." In cardiology, **fibrillation** refers to an incoordinate twitching of individual muscle fibers in the atria or ventricles. **Fibrin** is the product of plasma that forms the proteinaceous fibers that constitute the matrix of a blood clot. **Fibroid** is a hybrid term combining the Latin *fibra* + the Greek *eidos,* "like," and can refer to anything that appears to be composed of fibers. More specifically, "fibroid" was long used mistakenly as the name for a benign, smooth muscle neoplasm arising in the myometrium. This, of course, is a leiomyoma of the uterus and is now so called.

fibula is the Latin word for "clasp or brooch," particularly the needle of a brooch or the tongue of a buckle. Probably this was derived from the Latin verb *figere,* "to fasten." The relation of the two bones of the lower leg was likened to that of the bar and clasp of a brooch, the fibula being the clasp.

filariasis is the disease caused by *Filaria,* a genus of nematodes or "thread worms," which, in some areas, are common parasites of man and beast. The name comes from the Latin *filum,* "a thread." One manifestation of filariasis can be grotesque swelling of the affected leg consequent to lymphatic obstruction; hence the name **elephantiasis** also has been given to the disease.

filter began with the German *Filz,* "felt," that nonwoven fabric made from the hair or fur of animals by the application of heat, moisture, and pressure. It was of this fabric that the first efficient fine strainers were made, and *Filz* became Latinized in medieval times as *filtrum.* This term later became applied to any porous material through which a fluid mixture could be passed to remove its particulate matter.

fimbria is the Latin word for "fringe" and the name given to any fringe-like border, such as that of the distal end of the oviduct.

finger as the name for a digit of the hand is of Teutonic origin and possibly goes back to *pengros,* related to *penge,* "five." The Romans named rather than numbered the fingers: *pollex* (thumb), *index* (the pointing finger), *medius* (the middle finger), *annularis* (the ring finger), and *minimus* (the smallest finger).

fissure is taken from the Latin *fissura,* "a cleft," which was derived from the Latin verb *findere,* "to cleave." The postulated Indo-European root is said to have been *bheid,* "to split" (from which, incidentally, we get the words bit, bite, bitter, beetle, and boat). "Fissure" has been applied to the names of various cleft structures, particularly those of the surface of the brain. An anal fissure is a painful split in the mucosa or skin of that keenly sensitive area.

fistula is the Latin word for "pipe or tube." To the Romans, this usually meant a water pipe but could also mean the opening of an ulcer. It is in this latter sense that, in medicine, "fistula" has come to refer to any abnormal drainage tract. A related word is **fester,** an intransitive verb acquired from the Old French *festre,* "a draining or rankling sore."

fix is a contraction of the Latin *fixus,* the past participle of *figere,* "to fasten or make firm." This is the precise sense in which a fracture is "fixed." The common meaning of the word has been broadened to include repair or restoration to a normal, functioning state. By extrapolation, a drug addict, in a state of disrepair, demands "a fix."

flagella is the plural of the Latin *flagellum,* "whip." The whiplike appendages providing motility to various microorganisms are called flagella. The word is a diminutive of *flagrum,* "a scourge." This in turn came from the Indo-European root *bhlag,* "to strike." Through French we get "flail." A **flail** joint is one of unusual or abnormal mobility. This is an allusion to "flail" as the name of a tool for threshing grain, consisting of a staff or handle at the end of which is a freely swinging bar. The English "flog" has been said to be a schoolboy's (though perhaps it was a sailor's) abbreviation of "flagellate."

flatus is the Latin word for "blowing," as a breeze or a snort. Formerly, "flatulence" meant the disagreeable presence of "wind" or gas in the gut generally, but latterly "flatus" has come to be restricted to gas expelled through the anus. The Greek word for "breaking wind" was *perdomai,* and from this came *perdix,* the Greek name for the gallinaceous game bird we call the "partridge." Anyone who has flushed a partridge in the field can recognize the Greeks' allusion to the whirring sound as the partridge takes flight.

flex comes from the Latin verb *flectere,* "to bend or to turn." Muscles that bend a joint are "flexors" as opposed to "extensors," which straighten a joint. One can flex a joint but not a muscle, common parlance notwithstanding.

flocculation comes from the diminutive of the Latin *floccus,* "a tuft of wool." Particulate matter coming out of solution as a result of chemical or physical action may resemble little tufts of wool.

fluke in the descriptive sense of "flat" probably is related to the German *flach,* "flat." The fluke, or flounder, is a flatfish, and parasitic flatworms are also commonly called "flukes," according to their habitat, be it blood, the intestine, the lung, or the liver.

fluoroscopy is a means of viewing an image generated by X rays acting on a fluorescent screen. **Fluorescence** is a word coined in 1852 by Sir George Stokes, a British physicist, to denote glowing of the mineral fluorite, or fluorspar, when exposed to certain rays of the electromagnetic spectrum. Fluorite was used as a flux, hence its name from the Latin *fluere,* "to flow." Sir George chose to follow the custom of incorporating the names of other minerals in similar terms, such as "opalescence" and "phosphorescence." Actually, the "fluorescent" screen used to capture the image generated by X rays was coated with calcium tungstate (not calcium fluoride or fluorite). What is now called "fluoroscopy" in a modern radiology department employs a television screen.

focus is a direct borrowing of the Latin word that to the Romans meant "hearth, fireplace, or altar." The hearth, in a Roman home, was the place where most of the essential household activities converged. Now we use the word to refer to any point of convergence or center of attention. A focal pain, for example, is clearly where the patient's attention is centered.

folie à deux is a term used in psychiatry for the sharing of delusions simultaneously by two closely associated persons. It is obviously French and combines *folie,* "madness," + *à,* "in," + *deux,* "two." The French *folie,* incidentally, also can mean "playful, frisky, or extravagant" and in this sense gives us the show-business term "the follies."

follicle comes from the Latin *folliculus,* the diminutive of *follis,* "a bag or bellows." A follicle, then, is "a little bag" and an apt name for a host of saccular or encapsulated structures, usually occurring as aggregates, in biology and medicine.

fomentation is a quaint term for the application of hot packs. "Foment" as a verb, now usually used in a figurative way to mean "heat up," was derived as a contraction of the Latin *fovimentum,* "a warm application," from the Latin verb *fovere,* "to warm."

fomite comes from the Latin *fomitis,* the genitive of *fomes,* "tinder." In medicine, a fomite is an inanimate object that can be a source of infection. Often the risk of infection from such a source is exaggerated.

fontanelle is from the diminutive, through the Italian, of the Latin *fontana,* "spring or fountain." The term refers to the incompletely ossified junctions of the bones in a baby's skull, also known as "soft spots." The allusion to "a little fountain" may have arisen because of pulsations felt at the fontanelles.

foramen is the Latin word for "a hole or an opening." In anatomy, holes or openings in all sorts of structures have been called "foramina," which is the Latin plural.

forceps is a direct borrowing of the Latin name for an instrument used to grasp, pluck, or lift. Probably the term was derived from a combination of the stems of the rare Latin *formus,* "hot," + *capere,* "to take," thereby designating an instrument designed to pick up whatever is too hot to handle.

forensic is an adaptation of the Latin *forensis,* meaning whatever pertains to the forum. To the Romans, the Latin *forum* originally designated the marketplace where people gathered to conduct all sorts of transactions including the business of public affairs. Later, the word became more restricted in reference to courts of law. Now, forensic medicine relates to medical jurisprudence.

formalin is a 40% solution of gaseous formaldehyde and is used widely as a fixative for tissue specimens and as an embalming fluid. **Formaldehyde** (HCHO) is the aldehyde of formic acid, which was so called because it was first obtained, in the 17th century, by distilling, of all things, a mess of red ants. *Formica* is the Latin word for "an ant." In years past, diluted (1 : 200 to 1 : 2000) solutions of formalin were commonly used as disinfectants, and their pungency accounted for the peculiar odor that pervaded hospitals of a bygone era.

forme fruste describes an incomplete or atypical expression of a disease. These are French words which together mean "a defaced, rough, or unpolished form." In medicine, for example, a patient may exhibit sudden, intense epigastric pain and a rigid abdomen.

He is thought to have a perforated peptic ulcer. But at operation only a penetrating ulcer is found, sealed off by adhesion to the omentum or anterior abdominal wall. Such a patient is said to have a *forme fruste* of acute, free perforation as a complication of his peptic ulcer disease. A *forme pleine,* also French but seldom used by English-speaking clinicians, is a term for the complete or full-blown form of a disease.

fornix is the Latin word for "arch or vault." In anatomy, the fornix of the cerebrum is an arched fiber tract having two lateral halves that are united under the corpus callosum. The fornix of the vagina is the recess between the vaginal wall and the protruding uterine cervix. **Fornication,** as the term for sexual intercourse between a couple unblessed by holy wedlock, has a similar classical origin. In ancient Rome, prostitutes customarily loitered under the arches of certain public buildings, and an illicit dalliance therewith came to be known euphemistically as "going under the arches," or "fornication."

fossa is the Latin word for "ditch or trench." This, in turn, came from the Latin verb *fodere,* "to dig." In anatomy, a variety of concavities that resemble excavations are referred to as "fossae."

fovea is the Latin word for "a small pit" and is so used in anatomy to designate small depressions in various structures. The fovea of the eye is a tiny pit in the center of the retinal macula where the registration of vision is the most precise.

fracture is derived from the Latin verb *frangere,* "to shatter or to break in pieces." The term is aptly applied to the common injury to which bones are subject.

fremitus is the Latin word for "grumbling or growling." In physical diagnosis, the word denotes the vibration perceived by palpation, particularly over the chest as the patient makes a vocal sound. Fremitus is increased when there is consolidation of the underlying lung and is absent in pneumothorax.

frenulum is the diminutive of the Latin *frenum,* "a bridle." In anatomy, various ligamentous or membranous folds that have a restraining function and hence resemble a bridle are known by this term. An example is the frenulum of the tongue, a vertical fold of mucous membrane under the tongue that attaches it to the floor of the mouth.

friable is derived from the Latin *friare,* "to crumble into small pieces." Thus, Varro wrote of earth that crumbles easily, *terra quae facile frietur.* The word was used in English as early as the 16th century but applied mainly to mineral substances. The ancient meaning serves well in pathology to describe tissues that are readily fragmented.

frontal comes from the Latin *frons,* "forehead or brow," and hence describes whatever pertains to the forehead, such as the frontal nerve or the frontal sinus. The Latin meaning also encompassed "countenance or facade" in the sense of whatever was seen first, and thus "front" commonly is used in a figurative sense.

fuchsin is a brilliant red dye formerly used as a topical antiseptic agent, but now more widely employed as a stain for bacteria and tissue in the preparation of slides for microscopic examination. The dye was discovered as a product of coal tar in the mid-19th century and so named because its color resembles that of fuchsia blossoms. The plant, in turn, was named for Leonhard Fuchs (1501–1566), a famous German botanist. Fuchsin is not to be confused with **fuscin,** a brown pigment occurring in the retinal epithelium, or with **lipofuscin,** a fatty pigment observed as the intracellular product of certain degenerative processes. "Fuscin" comes from the Latin *fuscus,* "dark or indistinct." This Latin word also gives us "obfuscation," rumored to be a major course of study in law schools.

fulguration refers to the use of electrical energy in the form of sparks to desiccate and destroy unwanted tissue, such as that comprising small tumors. The term is derived from the Latin *fulgor,* "a flash of lightning." While it is perfectly proper to refer to a doctor who fulgurates a lesion as a "fulgurator," to the Romans a *fulgurator* was a person who interpreted the mystical significance of lightning.

fumigate comes from the Latin verb *fumigare,* "to expose to the fumes of smoke." In turn, this derived from *fumus,* "smoke," + *agere,* "to drive." The ancients knew that fire and smoke could have a disinfectant action. Homer's Odysseus called for burning sulfur to fumigate the palace in Ithaca. Our word "perfume" is related and is a combination of the Latin *per-,* "through," + *fumus,* "smoke." In the Middle Ages dwellings were "perfumed" to prevent or counteract the plague. Out of this evolved the idea that anything fetid would be cleansed if it was

made fragrant. Thus a substance that conferred fragrance came to be known as "perfume."

function is derived from the Latin *functio,* "a performance," which in turn comes from the Latin deponent verb *fungor,* "to perform or accomplish." Thus, physiology as a major arm of biomedical study concerns itself with how organs and organisms perform. "Functional disorders" are those in which there is a defect of performance or behavior in the absence of any known or recognized defect in structure.

fundus is the Latin word meaning "bottom." In anatomy, the term indicates that portion of a hollow structure that is farthest from its opening. Thus, the fundus of the gallbladder is the very bottom of the bag, and the fundus of the uterus is that part farthest from the cervix. The fundus of the stomach, being that portion superior to the entrance of the esophagus, is a little harder to explain, except that it is the most dependent part when the body is recumbent. Perhaps the meaning is that it is farthest from the pylorus.

fungus is a Latin word that means the same as in English, i.e., a class of vegetable organisms that includes mushrooms, toadstools, and various molds. The Latin word is said to have been derived from the Greek *spho-*[*n*]*ggos,* "a sponge" (the initial "s" having been suppressed in transition). The allusion, of course, is to the spongy texture of the various forms that the Romans came to call *fungi.*

funny bone is an expression used by an occasional patient to refer to his elbow or, more specifically, to the olecranon process of his ulna. Punsters have tried to explain this by pointing out that the ulna articulates with the humerus. The real explanation for "funny bone" is that the ulnar nerve lies in the exposed ulnar groove of the olecranon, which, when bumped, causes a strangely "electric" sensation in the forearm and hand.

furuncle is from the Latin *furunculus,* "a petty thief," being the diminutive of the Latin *fur,* "a thief," presumably of standard dimensions. Roman writers on agriculture used the term to mean a knob on a vine. A word of related origin is "furtive,"

meaning sly and stealthy, like a thief. What all this has to do with a small focus of suppuration in a hair follicle has baffled most medical linguists. A guess might be that extensive furunculosis can result in the loss or "theft" of hair. Another possibility is that since boils were once thought of as a form of corruption, little boils might be considered evidence of only petty corruption.

fusiform means spindle-shaped, and this is appropriate because the Latin word *fusus* means "spindle" or, as the past participle of *fundo,* "spread out."

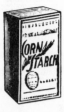

G

galea is the Latin word for "a helmet," particularly one made of leather or skin. According to Professor H. A. Skinner, the Latin word may have come from the Greek *galeē*, "a cat," inasmuch as head coverings once were commonly made of the hides of cats or other small furry animals. The galea aponeurotica is the tough, tendinous connection between the anterior and posterior bellies of the occipitofrontalis muscle, now called the epicranius. It covers the scalp as a cap.

gall as a name for bile is descended from the Old English *gealla*, which meant the same, being probably related to *geolo*, "yellow." Thus, the English word for bile seems to refer to its color. In all likelihood there was a primordial root word that also led to the Greek *cholē*, "bile." There happens to be another "gall," quite unrelated to bile, which comes from the Latin *galla*, meaning a nutlike deformity found on plants infected by the larvae of certain insects. Gallic acid, an astringent substance, was first found in a decoction of gallnuts. In Late Latin, *galla* became a word for tumor, particularly that which seemed to result from focal irritation. This also led to the verb "to gall," meaning to rub harshly or repetitively so as to produce a sore. A saddlesore on either a horse or its rider can be said to result from galling. One occasionally hears the word used figuratively, as in "His rude behavior galls me."

galvanometer designates an instrument for determining the strength and direction of an electric current. The name comes from that of Luigi Galvani (1737–1798), a professor of anatomy at Bologna, who was fascinated by the wondrous properties of the newly discovered electricity. The story is told that one day in 1786 Galvani was working with a machine that produced static electricity, while on a nearby table lay some skinned frog's-legs. Through a scalpel held by an assistant, an impulse of electricity was transmitted to the frog muscle, which thereupon jerked. Galvani seized on this curious observation and expanded it into a rather fanciful theory of "animal electricity," which later was discredited. Nevertheless, Galvani went on to invent a chemical battery to produce a flow of electric current, and on this his fame rests secure. By an interesting turnabout, Willem Einthoven (1860–1927), a Dutch physiologist, in 1902 invented a string galvanometer so sensitive as to detect the electrical impulse generated in the heart, and this became the basis for **electrocardiography.**

gamete means a germ cell, either an ovum or a spermatocyte, essential to sexual reproduction. The term comes from the Greek *gametēs,* "husband," or *gametē,* "wife." These, in turn, relate to the Greek verb *gamein,* "to marry." The biologic usage of "gamete" was advanced by Johann Gregor Mendel (1822–1884), an Austrian monk who gained belated fame as the naturalist who discovered the fundamental principles of genetics.

ganglion comes from the Greek *ga[n]gglion.* (The Greek letter gamma is pronounced as "n" in "ng" when it appears before certain consonants, such as gamma, kappa, chi, and xi; this explains the change of Greek "gg" to "ng" in Latin and modern languages.) In Hippocratic writings *ga[n]gglion* was used for any small subcutaneous nodule, and this sense has persisted in the use of "ganglion" to refer to a tendinous cyst, such as is found commonly at the wrist. Galen, the 2nd-century Roman physician, used the term to refer to nerve complexes, and in this usage "ganglion" has been most widely applied in anatomy.

gangrene comes from the Greek *ga[n]ggraina,* "an eating sore ending in mortification." The Greek root verb may have been *graō,* "I gnaw." The Greeks referred to the degeneration and necrosis of tissue in stages. That which led to mortification was *ga[n]ggraina;* the final stage of tissue death was *sphakelos.*

gargle is an imitative word that sounds like what it means, just as does the Greek *gargarizein,* "to wash the throat."

gargoylism is a rare familial condition characterized by a grotesque facies, a stunted and deformed body and limbs, an enlarged liver and spleen, and mental impairment. The term comes from "gargoyle," which is a type of rainspout affixed to the gutters of buildings of medieval architecture. Often the end of the spout was decorated with a caricature of a human or animal face. "Gargoyle" refers to the function of the spout, not to the face. The word comes from the French *gargouille,* "waterspout," as a sort of throat.

gas is a word invented by Johannes Baptista van Helmont (1577–1644), a Flemish physician and natural philosopher, who felt called upon to distinguish between carbon dioxide in its usual state and the ultrafine disposition of water which became a vapor when exposed to cold. Later, van Helmont explained that his invention of the word was prompted by the Greek *chaos,* meaning "space," particularly in the sense of a rude, unformed mass. To the ancients, *chaos* was the disordered mass of elemental substances that existed before creation. Hesiod, the Greek poet of the 8th century B.C., wrote:

> Light, uncollected, through the chaos
>   urged its infant way,
> Nor order yet had drawn his lovely train
>   from out of the dubious gloom.

This concept is echoed in the first chapter of the Book of Genesis:

> In the beginning God created the heaven and the earth. And the earth was without form, and void; and darkness was upon the face of the deep. . . . And God said, let there be light: and there was light. . . .

gastric comes from the Greek *gastēr,* "the paunch or belly." To the ancients, this could refer to anything roundly protruding. In modern medical terminology, "gastric" is used only as an adjective (pertaining to the stomach), as in gastric ulcer, or as the combining form "gastr-," as in gastrectomy or gastroscope.

gastrocnemius is the name of the large muscle forming the calf of the leg. Originally, the Greek *gastroknēmia* (from *gastēr,* "belly," + *knēmē,* "leg") referred generally to the calf, or "belly," of the lower leg.

gauze as the word for a light, loosely woven fabric is said to have originated in the name of Gaza, a town near the eastern Mediterranean shore in what is now the oft-disputed strip of land between Egypt and Israel. The Old French term was *gaze,* and supposedly the fabric was imported from Gaza, but this may be only a fabrication.

gene is the biologic unit of heredity through which certain characteristics are passed from generation to generation. The name was taken from the Greek *gennaō,* "I produce, I beget (of the father), or I bring forth (of the mother)."

genio- is a combining form used to designate that which pertains to the chin or, specifically, the mandible. Thus, the geniohyoid muscle connects the mandible and the hyoid bone. "Genio-" is derived from the Greek *geneias,* "a beard"; in the plural the word means "the cheeks."

gentian sounds like an adjective but really is a noun and the name of a plant with showy blue blossoms. An extract of the root of *Gentiana lutea* was long used as a tonic and an antidote to poisons. The plant is said to have been named after King Gentius, who ruled over Illyria in the 2nd century B.C. and supposedly discovered the plant's useful properties. Gentian violet is an aniline dye that has nothing to do with the plant other than reproducing the color of its flowers. The dye formerly was used as an antiseptic solution but now is used mainly as a stain for cytology, especially of bacteria.

genu is the Latin word for "the knee," being related to the Greek *gonu,* which has the same meaning. In the brain, the genu of the internal capsule is the point where the fiber tracts bend. **Geniculate,** being the diminutive, refers to whatever resembles a little knee and has been applied to knotty or nodal structures, especially when they are shaped in a knee-like bend, as the "geniculate ganglion" of the facial nerve. A related word is "genuflect," meaning to bend the knee or to bow down.

geriatrics is the treatment of disorders or diseases characteristic of old people. It was coined by combining the Greek *gerōn*, "an old man," + *iatreia*, "the treatment of disease." The primitive Indo-European root may have been *gar*, "to wear away," or *ger*, "to grow old, to mature." From this came the Latin *granum*, "grain," in the sense of grain being the product of the mature plant. The classical Latin *grandis*, "full-grown, great, aged," became favored in popular or Vulgar Latin over *magnus* and led to the French *grande* and the English "grand." In the sense of advanced age, this led to "grandfather" and "grandmother."

germ is a derivative of the Latin *germen*, "a sprout, bud, or offshoot." Thus, a **germinal** cell is so called because it is capable of proliferating into a more mature tissue, organ, or organism. The use of "germ" in the sense of bacteria carries the idea that these minute bodies are the origin of certain diseases, a concept now firmly established but at one time disputed as "the germ theory of disease."

gestation comes from the Latin *gestare*, "to carry or bear," and thus has been applied to pregnancy. Curiously, the Latin *gestare* meant also "to carry a tale, to blab," and there are few in the bloom of pregnancy who are not anxious to converse on their condition.

-geusia is an inseparable root term from the Greek *geuma*, "a taste of a thing." Thus, "ageusia" is an absence of the sense of taste,

"hypogeusia" is a diminished sense of taste, and "hypergeusia" is a heightened sense of taste, while "dysgeusia" is an altered or perverted sense of taste. A related word is "disgust."

giddiness is a common form of dizziness that is also described as light-headedness. "Giddy" in Old English was *gidig*, which meant "insane." This, in turn, can be traced back to the Teutonic *gudo* or "god." Thus, to be giddy once meant "to be possessed by a god." Incidentally, our word "enthusiasm" once meant much the same thing, from the Greek *enthusiastes*, which was formed from *en*, "in," + *theos*, "god."

gingiva is a direct borrowing of the Latin word for the gum of the mouth. It has been suggested that "gingiva" is a transposed derivative of the Latin *gignere*, "to bear or to produce," the allusion being to the observation that the teeth spring from the gums.

gland is a derivative of *glandulus*, being the diminutive of the Latin *glans*, "a nut or acorn," a term also applied, as **glans penis**, to the end of the male organ because of its shape. The Greeks referred to lymph glands as *adenos*, which apparently was derived from *adēn*, a word for "an acorn." **Adeno-** has become the combining form to designate whatever pertains to glands or glandlike structures, as in adenoid, adenopathy, adenoma, adenocarcinoma, and many other medical terms.

glaucoma is an almost direct borrowing of the Greek *glaukōma*, "a silvery swelling," being combined from *glaukos*, "gleaming or silvery, especially of the sea," + *-ōma*, "a swelling or tumor." The early Greeks used *glaukōma* to refer to any condition of degeneration wherein the eyeball was reduced to the appearance of a silvery-green globe, such as occurred with a dense opacity of the crystalline lens. Later, a distinction was made between lenticular opacities and deeper degeneration consequent to increased intraocular pressure. "Glaucoma" came to be the term for the latter condition.

glenoid refers to the shallow concavity in the scapula which serves for articulation with the humerus. But the word comes from the Greek *glēnē,* by which the ancients meant the eyeball and, particularly, its pupil. Perhaps the shiny cartilaginous concavity in the humerus suggested an appearance similar to that of the eyeball.

glia is a near borrowing of the Greek *gloia,* "glue." Presumably the supporting and connective tissue was looked upon as a sort of glue that held together the functional elements of the nervous system. A **glioma** is a tumor of the glial cells.

globulin is the diminutive of the Latin *globus,* "sphere," wherein the suffix *-in* denotes a derivative. Hence, the term "globulin" was applied in the early 19th century to the substance thought to originate in the "globules" (i.e., the particulate cellular elements) of the blood. Later, with a better appreciation of blood chemistry, "globulin" was reserved for certain plasma proteins of high molecular weight.

glomerulus is the diminutive of the Latin *glomus,* "a ball of yarn," related to the Latin verb *glomerare,* "to form into a ball." **Glomus** is directly borrowed from the Latin word as an anatomic term for an agglomeration of small arteries, veins, and neural elements that serves as a chemoreceptor responding to changes in blood content. The glomerulus of the kidney, a minute ball-shaped capillary tuft, was so named about 1670 by Marcello Malpighi (1628–1694), the great Italian anatomist, and formerly was called a "malphigian corpuscle."

glosso- is a combining form descended from the Greek *glōssa,* "the tongue." The glossopharyngeal (or ninth cranial) nerve serves the tongue and the pharynx. **Glossitis** is an inflammation or erythema of the tongue often seen in various states of nutritional deficiency. Incidentally, by the relation of "tongue" to language, we have "glossary" as a list of special terms.

glottis comes from *glōtta,* the Attic variant of the Greek *glōssa,* "the tongue." The Greeks also used their word for "tongue," as we do, to mean "a voiced language," and it is in this sense that "glottis," in anatomy, has been applied to the vocal apparatus. Incidentally, the related word "polyglot" means a mixture, and sometimes a confusion, of several languages.

glucose is a word contrived by a committee of the French Académie des Sciences in a report dated 16 July 1838. The purpose was to name the principal constituent sugar of the grape, of starch, and of diabetic urine. The committee settled on *glucose* as a Gallicized transformation of the Greek *glukus,* "sweet to the taste," + the Latin *-osus.* "Glucose" was the prototype term, and its last three letters, "-ose", became a biochemical suffix indicating a carbohydrate. Such a suffix, of course, already was used in a quite different way in English, where "-ose" was derived from the Latin *-osus,* by which adjectives were formed from substantives with the meaning "full of or abounding in," as in "bellicose" and "verbose." Glucose, as the term usually is applied, is a dextrorotary monosaccharide ($C_6H_{12}O_6 \cdot H_2O$) and, as such, really should be specifically designated as d-glucose or dextrose. The levorotatory counterpart is levulose, also called fructose ("the sugar of fruit," from the Latin *fructus*).

gluteal comes from the Greek *gloutos,* "the buttock," and refers specifically to that area of the anatomy.

gluten is the substance in wheat and other cereal flours that imparts a sticky consistency when moistened. The word is the same as the Latin *gluten,* meaning "glue." Of more concern in medicine is that gluten is responsible for impaired absorption of nutriments in patients with celiac disease.

goiter comes, through French, from the Latin *guttur,* "gullet, throat, or neck." However, the Romans referred to a swelling of the neck as a "bronchocele." According to Professor H. A. Skinner, the term "gutturosi" was used in reference to persons with visibly swollen thyroid glands by Gerolamo Fabrizio (1533–1619), better known as Fabricius ab Aquapendente, a famous Italian anatomist and surgeon. At that time, and for at least two centuries thereafter, the condition usually was called "struma," not being distinguished from scrofulous swellings. In the late 18th and early 19th centuries, the relation between thyroid enlarge-

ment and hypermetabolism was recognized and variously known as Parry's (after the Englishman C. H. Parry), Graves' (after the Irishman Robert Graves), or Basedow's (after the German Karl von Basedow) disease.

GOK is a flippant acronym for "God only knows." Neophyte doctors have been known to list GOK as their "diagnosis" when stumped by a perplexing and incomprehensible case. A seemingly more learned acronym, useful in the same way, would be "ygiagam," which sounds as though it might come from the Greek but, of course, does not. It stands for "Your guess is as good as mine."

gonad comes from the Greek *gonē,* which means, variously, "the offspring, the seed, childbirth, the womb, or a generation," all having to do with reproduction. In zoology, the gonads are the organs of sexual procreation, both in the male (the testis) and in the female (the ovary).

gonio- is a combining form taken from the Greek *gōnia,* "a corner or an angle." The Indo-European root was *genu,* "knee," the predecessor of the Greek *gonu* and the Latin *genu,* both terms designating that joint which is the "angle" of the leg. In medicine, "gonio-" refers to that angle in the anterior chamber of the eye between the iris and the cornea. Thus, gonioscopy (+ Greek *skopein,* "to observe") is the direct visual examination of that angle, and goniotomy (+ Greek *tomē,* "a cutting") is the operation performed in the anterior chamber of the eye to facilitate drainage as a remedy for the "open angle" type of glaucoma. However, a goniometer is an instrument used to measure the range of motion in a joint.

gonorrhea is a word contrived by the ancient Greeks by combining *gonē,* "a seed," + *rheos,* "a flowing," their idea being that the urethral discharge characteristic of gonorrhea was a leakage of semen. Though this idea was early known to be erroneous, the disease was so ancient and ubiquitous that the original name stuck. Even the causative organism, when discovered in 1879, was named **gonococcus.** Meanwhile, other people of other cultures have called it by a variety of names. Of particular interest are the French *clap* (whose origin is described under that heading) and *chaude pisse* ("hot piss," which is vividly descriptive of the chief symptom).

gout is attributed to the French *goutte* and the antecedent Latin *gutta,* "a drop of fluid." The term apparently grew out of the medieval belief that the concretions which characterize the malady were the result of a distillation, "drop by drop," of "bad humors" in the diseased part. A classic account of gout for the general reader, but also fascinating for doctors, was written by Berton Roueché and published in the 13 November 1948 issue of *The New Yorker* magazine.

gracilis is the Latin word for "slender," and became, in anatomy, the name of a long, thin muscle originating at the inferior ramus of the pubis and inserting along the upper medial aspect of the tibia.

graft sounds as if it might be related to "graph," and it is, though the uses of the word are quite different. The origin of both is the Greek *graphein,* "to write." The relation of this to "graph" as a recording is obvious. But what about "graft" as an implanted tissue? The explanation is that the Romans, in the propagation of trees, used a thin, sharpened shoot to affix to the rootstock, and this was called a *graphium,* from the Latin word for "a stylus." The principle of "grafting" in botany was later applied in medicine, as in skin or bone grafting.

Graham crackers are so named after the Reverend Sylvester Graham, a self-styled 19th-century American nutritionist who attracted a surprisingly large following in his crusade against refined white flour and in favor of brisk cold showers. He espoused the belief that eating natural cereal foods suppressed the baser passions. Graham advocated the use of only whole, coarse-grain flour for baking, and his name became attached to "graham bread" and "graham crackers," then known as "digestive biscuits." Doubtless Graham's ghost revels in the recent revival of the high-fiber diet.

granuloma is a swelling or tumorlike aggregation of granulation tissue, a form of inflammatory reaction. Its texture is like that of small grains. The word is derived from the diminutive of the Latin *granum,* "grain or seed," plus the Greek *-ōma,* "swelling."

gravid describes a pregnant uterus or a pregnant woman and comes from the Latin *graviditas,* "pregnancy." This, in turn, was derived from the Latin adjective *gravis,* "heavy or burdensome," which has numerous descendants, including "grave" (in the sense of weighty), "gravity," and "aggravate" (only distantly related to the Latin *gravidare,* "to impregnate").

grippe is French and more properly called *la grippe*, "a seizure or an attack," particularly by an acute febrile illness. Influenza, in bygone days, was commonly called *la grippe* or, in English, "the grip." The English verb "to grip" and the noun (and sometimes verb) "gripe" are related, being descended from the Anglo-Saxon *gripan,* "to clutch or grasp."

groin is of uncertain origin but may have originated as the Old English *grynde,* "a trench or abyss." That the groin is a depression or cleft between the lower anterior abdominal wall and the thigh, especially when the thigh is flexed, would support this supposition.

gtt. formerly appeared in prescriptions as an abbreviation of the Latin *gutta,* "a drop of fluid." Thus, "Rx: gtt V" meant "Take five drops." "Gutta serena" is an old term for ocular opacity, such as might be caused by cataract. In **guttate psoriasis,** the spots on the skin may resemble drops.

guaiac comes from the Spanish *guayaco,* derived from the Taino Indian name *(Waiacan)* for a tree originally found in the West Indies and South America. The tree was prized for its resin and became known as *lignum vitae* ("wood of life"). A preparation of the resin was once used as a tonic medicine and also was applied topically as a remedy for rheumatism and skin rashes. Now a tincture of the resin is used as a reagent to detect blood in stains or feces, as in the "guaiac test." A widely used form of this test is known as "Hemoccult," a trade name contrived by hybridizing the Greek *haima,* "blood," + the Latin *occultus,* "concealed."

gubernaculum is the name of two structures involved in developmental anatomy. One is the gubernaculum testis, a fibrous cord connecting the lower portion of the epididymis to the fold of skin that becomes the fundic portion of the scrotum. The other is the gubernaculum dentin, a band of connective tissue connecting the dental sac of an unerupted permanent tooth with the gingiva. In both cases, the *gubernaculum* (the Latin word for "rudder or helm") is thought to serve as a guide or "governor" to the testicle as it descends into the scrotum or to the tooth as it erupts from the gum.

gum as the name for the membrane covering the alveolar process of the jaws began with the Anglo-Saxon *goma,* "jaw." In Middle English this was *gome,* pronounced "goom." One may still, but rarely, near an elderly, provincial person complain, "Ay, an' me gooms hurt!"

gumma is a term for the circumscribed lesion of chronic granulation tissue, particularly that of tertiary syphilis. It comes from the Latin *gummi,* "gum," in the sense of a rubbery resin. A gumma is so called because its center has a gummy consistency.

gustatory in referring to the sense of oral taste comes from the Latin *gustatus,* "taste or flavor," and is related to the Greek *geuma,* "the taste of a thing." The Spanish and Italian *gusto* means both "a pleasing and appetizing flavor" and "pleasure," in a general sense. Taken into English, "gusto" means an even more exuberant relish. Incidentally, "relish" is derived from the Old French *relais,* "that which is left behind," which came to be used in the sense of aftertaste.

gut is an Old English word for "the entrails," being the contents of the abdominal cavity. Probably the term originated in the Anglo-Saxon *geotan,* "to pour." The Oxford English Dictionary says that *gut* "formerly, but not now, [was] in dignified use with reference to man." The OED notwithstanding, *Gut* is the name of the official journal of the prestigious British Association of Gastroenterology.

gynecology comes from the Greek *gynē, gynaikos,* "woman," + *logia,* "study." According to a strict etymologic definition, then, a gynecologist would be one steeped in the study of women. Those doctors who actually practice gynecology would rightly disclaim such a bold and sweeping purview. Their concern is limited to disorders of the female reproductive apparatus.

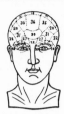

H

haggard as used to describe a person of gaunt, worn, and anxious appearance was also used in falconry to designate a wild female hawk caught only after it had attained adult plumage, presumably having already undergone the rigors of the hunt on its own. The pejorative "hag," meaning an ugly, malicious, old woman, is related and probably was the original term, coming from the Old English *haegtes(se)*, "witch."

hair is of Teutonic origin, through the Anglo-Saxon *hǽr*. Professor H. A. Skinner points out that Latin provides a variety of words denoting different kinds of hair. Some of them have been carried over into medical terms. *Capillus* means hair generally but, in particular, the fine hair of the head. The Latin term is a contraction of *capitis pilus*. From this we derived **capillary** as a name for the minute blood vessels connecting arteries and veins. The ancients had no idea these vessels existed. *Cirrus* means "curly hair" and now is used to describe a type of cloud formation. *Cilium* is "an eyelash," and *supercilium* is "the eyebrow." *Vibrissa,* from the verb *vibrare,* "to quiver," refers to hair in the nostrils. *Mystax* (related to the Greek *mustax*) refers to hair on the upper lip and led to "mustache." *Barba* is "a beard." *Pilus* (related to the Greek *pilos,* "carded wool") is hair generally. **Villus** refers to the shaggy hair of beasts and gave us the anatomic term for the slender mucosal projections lining the lumen of the intestine. *Seta* is "a bristle" such as is found on pigs, and *pappus* is the down on the cheeks of children and women.

haircut used to be heard as a dialect word for the primary lesion of syphilis. The allusion was to the former medical custom of shaving the pubic hair when applying topical therapy for venereal disease.

hale as in "hale and hearty," referring to a state of ebullient wellness, is descended

105

from the Old English *hāl,* meaning "whole" in the sense of all parts intact and functioning in good order.

halitosis comes from the Latin *halitus,* "breath or vapor." Strictly speaking, halitosis means "a condition of the breath." But, thanks to the gratuitous efforts of the advertising industry, everyone knows that halitosis is bad breath. One could hardly expect Madison Avenue to handle the full and proper Latin term: *halitus oris foetidus,* "breath of a stinking mouth."

hallucination comes from the Latin *hallucinari,* "to dream or to talk wildly." An earlier Latin deponent verb form was *alucinari,* "to engage in small talk or to ramble." This, in turn, is related to the Greek *aluō,* "to wander, as in mind, or to be distraught."

hallux is the Latin word for the big toe and is so used in terms referring to deformities, such as *hallux valgus. Hallux* came from the earlier form *allex,* which is thought to have been derived from the Greek *alomai,* a deponent verb meaning "to leap." The Latin adjective for bowlegged is *valgus,* obviously referring to the knee, as in *genu valgum.* But the metatarsophalangeal joint of the big toe could become bowed, too, and this came to be called *hallux valgus.* A better term is simply "bunion," from the Old French *buigne,* "a swelling or bump due to a blow."

hamartoma is derived from a combination of the Greek *hamartanō,* "I fail of purpose, I go wrong," + *ōma,* "swelling." The idea is that a hamartoma is a tumor resulting from something "gone wrong" in development.

The term is said to have been introduced by Karl Albrecht (1851–1894), a German anatomist, to denote a tumorlike nodule of superfluous tissue. The essential feature of a hamartoma is that it contains elements or variants thereof that are indigenous to the part involved, and that these have proliferated because of an ontogenetic defect. Hamartomas are thus distinguished from neoplasms that arise later in life and may or may not contain elements normally found in the part affected.

hamate comes from the Latis *hamatus,* "hook-shaped," and is the name of one of the carpal bones that has a hooklike process extending from its volar surface. **Hamulus** is the diminutive, and the pterygoid hamulus, a process of the sphenoid bone, is shaped like a little hook at the end of the medial pterygoid plate.

handicap is a disadvantage or burden that diminishes the chance of success and, when applied to a person, refers to a physical impairment. The term originated in sport in the 18th century, and is still used specifically to refer to added weight placed on the back of a favorite entry in a horse race. The custom was to place the wager money in the cap of an impartial umpire who decreed the extent of burden to be placed on the superior horse so as to assure a fair race. The challenged and the challenger each put his hand in the cap. If either withdrew his money, the race was off. If both pulled back an empty hand, the race was on. The gesture of the "hand in the cap" came to be called simply "handicap."

hangnail is the term for a tender, split cuticle at the edge of a fingernail or toenail, but it has nothing to do with hanging. It is derived from the Anglo-Saxon *ang,* "painful," + *naegl,* "nail." How or why "h" came to be the initial letter is a mystery. Perhaps "hangnail" seemed easier to pronounce, at least to cockneys.

haptin is derived from the Greek *haptein,* "to fasten or bind." The term, sometimes spelled "haptene," was introduced by Paul Ehrlich (1854–1915), the German bacteriologist and immunologist. Ehrlich's "side-chain theory" postulated the presence of receptors in cell membranes that served as binding sites for various antibodies. A haptin is not a whole antigen, but rather is that part of the antigenic molecule or complex that determines its immunologic specificity.

harelip is a congenital cleft in the upper lip consequent to failure of the median nasal and maxillary processes to unite in the course of embryo development. It is so called because the hare normally has a divided upper lip.

hashish is the dried, flowering tip of the hemp plant which is smoked, chewed, or brewed as a potent source of the intoxicant drug cannabis. *Hashish* is the Arabic word for dried vegetation, such as hay. Thus, "hashish" is analogous to "grass," the common street word for marijuana in the U.S. **Cannabis,** incidentally, is a direct borrowing of the Latin word for hemp, being related to the Greek *kannabis.* The ancients were acquainted with the psychotropic property of hemp. Smoking for pleasure is by no means a recent discovery.

haustrum is the Latin word for "a scoop or bucket" and, as the neuter plural *haustra,* has been applied to the bucket-like pouches that characterize the wall of the colon.

hay fever was first described in 1819 by John Bostock (1773–1846), an English physician who himself suffered from the condition that he called "summer catarrh," because it recurred perennially in the late summer season. Shortly thereafter it was correctly surmised that the cause was the inhalation of irritating pollen, but the source was mistakenly thought to be the ripening grasses mown for hay. Only later was pollen ragweed properly indicated. And, of course, the allergy is not marked by fever. So "hay fever" is a misnomer all around, but its common use persists.

heal comes from the Old English *haelan,* "to make sound or whole," and has its similar counterparts in most Teutonic languages. **Health,** also derived from Old English, is a state of soundness or wholeness or, as might be said today, "to have it all together." Related words are "hail," a greeting, and "hale," a poetic or dialect word for "health."

heart is descended from the Anglo-Saxon *heorte.* Through the ages, despite an ignorance of the circulation of the blood, the heart was somehow associated with the essence of life and vigor and was looked upon as the seat of courage, hence the use of words such as "hearty" and "to hearten" or "to dishearten."

helix is borrowed from the Greek *hēlix,* "a coil," and is related to the verb *hēliō,* "I roll or twist." The helix of the ear is the curved superior and posterior margin of the pinna of the ear. In modern biology, the "double helix" is the paired, spiral structure of DNA (deoxyribonucleic acid) that enables reproduction of genetic information in living cells.

hema-, hemo- are combining forms indicating a relationship to blood and are derived from the Greek *haima,* "blood." By centrifugation of blood, the plasma is separated from the cellular and other formed elements, and the percentage volume of the latter, consisting mostly of red blood cells, is known as the **hematocrit** (+ Greek *krinein,* "to separate"). **Hemangioma** (+ Greek *aggeion,* "vessel," + *ōma,* "tumor") is an abnormal proliferation of blood vessels, often as a **hamartoma.** The vomiting of blood is **hematemesis** (+ Greek *emein,* "to vomit"), whereas to pass recognizable, usually fresh blood at stool is **hematochezia** (+ Greek *chezō,* "to defecate"). The process of forming blood is **hematopoiesis** (+ Greek *poieō,* "I produce"). Originally the liver and spleen were thought to be the principal blood-forming organs. It was not until the mid-19th century that the hematopoietic role of the bone marrow was recognized. **Hematoxylin** is a common tissue stain, often combined with eosin, as in the familiar "H & E" preparation of histologic sections. The heavy, reddish-brown heartwood of a West Indian and Central American tree, called "logwood," is used as a source of the dye. The generic name for the tree is *Haematoxylon* (+ Greek *xylon,* "wood"). The name presumably was suggested by the color of the wood. The dye, extracted from the wood by ether, became known as "hematoxylin" and has been applied to tissue sections since the mid-19th century. **Hemoglobin** is a word that can fool the armchair etymologist. Professor Alexander Gode points out (*JAMA* 192:1066, 1965) that, when dissected, "hemoglobin" seems to be a combination of *hemo* + *glob,* "ball," + *in,* "substance"; this would add up to "blood-ball stuff," which sounds silly. Actually, the original form of the word probably was "haematoglobulin," corresponding to the German *Blutkügelchenstoff,* and for convenience became "hemoglobin." Only later, when the chemical composition of hemoglobin was better understood, did the word make sense as indicating a composition of "heme," the pigment component, and "globin," the protein moiety. **Hemolysis** (+ Greek *lysis,* "a solution or breaking up") refers to the consequence of a disruption of red blood cells and the dispersion of their contents into whatever medium they were suspended. **Hemophilia** has been recognized since biblical times as a familiar condition, being mentioned in the Talmud, the collection of Jewish law, as exempting the sufferer from the rite of circumcision because of the hazard of hemorrhage. The term combines *hemo-* with the Greek *philos,* "loved or dear." The idea is not that blood is loved or that a condition of the blood affects loved ones; "*-philia*" means a tendency, in this case to bleeding. **Hemoptysis** incorporates the Greek *ptysis,* "a spitting" (an onomatopoeic word if there ever was one). The ancients used "hemoptysis" to refer to the spitting of blood from any source. Only later was it restricted to the coughing up of blood from the respiratory tract. **Hemorrhage** (+ Greek *rēgnumai*, "to break forth") means a free and forceful escape of blood. **Hemorrhoid** comes from the Greek *haimorrhoia*, "a flow of blood," being a combination of *aima* + *rheein*, "to flow"); in this case the ending "-oid" does not originate in the Greek *eidos*, "like." Rather, our word came through the Old French *emoroyde*. Apparently the flow of blood from distended, prolapsed anal veins was familiar to the ancients. Because the condition was frequent, the source of the bleeding was referred to as "the hemorrhoidal veins." In other words, the bleeding was named first and then the source.

hemi- is a combining form derived from the Greek *ēmisus*, "half," and is equivalent to the Latin *semi-*. As a rule, which is not always followed, "hemi-" is attached as a modifier to words of Greek origin and "semi-" is attached to those of Latin origin.

hepar is borrowed from the Greek *hēpar*, "the liver," and is now modified and used only as a combining form, as in **hepatitis**, an inflammation of the liver. **Hepatic,** of course, refers to the liver, being derived from the Greek *hēpatikos*, "of the liver." Not so many years ago there was a once-popular, proprietary, over-the-counter medicinal known as "Sal Hepatica," literally "the salt of the liver." According to the rules of Latin syntax it should have been "Sal Hepaticum." It was a saline laxative containing magnesium sulfate and purportedly stimulated the flow of bile, which doubtless it did to some extent. Touted as a tonic, it was supposed "to get the juices going."

heparin was the name given by William Henry Howell (1860–1945), an eminent American physiologist, to an anticoagulant phospholipid substance extracted from canine liver. The name was concocted from the Greek *hēpar*, "the liver," + *-in*, "substance of." Howell thought this substance was equivalent to what he had postulated as the "antiprothrombin" principle that prevented circulating blood from clotting. The hypothetical "antiprothrombin" figured in a mistaken theory of blood coagulation that was propounded in Howell's *Textbook of Physiology* through several editions from 1911 to 1921. It was in the 1930s that a quite different substance having potent anticoagulant activity was extracted from beef lung by A. F. Charles and D. A. Scott, in Toronto. But the original name "heparin" stuck. The refined substance used in clinical practice today is a mucopolysaccharide prepared from beef lung or from beef and hog intestinal mucosa; it has nothing to do with the liver.

hermaphrodite is a person or animal whose body exhibits anatomic features of both sexes. The word comes from Hermaphroditus, so named in Greek mythology because he was the son of Hermes and Aphrodite. Hermaphroditus was beloved by a nymph, Salmacis, who pursued and embraced him, imploring the gods to unite them "so the twain might become one flesh." Her fervent prayer was not only heard but granted, one might think to the dismay of Hermaphroditus. Sailors know a "hermaphrodite brig" as a two-masted vessel that is square-rigged forward and schooner-rigged aft.

hernia probably comes from the Greek *ernos,* "a sprout or shoot," as it referred to the protruding bud of a plant. The allusion originally was to any unsightly bulge from the body. Only later was the essential definition established as a protrusion through an abnormal opening.

heroin was first described in 1874 as a semisynthetic derivative of morphine, but it gained attention in 1898 when commercially introduced by the Bayer company of Germany. The name "heroin" was purportedly bestowed on the drug by Dr. Heinrich Dreser, then head of Bayer's drug research department, who adapted the name from the German *heroisch,* "heroic, strong." The claim was that heroin was both strong (true: the drug has more than twice the potency of morphine) and benign (false: the malignant addicting property of the drug was soon apparent but slow to be believed). Curiously, heroin was at first touted as a cure for morphine addiction. Whoever believed that must have forgotten that morphine was once touted as a cure for opium addiction. Some lessons are hard to learn.

herpes is a borrowing of the Greek *herpēs* that appears in Hippocratic writings as a term for a spreading cutaneous eruption. The root word is the Greek *herpein,* "to creep." The Latin equivalent is *serpere,* "to crawl, to move or spread slowly." To the Romans a *serpens* was a creeping thing, a snake. The Greek *zōstēr* denotes "a girdle." Hence, **herpes zoster** is an eruption that tends to creep around the torso. But it is only "half a girdle," because the eruption of herpes zoster (or **shingles,** as it is popularly known, this term being hobson-jobsoned from the Latin *cingulum,* "a girdle") almost never crosses the midline from one side to the other. **Herpes simplex** (Latin *simplex,* "simple or plain") is the name given to a virus that occurs in two types. Type 1 causes ordinary "cold sores," such as erupt around the mouth, sometimes in response to fever, but Type 2 causes recalcitrant genital sores that are anything but simple for the sufferer.

hetero- is a combining form taken from the Greek *heteros,* "different, or the other of two." This is in contrast to the Greek *homoios,* "like or resembling," from which is derived the combining form **homo-.** Whatever is **heterogeneous** (+ Greek *gennaō,* "I produce") is made up of different things, particularly of things from different sources. Whatever is **heterotopic** (+ Greek *topos,* "place") is in a location other than where it should be.

hiatus is the Latin word for "an opening, a gaping mouth, or a chasm." The Latin verb *hiare* means "to yawn or gape." The word has been incorporated into various medical terms, such as "hiatus semilunaris," which refers to the crescentic groove anterior and inferior to the bulla of the ethmoid bone into which the paranasal sinuses drain. What is commonly called "hiatus hernia" is a protrusion of the cardial portion of the stomach superiorly into the opening in the diaphragm that is normally occupied by the esophagus.

hiccup is an imitative word that when pronounced sounds like what it means. Similar sounding words of the same meaning occur in most European languages, as, for example, the Spanish *hipo* and the French *hoquet* (the German *Schlucken* has a juicier sound). Occasionally there comes along a pseudosophisticated pedant to whom "hiccup" looks inelegant. He then insists on spelling it "hiccough," which is nonsense. **Singultus** is highfalutin "medicalese" for hiccup. It is a Latin word meaning "a gasp or sob," especially those that occur repetitively. *Singultus,* in turn, is related to the Latin adjective *singuli,* "one at a time."

hidro- is a combining form taken from the Greek *idros,* "sweat." Hence, **anhidrosis** is an absence of sweating, and **hidroadenosis** is an inflammation of the sweat glands. "Hidro-" is not to be confused with "hydro-," a pitfall for the unwary misspeller.

hilum is the Latin word for "a little something, a trifle." The Romans used the word to refer to the small spot on a seed or bean that marked its point of attachment to a stalk. Hence, in anatomy, the hilum of the lung or of the kidney is the point of apparent attachment by the serving vessels. *Hilum* is a neuter singular noun; "hilus" would be imputing an incorrect gender, and the proper plural is *hila.* The Romans are said to have had an expression *ne hilum,* meaning "not worth the spot on a bean." From this comes our "nihilism" and "nil." It would seem that the old English expression "not worth a hill of beans" is a miscarriage. At today's

prices a hill of almost any kind of beans would be valuable. The phrase probably should be "not worth the hilum on a bean."

hip is a word of Anglo-Saxon origin that in its earliest form may have meant "a bump or lump," the humps on either side of the pelvis being sufficient to hang one's pants on. The same word appears in "rose hips," meaning the fruit of the rose plant, now purveyed in so-called natural-food stores as a source of vitamin C.

hippocampus is a curved gyrus in the medial part of the floor of the inferior horn of the lateral ventricle of the brain. Functionally, it is part of the olfactory cortex. Its shape suggests that of the seahorse, which exists both in mythology, as a sea monster with the head of a horse and the tail of a fish, and as an actual sea creature, a member of the pipefish family. The name comes from a combination of the Greek *hippos,* "horse," + *kampos,* "a sea monster."

histo- is a combining form that refers to any biologic tissue or composite of cells. The Greek *histos* means "a ship's mast," but it came to be used also for the upright pole supporting the web of a loom (the warp of ancient looms was stretched horizontally rather than suspended vertically). Later, the term was applied to the web as well. Building on "histo-," we have **histology** (+ Greek *logos,* "a treatise"), **histamine** (an amine occurring in tissues), and **histolytic** (+ Greek *lysis,* "a dissolution"). **Histio-** is a variant of "histo-" and used in the same sense of pertaining to tissues. The Greek *histion* means "anything woven, particularly a sail." By convention we use **histi-**

ocyte to refer to a particular type of tissue cell, but it could as well be "histocyte."

hive as a localized swelling of the skin (and, because multiple, usually referred to as "hives") traditionally is related to the verb "to heave," in the sense of raising up. However, it would seem more likely that the bump in the skin suggested the shape of a beehive, a conical or domed structure. This kind of "hive" is descended from the Icelandic *hūfr,* "a ship's hull."

homeopathy is a concept of medical therapy promoted by Christian Friedrich Samuel Hahnemann (1755–1843), a German physician. The concept did not originate with Hahnemann but was embodied in the ancient aphorism *Similia similibus curantur* (Like things are cured by like things). According to this notion, symptoms are best treated by agents believed to induce the same reaction. An example would be an attempt to combat fever by administering pyrogenic agents, thus to "fight fire with fire." In this sense, "homeopathy" was derived from the Greek *homo-,* "the same," + *pathos,* "suffering or disease." Hahnemann himself suggested the contrasting term **allopathy** (concocted from the Greek *allo-,* "other," + *pathos*) to refer to the use of medications having effects antagonistic to symptoms, then and still now the prevalent view. To Hahnemann's credit, he advocated the use of minute doses of drugs synergistic to symptoms. Some wag derisively suggested that Hahnemann would make coffee by plugging the cloaca of a duck with a coffee bean and chasing the duck across a lake. Ambrose Bierce, in his *Devil's Dictio-*

nary, defined homeopathy as "a school of medicine midway between allopathy and Christian Science. To the last, both the others are distinctly inferior, for Christian Science will cure imaginary diseases, and they cannot."

homo- is a combining form taken from the Greek *homos,* "like or similar." The Greek *homologos* (+ *logos,* "a statement") means "an agreement or being in accord with." In biology, a **homolog** is a part having the same structure and origin in different organisms, while an **analog** (Greek *ana,* "against") is a part having the same function but a different origin in different organisms. "Analog" is not to be confused with the German **anlage,** a term meaning "a laying on" but in biology referring to a primordial structure or rudiment. **Homogeneous** (+ Greek *genos,* "race or tribe") denotes whatever is made up of the same elements or is of the same quality throughout. A **homozygote** (+ Greek *zygōtos,* "yoked together") is an individual organism possessing an identical pair of alleles in regard to a given phenotype.

hordeolum is a polysyllabic term for a sty, an inflamed meibomian gland in the eyelid. It comes from the diminutive of the Latin *hordeum,* "barley"; the lesion was fancied to resemble a little barleycorn. **Meibomian** comes from the name of Heinrich Meibom (1638–1700), a German anatomist who described the tarsal glands of the eyelid in 1666.

hormone is derived from the Greek *hormaō,* "I set in motion or I stir up." The Greek word appears in Hippocratic writings to denote the action of supposed "vital principles," the idea of "getting the juices going" being an ancient one. The term was revived in 1902 by W. M. Bayliss and E. H. Starling when they described the stimulus to pancreatic secretion (*J Physiol* 28:325) as mediated by a humoral agent they called **secretin,** taken from the Latin *secretus,* "that which is separated." This marked the discovery and recognition of the first true hormone.

hospital is from the Latin *hospitalia,* "apartments for strangers or guests." This, in turn, was derived from the Latin *hospes,* which could mean either "a visitor" or "one who entertained a visitor." Related words are hospital, host, hostel, and hotel, all in the sense of contributing to the congenial accommodation of guests. A time-honored French proper name for a hospital is "Hôtel-Dieu." But, as Professor Alexander Gode points out (*JAMA* 194:1230, 1965), all visitors are not friendly, hence the use of the word "host," from the Latin *hostis,* "enemy," to mean a confronting army, and also the word "hostile."

human is said to have originated in the postulated Indo-European root *ghdhem,* which referred to "earth or soil." From this comes the Latin *humus,* "earth or land"; *humilis,* "common or colloquial"; *homo,* "a person" (*Homo sapiens* is "a wise, knowing, or sensible person"); and *humanus,* "kind or compassionate." Also, presumably from this root came the Anglo-Saxon *guma,* "man," which in Old English was incorporated into *brydguma,* "a bride's man," and later became "bridegroom."

humerus is derived from the Latin *umerus,* related to the Greek *ōmos,* both meaning "shoulder." To ancient anatomists, the scapula, the clavicle, and the humerus were known collectively as the *ossa humeri,* "bones of the shoulder." Later, "humerus" came to denote the bone of the upper arm alone. Exhaustive research yields no evidence supporting the notion that the humerus is so called because it is connected to the funny bone.

humoral comes from the Latin *umere,* "to be moist," which seems close to the modern sense of "humoral" as denoting those regulatory effects transmitted by internal (endocrine) secretions. This is in contrast to neural regulatory effects transmitted by nerve pathways. The action of insulin, secreted by the islet cells of the pancreas, on tissues involved in carbohydrate metabolism is an example of a humoral effect. Of course, "humoral" was used historically to characterize a concept of physiology and pathology that entailed four "humors" contained in the body: blood, phlegm, yellow bile, and black bile. Health was a state in which these four were in proper balance. Disease resulted from an imbalance, and treatment required the purging or strengthening of such "humors" as were considered excessive or deficient.

hyaline comes from the Greek *hyalos,* "a transparent stone (as a crystal) or glass." The word used by the Greeks is said to have originated in ancient Egypt, where the making of glass began. Hyaline cartilage is so called because of its glassy appearance.

hybrid apparently did not originate with the Greek *hybris,* "wanton violence or insolence," but probably is derived from the

Latin *hibrida,* the word for an untamable offspring of a domestic sow and a wild boar. Later the term was applied to any mongrel, especially to a child born of a Roman father and a barbarian mother. **Hybridoma** is a newly contrived term to designate the product of an amazing technologic feat wherein certain components of antigen-bearing cells and antibody-producing cells are genetically combined. (Here the suffix "-oma" presumably is used in the sense of "body" rather than "swelling.") The combination can result in a **monoclonal** (Greek *mono-,* "single," + *klon,* "twig") antibody of incredible specificity. Such hybridomas give promise of more precise diagnosis and treatment of disease than heretofore possible.

hydatid comes from the Greek *hydatoeis,* "watery," and refers to a watery cyst or vesicle. Hydatid cysts, often of large size, can occur in the liver, lungs, and other organs as a consequence of infection by the *Echinococcus* genus of tapeworm. Incidentally, "echino-" is from the Greek word for "a prickly husk," and "-coccus" suggests its berrylike appearance.

hydro- is a combining form derived from the Greek *hydōr,* "water." A **hydrocele** (+ Greek *kēlē,* "hernia") was so called originally because it was thought to be a serous sac from the peritoneum protruding into the scrotum. **Hydrocephalus** (+ Greek *kephalē,* "head") is literally "water in the head" or, more specifically, in the brain. **Hydrogen** (+ Greek *gennaō,* "I produce") is so named because the gas was observed to form water when burned in the presence of oxygen. **Hydrolysis** (+ Greek *lysis,* "a dissolution") is the splitting of a compound by the addition of water, wherein the hydroxyl group (-OH) attaches to one fragment and the hydrogen atom (H-) attaches to the other. **Hydrophobia** (+ Greek *phobos,* "fear"), a popular name for rabies, is explained by the intensely painful spasm of the throat muscles felt by the victim of the disease when he attempts to drink water. Incidentally, the Greek *hydro-potēs* was literally "a water drinker" but actually meant "a drinker of thin potations," in contrast to a drinker of more robust beverages, and hence to the Greeks it meant "a thin-blooded fellow." This notion survives in the present-day description of a lean, asthenic person as "a long drink of water." "Hydro-" is not to be confused with "hidro-," which is borrowed from the Greek *idros,* "sweat."

hydrops is derived from the Greek *hyderos* or *hydrops* as used by ancient writers to refer to an abnormal accumulation of serous or watery fluid in the tissues or in a body cavity. A colloquial rendering of "hydrops" became **dropsy,** a now archaic term for serous swelling of a part. "Hydrops" now is restricted to mean an accumulation of serous fluid, particularly in a chronically obstructed yet distensible gallbladder.

hygiene is the science of preventive medicine and the practice of healthy habits and is so called from Hygieia, the name of one of the two daughters of Asklēpios (in Latin, Aesculapius), the Greek god of medicine. The other daughter, Panaceia, became the goddess of healing. Hygieia, as the goddess of health, was credited with supplying a wholesome environment, thus promoting sound growth and with it the ability to ward off diseases. It is perhaps understandable that a somewhat acrimonious competition arose between the two legendary sisters. After all, if Hygieia had her way, Panaceia would have little to do.

hygroma is an endothelial-lined cyst filled with serous fluid. The word is derived from a combination of the Greek *hydros,* "wet or moist," + - *ōma,* "a swelling." In modern medicine, a hygroma is a lymphatic cyst, usually found in the neck of infants or children.

hymen comes from the Greek *hymēn,* "a skin or membrane." The Greek word was used for all sorts of membranes, including the pericardium and peritoneum. Later Hymen became the name of the god of marriage, a sort of overgrown Cupid. It was not until the 16th century that "hymen" was restricted to denote the vaginal (or virginal) membrane.

hyoid is a classical way of saying "U-shaped." The "hy-" is derived from the Greek equivalent of "h" (which was written not as a letter but as aᶥ, called "a rough breathing"), followed by the letter upsilon. The suffix is from the Greek *eidos,* "like." The hyoid bone is shaped like a U.

hyoscyamine is an anticholinergic alkaloid originally obtained from the henbane plant, which was so called because its poisonous substance was the bane of domestic fowl. It often killed the birds. The hairy beans of the plant were known to the ancient Greeks as *huskyamos,* "hog bean," either because swine ate it or its bristly surface appeared to resemble the hide of swine.

hyper- is a combining form signifying "over, above, beyond, or exceeding." It is said to have originated with the postulated Indo-European root *uper,* "over." This became the Greek *hyper,* the Latin *super* or *supra,* and the Anglo-Saxon *ofer,* the predecessor of the English "over." The list of biomedical terms in which "hyper-" has been incorporated as a prefix is almost endless. In vernacular speech, "hyper" has almost become a word in itself when used to mean an excessively animated state. The exaggerated and extravagant manner in which some patients describe their symptoms is called "hyperbole," an almost direct borrowing of the Greek *hyperbolē,* "a throwing beyond." This word meant the same to the ancient Greeks as our modern expression "to lay it on thick" or "to pile it on."

hypnosis comes from the Greek *hypnos,* "sleep," and was introduced in 1843 by James Braid, a Scottish surgeon, to refer to an induced, "nervous" sleep. "Hypnosis" became the preferred term for the state induced supposedly by a mysterious force called "animal magnetism" by Anton Mesmer (1734–1815), a Swiss physician. More is told of Mesmer under **mesmerism.**

hypo- is a combining form signifying "below, under, or deficient" and is the same as the Greek *hypo.* The prefix has been attached to a host of chemical and biomedical terms. **Hypochlorite** was so named because it contained less, or was deficient in, oxygen when compared with the chlorate. **Hypochondrium** (+ Greek *chondros,* "cartilage") designates the anatomic area beneath the cartilaginous costal margins. The ancients looked upon the spleen as the seat of melancholy, and even today a "splenetic" person is irritable, peevish, or spiteful. The spleen being located in the left hypochondrium, **hypochondriac** came to be applied to patients whose complaints seemed to have no organic basis. We now know that, in many cases, this is because of the "splenic flexure syndrome," a common expression of functional bowel disorder often seen in nervous persons. The **hypophysis** (+ Greek *physis,* "growth"), now better known as the pituitary gland, was so called because it seemed to "grow below" the brain. **Hypospadias** (+ Greek *spaein,* "to draw") is a condition wherein the urethral orifice appears to be "drawn under" the penis. A **hypothesis** (+ Greek *thesis,* "a placing") is "placed under" an idea as its foundation, just as "supposition" is derived from the Latin *sub-,* "under," + *positum,* "to place."

hysterectomy is derived from a combination of the Greek *hystera,* "the womb or uterus," + *tomē,* "a cutting." To the Greeks, *hysterikos* meant "a suffering in the womb." Professor H. A. Skinner tells us: "Plato and his followers described the uterus as an animal endowed with spontaneous sensation and motion, lodged in a woman, and ardently desiring to bear children. If it remained sterile long after puberty, it became indignant, dissatisfied, and ill-tempered and caused a general disturbance of the body until it became pregnant, when it became normal again." This is in keeping with the age-old proclivity to attribute various abnormal manifestations to specific organs of the body. Emotional instability, thought to be more characteristic of women than men, was attributed to the uterus. A safe assumption is that this notion was proclaimed and promoted, in the main, by men. From this anatomic assignation comes the term **hysteria,** doubtless conceived by a confirmed male chauvinist.

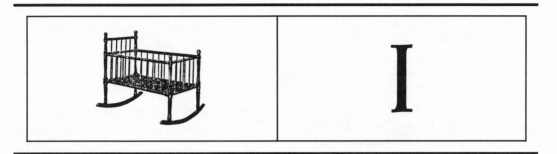

iatros is the Greek word for "healer" and is related to the verb *iaomai,* "to heal." We use this derivation to describe a special branch of healing, as in **pediatrics** or **geriatrics,** and we use it as a combining form, as in **iatrogenic** (+ Greek *gennaō,* "I produce"), although in this term the idea is not that healing is being produced but rather that whatever is "iatrogenic" is the consequence of or produced by therapy. To the Greek *iatros,* the Roman counterpart was *medicus,* derived from the Latin verb *medeor,* again, "to heal." Modern Romance languages have followed suit, witness the Spanish *medico.* The Swedish *läkare* is derived from *läka,* "to heal." The German *Arzt* is said to have descended from the Greek as a contraction of *archi-iatros,* "the master healer." The concept that one who ministers to his fellows' illness or injury is a "healer" is heartening and inspiring. The pity is that in English we do not say "healer." For some reason, we prefer **doctor** (which, of course, means "teacher") or **physician** (one who is steeped in "physic"). Several obscure but intriguing terms have been made up from *iatros.* **Iatromelia** (+ Greek *meleos,* "fruitless or vain") refers to ineffective or negligent medical treatment. **Iatrapistic** (+ Greek *a-,* "lacking," + *pisteuō,* "I trust in") refers to a lack of faith in doctors. **Iatromisia** (+ Greek *miseō,* "I hate") is an intense dislike of doctors.

ichthyosis comes from the Greek *ichthys,* "a fish," and refers to a rough, scaly skin resulting from overgrowth of the keratin layer.

icterus is a Latinized form of the Greek *ikteros,* which, to the ancients, meant both "jaundice" and "a yellow bird," probably the oriole, the familiar small bird with golden-yellow plumage. "Oriole," incidentally, comes from the Latin *aureum,* "golden." According to Professor Alexander Gode

(*JAMA* 184:615, 1963), the connection between the bird and the disease is explained in Pliny. The disease purportedly could be cured by having the patient gaze on the bird. Through a mysterious transmigration, the disease was supposed to pass from the patient to the hapless bird.

idio- is a frequently applied prefix that comes from the Greek *idios,* meaning that which is "personal, private, or one's own." In the sense of being the opposite of public or popular, *idios* might also mean "peculiar." **Idiolalia** (+ Greek *laleō,* "I chatter or babble") is the use of an invented language peculiar to the prattler himself. **Idiopathic** (+ Greek *pathos,* "disease") has come to be a useful word to describe a condition of which one is ignorant of the cause, yet it is a high-sounding word that seems to mask that fact. Originally, an idiopathic condition was thought of as arising in the patient himself rather than occurring as a consequence of any recognized outside cause. Later, the sense shifted slightly to that of a condition peculiar to a given individual, in contrast to that being representative of a widely recognized disease. Now, when the doctor says "It's idiopathic," probably he really means, in effect, "I don't know what it is." **Idiosyncrasy** (+ Greek *sy*[*n*]*gkrasis,* "a mixing together or blending") in common parlance is an expression of a temperament peculiar to a given individual. Medically, it is an abnormal susceptibility or allergy, peculiar to an individual, to a drug or chemical agent. **Idiotropic** (+ Greek *tropos,* "a turning") refers, in psychology, to a type of personality satisfied with its own inner intellectual or emotional experiences. **Idioventricular** (+ Latin *ventriculus,* "little belly [of the heart]") refers to an impulse, conduction, or rhythm originating within the cardiac ventricle alone.

idiot is derived from the Greek *idiōtēs,* which originally was the word for a man engaged in private pursuits, as contrasted with a man who holds public office. From the assumption that such a man was ignorant of public affairs, the term became restricted to a deprecatory sense and was applied to persons judged to be of less than normal intelligence. To the laity, an idiot is any utterly foolish or senseless person. To psychologists, an idiot is an adult whose intellect has become arrested at a mental age of less than three years. A **mongolian idiot** is a mentally retarded person with a mongoloid facies, a condition now known to result from a chromosomal aberration. The term was suggested by Langdon Down (1828–1896), an English physician. What was called "mongolism" is now more properly known as "Down's syndrome."

ileum is derived from the Greek *eileos,* "twisted." When the abdomen is opened at operation or at necropsy, all of the small intestine appears twisted. So why should only the distal portion be called "ileum"? One explanation is that, insofar as the distal small intestine is more often the seat of obstruction, the ancients may have used *eileos* also as a pathologic term. This also could account for the surviving use of **ileus** as a reference to an apparent obstruction due to paralysis of the gut. The British, classical scholars that they are, pronounce "ileum" as "eye-leum."

ilium is the Medieval Latin term for the hipbone, and it is so used today. But to the Romans the *ilia* (the plural noun) referred generally to the belly, groin, and guts. Possibly the later connection was that the hipbones were looked upon as delimiting and protecting the flanks of the belly. "Ilium," of course, is not to be confused in spelling or in meaning with "ileum."

imbecile comes from the Latin *imbecillus,* "weak or feeble." It has been suggested that this might have been derived from a combination of the Latin *in-,* used in the sense of "on," + *baculum,* "a rod or staff," thus referring to one who was obliged to lean on a crutch. Before long the meaning was transferred from weakness in body to weakness in mind.

immunity is an almost direct borrowing of the Latin *immunitas,* which to the Romans meant "an exemption from taxes or from public or military service." The Latin word comes from combining *in-,* "not," + *munus,* "tribute or service." The legal sense, both lay and judicial, was the principal meaning of the word in English, too, until the 19th century, when knowledge of toxins and infection evolved and persons "exempt from" or protected against the onslaught of foreign substances were said to be "immune."

impetigo comes from the Latin *impetus,* "a vehement attack or assault," which also is the origin of "impetuous." Originally, "im-

petigo" was given as a name for a variety of inflammatory skin afflictions. Currently, the term usually refers to an infectious, pustular dermatitis.

inanition comes from the Latin *inanire,* "to empty," which is akin to the Latin *inanis,* "empty." "Inanition" is used especially with reference to that which has been rendered void or hollow by depletion. In medicine, "inanition" describes the condition of a patient who has been depleted by lack of nourishment. From the same source comes "inane," meaning whatever is empty, void, or worthless.

incarcerated describes a hernia wherein the protruding tissues are stuck or held fast and hence cannot be restored to their normal location. To the Romans, *incarceratus* meant "imprisoned," the word being a combination of the Latin *in-* + *carcer,* "prison."

incise comes from the Latin *incidere,* "to carve or cut into." An **incisura** is "a notch or cleft," as if the result of cutting into, and an **incisor** tooth is one capable of cutting into anything that is bitten (as compared to a molar or grinding tooth).

incubate is taken from the Latin *incubare,* "to lie in or on; to brood," this being, in turn, a combination of *in-* + *cubare,* "to lie down or to recline." While an **incubator** is usually warm, it is the idea of the "lying in" rather than the heating that is essential. The **incubation period** of any infectious disease is the time during which the causative organism "lies in" before the disease is "hatched."

incus is the name of one of the little bones in the middle ear. The name is the Latin word for anvil, related to the verb *incudere,* "to strike upon." Thus, to transmit sound in the ear, the *malleus* (or "hammer") strikes upon the *incus* (or "anvil").

index is the Latin word for "a sign or mark of something." It is related to the verb *indicare,* "to point out or disclose." The index of a book, thus, is supposed to disclose its contents, and the index finger is that used to point out whatever merits attention.

indolent has changed its meaning in common usage but has retained its original sense when used as a medical adjective. The Latin *indolentia* means "freedom from pain," being a combination of *in*-, "not," + *dolens,* "painful or distressing." The Latin *dolor* is preserved intact in the Spanish word for pain. Hence, an indolent ulcer is a painless ulcer. While most such ulcers also are of long standing, the true meaning of the term emphasizes lack of pain, not chronicity. In common usage, "indolent" has come to mean "lazy or slothful." Presumably a person so disposed feels little or no pain.

induration comes from the Latin *indurare,* "to harden," and refers to tissues that have become stiff and firm as a consequence of inflammation, hyperplasia, or neoplasia.

inexorable sometimes is used to describe the unalterable progress of a disease. The word is an almost direct borrowing of the Latin *inexorabilis,* which, to the Romans, meant "not to be moved by prayers." This, in turn, is a combination of *in*-, "not," + *ex*, "out of," + *orare*, "to pray or beg." Whatever is inexorable, be it disease or taxation, is beyond getting out of by prayer.

infant comes from the Latin *infans,* "speechless," which, in turn, is derived from *in*-, "not," + *fari,* "to speak." Because an ability to speak usually becomes evident at the age of two years, all those younger are generally considered to be infants. By an odd twist, some adults only betray their infantile attitudes when they open their mouths to speak.

infarct is derived from the Latin *infarcire,* "to stuff or cram." The original use of the term, in pathology, referred to consolidation or stuffing of "humors" in the affected part. We now recognize an infarct as a necrotic lesion that results from acute deprivation of circulating blood. The swelling is due to transudation of fluid and inflammatory infiltration. The process of infarction is in the affected tissue. The emphasis was originally, and should be now, on the reaction and not on its cause. To refer to a myocardial infarct is to designate the pathologic changes occurring in the heart muscle; the cause of these changes is another matter.

infection comes from the Latin *inficere,* "to dye or stain" but also "to corrupt or spoil." The ancients conceived that disease could result from the entrance of invisible agents into the body, hence a sort of "tainting." But it was not until the latter part of the 19th century that the germ theory of disease gained currency and the true nature of infection was appreciated.

inferior is a comparative form of the Latin *inferus,* "low or beneath." In anatomy, the meaning is confined to a spatial relation, as in the statement that the liver is inferior to the heart. This implies no value judgment in comparing the merit of the liver with that of the heart.

infestation is the invasion of the body by arthropods, such as insects, mites, and ticks. The word comes from the Latin *infestare,* "to annoy," as is the wont of bugs. Invasion of the body by parasites is often referred to as "infestation." This is incorrect. Invasion by amebas or any other animalcules which do not have jointed legs is an infection, not an infestation.

infirmary comes from the Latin adjective *infirmus,* "weak, feeble, or sick," and hence is a place where persons so afflicted are cared for. In former times the term designated places of treatment for the destitute poor, in contrast to private hospitals.

inflammation is derived from the Latin *inflammare,* "to set on fire, to kindle." It was Celsus, in the 1st century A.D., who set down the four cardinal features of inflammation in his celebrated *De Medicina: rubor* (redness), *tumor* (swelling), *calor* (heat), and *dolor* (pain). Naturally, these features suggested those of a smoldering fire.

influenza is an Italian word meaning, as it sounds, "influence," but including the further sense of "a visitation," as by an epidemic disease. It was in this way that *influenza* came to be used in the 14th century. Possibly the thought was that episodic and devastating illness were due to the "influence" of an ominous configuration of the planets and stars. Only in recent times, when infectious diseases have been more properly sorted out, has "influenza" been restricted to a viral disease of notorious contagion. Curiously, through the years, epidemics occurring in one place have always been blamed on some other place. In Russia influenza was called "the Chinese disease," in Germany "the Russian pestilence," in Italy "the German disease," and so on. Even today, in the U.S. we claim to suffer from the "Hong Kong flu." What the people in Hong Kong suffer from is not recorded.

infra is the Latin preposition meaning "below or beneath" and, by extension, "less than." Infrared rays or waves that generate heat are so called because their wavelength falls below that of the red end of the spectrum. An infradiaphragmatic abscess is situated below the diaphragm.

infundibulum is the Latin word for "funnel" and comes from the verb *infundere,* "to pour into." Hence, "infundibulum" has long been used to describe any funnel-shaped structure or passage. The infundibulum of the Fallopian tube refers to its funnel-shaped distal end.

infusion also is derived from the Latin *infundere,* "to pour into." The term currently is used for the administration of fluids through a catheter, as into a vein, usually by means of gravity. There is an older meaning of "infusion" that accounts for the name "Infusoria" as the class of protozoa characterized by the presence of cilia. The older meaning was "to soak or steep" in water for the purpose of extracting some constituent, as in the steeping of tea from a bag of crushed tea leaves. Antonj van Leeuwenhoek (1632–1723), the Dutch pioneer microscopist, observed tiny organisms in stagnant water, and to these organisms was applied the term "infusoria."

inject comes from the Latin *injicere,* "to throw into," being a combination of *in-* + *jactare,* "to toss, throw, or hurl." In the scientific sense, "to inject" means to put something in under pressure, as compared with the gentler forms of "infuse" or "instill."

innominate is a near borrowing of the Latin *innominatus,* literally "without a name." The innominate artery was described by Galen, but he gave it no name. Later, Vesalius simply called it "the unnamed artery." The pelvis is made up of three bones: the ilium, the ischium, and the pubis. Each of the three components was named, but the whole structure was not, and so Galen referred to it as the "innominate" or unnamed bone. Actually, Celsus did call it the *os coxae,* "the bone of the hips."

inoculate comes from the Latin *inoculare,* "to ingraft," being derived from *in-* + *oculus,* "the eye." That seems a strange connection until one recalls how the ancients accomplished grafting. An emerging sprout or bud, which resembled an eye, was taken from one plant and inserted into a niche cut into another plant. Thus, the process was "putting in the eye." When the idea was evolved of inducing immunity by "grafting" vaccine onto or into a person's body, the procedure was called inoculation. Even closer to the ancient meaning is the inoculation of a culture medium for the purpose of inducing the growth of whatever is inoculated.

insanity is a near borrowing of the Latin *insania,* "madness or mania" beyond the bounds of normal mental composure. The term combines *in,* "not," + *sanus,* "sound or rational." "Insanity" has been and is a legal term. It never has been given the status of a medical diagnosis.

insemination is contrived by the combination of *in-* + the Latin *semen,* "seed," and refers to the deposition of the male sperm into the reproductive tract of the female, usually by what comes naturally but sometimes, if needed, by artificial means. **Sperm** is derived from the Greek *sperma,* "seed."

insidious when referring to a symptom of a disease means one that lurks inconspicuously, being deceptively quiescent. The word is borrowed from the Latin *insidiae,* "deceitful" in the sense of "ambush." This, in turn, is a combination of *in-* + *sedere,* "to sit." So, an insidious disease is one that is "sitting in," waiting to wreak havoc. "Ambush," incidentally, comes through the Old French from the Late Latin *imboscare,* "in the woods or among the bushes."

in situ is a Latin term combining *in-* + the ablative of *situs,* "position or place." The anatomic reference is to something "in place" and not wandering around.

inspissate is a near borrowing of the Latin *inspissatus,* being a combination of *in-* (here used as an intensive) + *spissatus,* "condensed, concentrated, or thickened." A liquid becomes inspissated by the loss of water or other fluid by evaporation or by absorption. Dehydrated, hardened fecal fragments lying in the bowel are said to be inspissated.

insufflation comes from the Latin *insufflatio,* "to blow into or to inflate," being a combination of *in-* + *sufflare,* "to blow or puff." The word provides still another example of polysyllabic inflation encountered in the language known as "medicalese." A doctor would insufflate a balloon, while an ordinary mortal would only blow up a balloon.

insula is Latin for "island." A triangular area of the cerebral cortex forming the floor of the lateral cerebral fossa was described by the German anatomist Johann Christian Reil (1759–1813) and is known as the insula of Reil. **Insulin,** the hormone essential to glucose metabolism, was so named because it was found in the pancreatic islets of Langerhans.

integument is a near borrowing of the Latin *integumentum,* "a covering," this being derived in turn from the verb *tegere,* "to cover." *Tegere* originated in the Indo-European *teg,* "to hide or to cover," which through the Dutch gives us "deck."

inter is the Latin preposition meaning "between or among" and serves a host of medical terms, such as "intercostal," between the ribs, and "interosseous," between the bones. Whatever is **intercalated** is "inserted between," which is what the Latin *intercalaris* means. This, in turn, is a combination of *inter-* + *calare,* "to proclaim." Originally, the Latin term referred to an extra day that was inserted in the calendar by proclamation. ("Calendar" comes from the Latin *calends,* the first day of the Roman month, on which proclamations customarily were made.) Intercalated disks are the stripes ex-

tending across fibers of heart muscle, and intercalated neurons are those situated between primary afferent and efferent nerve cells. **Internuncial** (+ Latin *nuntius,* "messenger") also refers to certain connecting neurons. **Interdigitate** (+ Latin *digitus,* "finger") refers to the configuration produced by the ten fingers when placed between one another. **Intermediate** (+ Latin *medius,* "middle") means literally "in the middle." **Intermittent** (+ Latin *mittere,* "to send") refers to the result of something "sent in between," hence not continuous. **Interstitial** (+ Latin *sistere,* "to put or to place") means whatever is placed between, such as "interstitial" fibrosis. **Intertrigo** (+ Latin *terere,* "to rub") is the chafing that occurs between opposing skin folds that rub on each other, such as under a pendulous female breast.

intern is an obsolete term because the internship, by that name, no longer exists. The first year of postgraduate training for new M.D.'s is now known as "PGY-I." In years gone by, the word was spelled *interne,* befitting its French origin, and referred, literally, to one who was confined within a certain geographic limit. To put it another way, the neophyte physician was stuck in the hospital. The custom, while restrictive, was instructive.

internal medicine is a term of somewhat disputed origin. Obviously it refers to the practice of those specially trained physicians who deal with the diagnosis and nonsurgical treatment of diseases affecting the internal organs. One explanation is that its use arose in 19th-century Germany as *innere Medizin* to distinguish internists from the large number of doctors whose specialty was dermatology and the external manifestations of various diseases, especially those of venereal origin.

intestine is a near borrowing of the Latin *intestinus,* which, as the adjective, generally means "internal" and, as the plural noun, means "the guts." The latter usage is analogous to the colloquial "innards" as a term for the viscera.

intima is the Latin word for "innermost." In anatomy, the term refers to the innermost lining of blood vessels, composed of a cylindrical sheet of endothelial cells surrounded by elastic and collagen fibers.

intoxication is derived from the Latin *intoxicare,* "to smear with poison." The Latin *toxicum,* "poison," is related to the Greek *toxon,* "a bow" as used by an archer. The connection between the Greek and the Latin words is that the arrow shot from a bow might be tipped with poison. This is unfair to the Greeks, whose principal weapon was the spear, whereas bows and arrows were favored by the Persians. Be that as it may, intoxication was, and still is, viewed as a form of poisoning, most commonly by alcohol.

intra is the Latin preposition meaning "within or inside" and serves as a prefix for numerous medical terms. As an example, **intramural** (+ Latin *murus,* "wall") refers to whatever may be contained within the walls of an organ, such as the intestine or heart. In common usage, the reference to wall is in the plural sense; hence, "intramural" sports

are those enjoyed within the walls of a given institution. **Intrinsic** is a near borrowing of the Latin *intrinsecus,* "on the inside," being derived from a combination of *intra-* + *sequi,* "to follow or accompany." Thus, the reference is to whatever "goes on" inside. **Extrinsic,** from the Latin *extrinsecus,* by the opposite token, is whatever goes on outside.

introvert is derived from a combination of the Latin *intro-,* "inward," + *vertere,* "to turn." In psychiatry, an introvert is a self-centered person who is more interested in his own emotions than in other people or external events.

intussusception was made up by combining the Latin *intus-,* "within," + *suscipere,* "to pick up, to take up, or to receive." John Hunter (1728–1793), the renowned English anatomist and surgeon, gave the name to a condition wherein a proximal segment of intestine is telescoped or "taken up" into a succeeding segment, thus causing an obstruction.

involution comes from the Latin *involvere,* "to roll up or to wrap up," particularly in the sense of concluding something. The Latin *volvere,* among its various meanings, could refer to the rolling along of a river. Thus, *involvere* could refer to a river not rolling along or to one drying up. It is in this sense that "involution" is used in pathology as a word for the process whereby an organ withers in old age. An example is the involuted ovary of the postmenopausal woman.

ion was so named from the Greek *iōn,* the present participle of *ienai,* "to go." Michael Faraday (1791–1867), the celebrated English physicist, named the particle set free by electrolysis "to go" to either the positive or negative pole of an electrically charged system (though some say it was Faraday's contemporary William Whewell who originated these neologisms). Faraday proposed the term **anion** (Greek *ana,* "up") for the negatively charged particle that is attracted to or "goes up" to the positively charged **anode** (Greek *odos,* "track or course"); bicarbonate (HCO_3^-), chloride (Cl^-), and sulfate (SO_4^-) are examples of biologically important anions. Incidentally, the Greeks had a word of their own, *anodos,* which to them meant "the upward way" and was used to refer to the path of the rising sun. The name **cation** (Greek *kata,* "down") was given to the positively charged particle that is attracted to or "goes down" to the negatively charged **cathode** (Greek *kata + odos*); hydrogen (H^+), potassium (K^+), and sodium (Na^+) are examples of biologically important cations.

ipecac is a shortened form of a native Brazilian word *ipecacuanha.* In the Guarani language, this is said to be a combination of *pe,* "flat," + *kaa,* "an herb," + *quana,* "to vomit"; hence "a small creeping plant that makes one throw up." The ending *-nha* indicates the passage of the word through Portuguese. In the 17th century, ipecac was touted as a remedy for dysentery.

iris is a direct borrowing of the Greek word for "rainbow" and is derived from *eirō,* "I announce." To the ancient Greeks, a rainbow was a sign from the gods and was personified as Iris, their messenger. Later the name was given to a genus of varicolored flowers. Because of the association with different colors, Jacob Benignus Winslow (1669–1760), a Dane who served as a professor of anatomy in Paris, applied the same name to the circular membrane that surrounds the aperture of the eye.

ischemia is derived from the Greek *ischanō,* "I hold in check" (a related verb, *ischainō,* means "I make dry"), + *aima,* "blood." The Greek *ischaimos* means "quenching the flow of blood," as a styptic substance would do. Rudolf Virchow (1821–1902), the famed German pathologist, used the term in referring to focal deprivation of blood.

ischium is from the Greek *ischion,* a word that appears in Homer and means "the socket in which the thigh bone turns." Ancient Greek anatomists extended the meaning to include the bone in which the socket sits (and on which we sit). The Greek source of the term (and **ischio-,** its combining form) dictates its pronunciation as "isk-," not "ish-."

iso- is a combining form derived from the Greek *isos,* "equal to, the same as, or like." Thus, an **isomer** (+ Greek *meros,* "part or share") is one of two distinct compounds having the same atomic composition, but in different molecular configuration and exhibiting different properties. **Isotonic** (+ Greek *tonos,* "tension") describes solutions of equal osmotic pressure, the standard of reference, in physiology, usually being serum. An **isotope** (+ Greek *topos,* "place") is one of two or more forms of an element, all occupying the same place in the atomic table.

-itis is a Greek suffix that converts a noun into an adjective. When used as such, the Greek *nosos,* "disease," is understood as following the adjective but is not stated. In other words, by adding "-itis" to the name of any anatomic structure, it is understood that reference is being made to a disease affecting that structure. For example, *nephro-,* "kidney," + *-itis* means a condition affecting the kidney; if completely spelled out, this would have to be *nephritis nosos,* "disease of the kidney." Thus, "-itis" saves a lot of effort and space. Originally, "-itis" meant any sort of disease, but later it became restricted to denoting inflammation in the structure to whose name it was added.

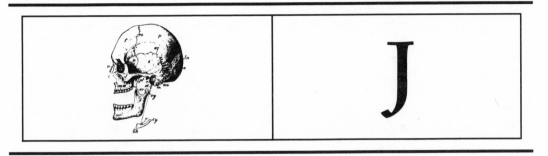

J

jade is a highly esteemed ornamental stone, so called because it was once thought to be a remedy for colic or flank pain. The ancient Spaniards called it *piedra de ijada,* "stone of the side." The French shortened this to *jade.* The adjective **jaded,** as in "jaded appetite," comes from quite a different source. In Old Norse *jalda* meant "a mare." In English, "jade" became a contemptuous term for a horse, particularly one of inferior breed or one that was old and decrepit. Hence, a jaded appetite is one which is weakened by fatigue, perhaps by overwork.

jaundice is considered to be ultimately derived from the Latin *galbinus,* an adjective meaning a light greenish-yellow. In French this became *jaune* and in German *gelb.* Non-medical persons use the word in an interesting way when they refer to regarding something with "a jaundiced eye." In this sense the allusion is to an attitude of distaste or satiety tinged by prejudice. This use is un-derstood by the clinician who knows that a person ill with a disease characterized by jaundice often has lost his appetite, often is disturbed by nausea, and is generally dis-comfited.

jaw originated in the Anglo-Saxon *ceowan,* "to chew," which led to *chawe* or *jawe* (the con-version of "ch" to "j" being not unusual). Chaucer spelled the word "jowe," and this suggests the current "jowl." The old form is preserved in the colloquial "chaw," as in "a chaw of tobacco."

jejunum is a near borrowing of the Latin adjec-tive *jejunus,* "fasting or hungry," in the sense of being empty and devoid of food. The ancient Greeks, impressed by their ob-servation at necropsy that the lumen of the proximal small intestine was always empty, used the descriptive term *nēstis,* "fasting," and this was translated into Latin as *jejunus.* In his treatise on the function of different parts of the body, Galen says that this part of the intestine is always found to be empty. In lay language, a jejune argument is empty, devoid of substance.

journal comes from the Old French word meaning "daily." This, in turn, was taken from the Latin *diurnus,* "of the day," the adjectival derivation of *dies,* "day." Obviously, our word **diurnal** is closer to the origin. Before A.D. 1500, "journal" was used as an adjective, as in "journal account." Then the modified noun was dropped, and the account that was kept daily was referred to as simply "a journal." Strictly speaking, every medical "journal" should be a daily publication. But no matter. The *Annals of Surgery* is a journal, but it comes out monthly, not just once a year as its name implies.

jugular comes from the Latin *jugulum,* "the throat," which is related to jugum, "a yoke or collar." Thus, the jugular vein is "the vein of the neck." Galen referred to this structure as *phleps sphagitis,* "the sacrificial vein," an ominous allusion.

jupe is an old dialect word for tuberculosis. "Jupe" was once commonly used among poor blacks as a name for the dread "consumption." Its origin is not known, but a source in an African tribal language would be a good guess.

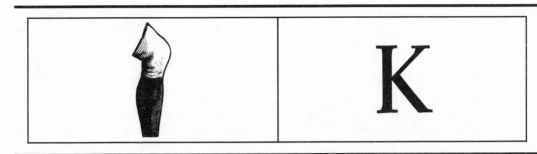

kala-azar is the Hindu name for "black fever," so called by the people of the Assam province, in northeast India, where the disease is endemic. The common name was given because of the dusky hue of the skin assumed by victims in the later phase of the disease. The cause is infection by a protozoon now known as *Leishmania donovani*. It was Sir William Leishman (1865–1926), of Her Britannic Majesty's Indian Medical Service, who first discovered the parasite in a spleen at necropsy in 1900, a finding later confirmed by his colleague, Dr. Charles Donovan (1863–1951).

kallikrein was the name given by H. Kraut, E. K. Frey, and E. Werle (Hoppe Seyler's *Z. physiol. Chem.* 189:97, 1930) to a hypotensive substance of which they found the pancreas to be a major source. The name is contrived from a Greek word for the pancreas. It is possible that the Greeks may have referred to the pancreas (which they usually called *pa[n]gkreas*) as *kallikreas,* this being a combination of *kalli-,* "beautiful, delectable," + *kreas,* "a piece of meat."

kaolin is a near borrowing of the Chinese *kauling,* "a high ridge," which describes the place where the clay-like silicate of aluminum was first found. Originally it was used by the Chinese in the manufacture of fine porcelain. Later, it was utilized in pharmacy as a coating for pills and then as a medicine itself in the treatment of diarrhea because of its adsorptive properties.

keloid is usually attributed to the Greek *kēlē,* "a rupture, as a hernia," though it could also come from the Greek *kēlis,* "a blemish." Professor H. A. Skinner has suggested still another origin: the Greek *chēlē,* "a hoof, claw, or talon." Any or all of these could describe the tough, tumorlike scar that occurs after the healing of skin wounds in certain susceptible persons. Such a scar was called "keloid" by Jean Louis Alibert (1768–1837), a French dermatologist, in 1835.

keratin is the name for the protein constituent of skin, hair, nails, and horny excrescences. It is attributed to the Indo-European *ker,* "horn," which led to the Greek *keras.* The rhinoceros gets his name from his nose-horn.

keto- is a prefix denoting the presence of a carbonyl group (=C=O) in an organic chemical compound. Such compounds are generically known as **ketones.** The proto-type was **acetone** (dimethyl ketone), so named from the Latin *acetum,* "vinegar," + the Greek *-ōne,* "a female descendant," in the sense of a weaker derivative. One might conclude that acetone was first thought to be a "weak sister" of acetic acid. The German word for acetone is *aketon,* and the generic term "ketone" emerged by simply dropping the initial "a."

kidney as a term for the paired, retroperitoneal organs of urinary excretion is hard to track down. In Middle English, says the Reverend Skeat, the spelling was variously *kidneer, kidnere,* or *kidenei.* The second syllable of the first two forms would seem to be related to a common Indo-European root from which the Greek *nephros,* the Old Icelandic *nyra,* and the German *Niere* are derived; all mean "kidney." *Kidenei* has been pos-tulated as a combination of the Anglo-Saxon *cyd,* "pod or husk," + *(n)ei,* "egg." Apparently there was confusion in ancient times as to whether the testis or the kidney was the source of sperm. The Romans gave up and called the kidneys *renes,* from which we take our adjective "renal." The Latin *rigare* means "to convey water." "Kidney" also has been used as a figure of speech to refer to a sort of temperament or nature. This is in keeping with the ancient proclivity to ascribe temperamental characteristics to certain organs of the body. Two fellows who take much the same view of things might be referred to as "men of the same kidney." The ancient Hebrews believed the kidneys were the seat of affections or passions. Solo-mon proclaimed, "Yea, my reins [kidneys] shall rejoice when thy lips speak right things" (Proverbs 23:16).

kine-, kinesio- are prefixes denoting a sense of movement and come from the Greek *kinē-sis,* "motion." Thus, **kinesthesia** (+ Greek *aisthēsis,* "feeling") is the sense by which movement of a part is perceived. A deriva-tive in common use is "cinema," as a name for the movies. **Kinins** are so called because they are endogenous peptides having an effect on the movement of smooth muscle. **Bradykinins** (from the Greek *brady,* "slow") cause a slow movement or contrac-tion of the gut muscle.

king's evil was a medieval term for scrofula or cervical lymphadenopathy, which in most cases probably was tuberculous adenitis. The original Late Latin term was *regius morbus,* the reference being not to a king afflicted with the disease but rather to the fact that a "laying on" of the royal hand was believed to be a sure cure. England's Ed-ward the Confessor, in the 11th century, was a foremost practitioner of the royal touch, and Charles II is said to have "laid hands" on a hundred thousand of his subjects, doubtless in an effort to bolster his shaky reign (1660–1685). The ancient practice of "laying on of hands" persists today. One professor of medicine wisely advised, "Always put your hand where the patient says it hurts."

knee originated in the Indo-European *gneu* or *genu,* "the knee," the latter being taken directly into Latin and into Greek as *gonu.* In Anglo-Saxon this became *cneow,* from which "knee" eventually emerged. The names of geometric figures are derived from the Greek *gonu.* A pentagon has five angles, or "knees."

knuckle began as the Anglo-Saxon *cnucl* and is related to the Dutch *knokkel,* the diminutive of *knok,* "bone"; hence a little bone.

koilo- is a combining form taken from the Greek *koilos,* "hollow or concave." A **koilocyte** is a hollow or empty cell, devoid of its normal cytoplasmic content. **Koilonychia** (+ Greek *onyx,* "nail") is a condition wherein the fingernails (and, in some cases, the toenails) assume a concave shape and are sometimes called "spoon nails."

kyphosis comes from the Greek *kyphos,* "bent or bowed," and usually refers to a bowing of the dorsal spine. Commonly it is a sign of osteopenia or bony depletion in postmenopausal women and sometimes is referred to as "dowager's hump."

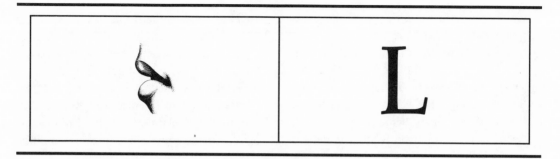

labium is the Latin word for "lip." It is a neuter noun, so the plural (for a pair of lips) is *labia.* But here is where it gets confusing. There is also a Latin feminine noun for "lip": singular *labia,* plural *labiae.* In anatomy, the neuter noun is used, so that the two sets of opposing lips of the vulva (even though this is strictly a female organ) are properly called the labia majora and the labia minora. A related Greek verb is *laphyssein,* "to swallow greedily, to devour." It would seem that these words, all pertaining to lips, originated in imitation of the sound produced by the act of lapping fluid into the mouth.

labor is another word for parturition, the process of giving birth to a baby, and comes closer in meaning to the Latin noun *labor,* "a troublesome effort or suffering," than the common use of the word today. The ancient meaning was implied in Jesus' entreaty, "Come unto me, all ye that labor and are heavy laden, and I will give you rest" (Matthew 11:28).

laboratory sounds as though it was conceived as a name for any place where work was done. But this is not the sense in which the word was used in ancient times, or, in fact, is used now. A place where people work at plucking chickens or at hammering out horseshoes is not a laboratory. The word comes from the Latin *elaborare,* "to work out, as a problem, and with great pains." An old English spelling was "elaboratory" and designated a place where learned effort was applied to the solution of scientific problems. We have simply dropped the "e."

labyrinth is a near borrowing of the Greek *labyrinthos,* "a large building with intricate passages intersecting each other." In Greek mythology, the Athenians were at one time sorely oppressed by Minos, the king of

Crete, who exacted from them an annual tribute of seven youths and seven maidens. These unfortunate youngsters were condemned by Minos to be devoured by the hungry Minotaur, a monster with a bull's body and a human head. That the Minotaur was fed but once a year accounts for his appetite. The victims were placed in a labyrinth, where the Minotaur roamed and from which there was no escape. A stop was put to this egregious practice by Theseus, the heroic son of the king of Athens. In anatomy, "labyrinth" designates the lateral mass of the ethmoid bone and also the internal ear, both of which contain intricate passages.

lac- is the Latin word for "milk." From this, in its combining form, have been derived **lacteal** (a vessel conducting a milky fluid, such as in lymphatic channels in the intestine where the fluid is fat-laden lymph), **lactic** acid (originally discovered in sour milk), and **lactose** (the sugar naturally occurring in milk).

laceration is a near borrowing of the Latin *laceratio,* "a tearing or a mangling." The word now serves for any cut incurred as an injury, but it retains its sense of forceful trauma. A cut made by a surgeon is an "incision," not a "laceration."

lacertus is a Latin word that to the Romans meant both "a muscle" and "a lizard," presumably because of the fancied resemblance in shape. More specifically, the reference was to the biceps muscle in the upper arm. Now, in anatomy, "lacertus" designates the fibrous expansion or attachment of certain muscles, particularly the biceps brachii and the lateral rectus muscle of the eye.

lacrimal originated in the Indo-European *dakru,* "a tear, as from a weeping eye." The same word was used by the Greeks. In archaic Latin this became *dacruma,* but in classical Latin the "d" was changed to "l" under Sabine influence, and to the Romans "a tear" was either *lacruma* or *lacrima.* The Anglo-Saxon derivative was *taehher,* whence the English "tear." In anatomy we put this together when we say, "The lacrimal duct conveys the tears." An alternative spelling is **lachrymal,** which is an aberration arising from the Medieval Latinists' custom of changing "c" to "ch" preceding an "r" (as in "pulchritude"); the "i" became "y" simply as a graphic variant. So "lacrimal" is the correct spelling, even though we persist in using "lachrymose" to describe a person given to weeping.

lacuna is the Latin word for "ditch, hole, pit, pond, or pool." In anatomy, the term is used to refer to any similar structure as, for example, the lacunae of bone. These minute apertures in bones, having been first described in 1691 by Clopton Havers (1657–1702), an English physician and anatomist, are also known as "Haversian canals."

lambdoid refers to whatever may be fancied in the shape of the Greek letter lambda, Λ, or an inverted V. Thus, the lambdoid suture of the skull and the lambdoid incision for gaining access to the epigastric viscera were so named.

lamina is the Latin word for "a thin plate," and **lamella** is the diminutive form meaning "a little, thin plate." A host of anatomic structures incorporate these terms in their names. The plate-like dorsal arches of the vertebrae are called "laminae," and the operation whereby they are removed is called a **laminectomy.**

lancet is a slightly shortened form of the French *lancette,* which was derived from the Latin *lancea,* "spear," and therefore is "a little spear." To lance a lesion, such as a boil, is "to spear" it.

lanolin is a fatty substance obtained from the wool of sheep. The name was concocted by combining the Latin *lana,* "wool," + *oleum,* "oil." As an emollient or unguent it usually is made up as a hydrous emulsion. It is commonly incorporated in cosmetic lotions aimed to soften or "moisturize" the skin.

lanugo is the Latin word for "down, meaning the small, fine hairs of plants." The lanugo hair of the fetus is the downy excrescence that appears about the fifth month of gestation.

laparotomy comes from the Greek *lapara,* "the soft parts of the body between the rib margins and the hips," that is, the flanks or loins. This, in turn, is related to *laparos,* "slack, loose, or relaxed." The ending of "laparotomy" comes from the Greek *tomē,* "a cutting." The term "laparotomy" was introduced as an operating term in 1878 by Thomas Bryant, an English surgeon. Purists argue that "laparotomy" should be used only for incisions in the flanks and not for incisions elsewhere in the abdomen, but the currency of usage has drowned out their cries. Similarly, **laparoscopy** (+ Greek *sko-*

pein, "to view") has been disdained, in some circles, as an improper term for looking into the abdominal cavity by means of an optical instrument, even though this instrument is inserted through the "soft parts" of the abdomen. This procedure was long known in the U.S. as "peritoneoscopy." But "laparoscopy," as it is widely known and used in Europe and Japan, is rapidly gaining currency.

larva is Latin for "mask or ghost." The Romans used the word to designate the specter of the dead, which they conceived as having a spirit but not the actual form of that which it represents. In this sense, the term became applied to an early phase in the life of an insect or parasite before its true form became apparent. Regressing to its figurative sense, we may make reference to a "larval" form of a disease when we mean an early, undefined phase in its development.

larynx is a direct borrowing of the Greek term for "the upper part of the windpipe." This is related to the Greek verb *lary*[*n*]*ggixō,* "I bawl or bellow," from which the term **laryngismus** was derived, as an allusion to the crowing sound issuing from a spastic larynx.

latent is a slightly abbreviated form of the Latin adverb *latenter,* "secretly," and is related to the intransitive verb *latere,* "to lie hidden or concealed." Thus, latent syphilis is a "hidden" form of the disease.

laudanum is an old designator of tincture of opium. Some scholars assert that the name is a derivative of the Greek *ladonon,* the resin obtained from an oriental shrub (not the poppy plant) that was known to the Persians as *ladan.* The claim is that this substance was confused with poppy juice. There is a more plausible (if not laudable) explanation. "Laudanum" was introduced into the pharmacopoeia by Aureolus Theophrastus Bombastus von Hohenheim (1493–1541), a Swiss physician who named himself Paracelsus to indicate that he was on a par with, if not superior to, the renowned Celsus. He claimed he had a secret remedy (which may or may not have contained opium) that he considered *laude dignum,* "worthy of praise." It is curious to note that, much later, "heroin" was given its name because it was thought to have special merit.

laughing gas was the name given to nitrous oxide in 1800 by Humphrey (dubbed "Sir" in 1812) Davy (1778–1829), the remarkable English surgeon-apothecary-chemist who investigated the curious psychotropic properties that became apparent when the gas was inhaled. Davy went on to discover and isolate numerous elements, among them sodium, potassium, chlorine, and fluorine. Some say Sir Humphrey's greatest discovery was his assistant, Michael Faraday.

lavage comes from the Latin *lavare,* "to wash." Gastric lavage is another way of saying "a stomach washing." A lavatory, of course, is "a place for washing."

laxative comes from the Latin *laxare,* "to extend, widen, open, or release." In the sense of "loosening or relaxing" the bowel, the term was not used by the Romans but came out of the Middle Ages, perhaps because those were such costive times.

lecithin comes from the Greek *lekithos,* "the yolk of an egg." This name for the mono-amine-monophosphatide was suggested by its early discovery in carp eggs.

leech is the common name for a bloodsucking worm of the class Hirudinea, but it also is, or was, used to designate a physician. In fact, the latter meaning came first, being derived from the Anglo-Saxon *lǽce,* "one who heals." Today, in Iceland, a physician is a *laeknir,* and in Finland a *lääkari.* The Dano-Norwegian term is *laege,* the Polish is *lekarz.* The bloodsucking annelid worm, in former times, was used medicinally, the idea being that the worm would consume corrupting substances from an inflamed lesion. Hence, the worm was given the name of "the healer." Later, "leech" became an epithet for a person who clung to and extracted sustenance from another. It is possible that "leech" (physician) and "leech" (worm) are words of separate origin that became assimilated.

leiomyoma is contrived by a combination of the Greek *leios,* "smooth," + *mys,* "muscle," + *ōma,* "swelling"; hence "a smooth muscle tumor." By mistake, such tumors as occur commonly in the muscular wall of the uterus were, and sometimes still are, called "fibroids."

lemniscus is derived from the Greek *lēmniskos,* "a woolen ribbon or bandage," related to *lēmnos,* "wool." In anatomy, a lemniscus is a band or bundle of neural fibers.

lens is the Latin word (the genitive is *lentis*) for the bean-like seed that we call "lentil." The only lens familiar to the ancients was that of the eye, and it was given the name of the bean because of its shape and not because of its transparency. The **len-**

ticular nucleus, a part of the corpus striatum of the brain (which has nothing to do
with the eye), was so named because of its
shape.

lenta is the feminine form of the Latin adjective meaning "slow or sluggish." Hence,
subacute bacterial endocarditis was once
known as "endocarditis lenta" because of its
typically slow, lingering course.

lentigo is the Latin word for "freckle." Indeed,
what the dermatologist calls "lentigo" looks
a lot like a freckle. It is a small, brown spot
in the skin, resulting from the deposition of
melanin by an active focus of melanocytes
near the basal layer of the epidermis. But to
the dermatologist there is an important distinction. A freckle comes from exposure to
the actinic rays of the sun, whereas **lentig-
ines** (the plural) can be the result of various
other causes. Incidentally, the suffix **-igo,** of
Latin origin, once was used in a number of
terms denoting conditions of disease in man,
animals, plants, and even metals. Those
medical terms that have survived are mostly
related to dermatology, e.g., vitiligo, intertrigo, and impetigo. Exceptions are vertigo
and, as a slight variant, lumbago.

leontiasis is a rare form of hyperostosis of uncertain cause affecting young persons,
wherein the facial bones enlarge, giving the
face a resemblance to that of a lion. *Leo,
leonis* is the Latin for "lion."

leprosy comes from the Greek *lepros,* "scaly,
rough, or mangy," hence "the scaly disease." Gerhard Hansen (1841–1912), a
Norwegian physician, correctly described
the causative organism, *Mycobacteriae le-*

prae, and the condition is now properly
known as Hansen's disease. In ancient
Greece, what we know as leprosy probably
did not exist. The "scaly disease" of the
Greeks more likely was psoriasis. Aretaeus
the Cappadocian described leprosy accurately in the second century A.D., but he
called it "leontiasis." There then followed a
confusion of names, and in the translation of
Arabic writings the Greek *lepra* became attached to what is now called Hansen's disease. The term "leprosy," then, doubly deserves to be abandoned, not only because of
its unjust connotation of despicability, but
also because it had been misplaced nosologi-
cally.

lepto- is a combining form taken from the
Greek *leptos,* "fine, slender, or delicate."
Thus, the **leptomeninges** (+ Greek *mē-
ni[n]gx,* "membrane") are the thin, delicate
membranes (comprising both the pia and
the arachnoid) that envelop the brain and
spinal cord. The *Leptospira* (+ Greek
speira, "coil") is a genus of finely coiled
spirochetes.

lesion comes from the Latin *laesio,* "an attack
or injury," which is related to the verb *lae-
dere,* "to strike, hurt, or wound."

lethargy is a state of overpowering drowsiness
or apathy, and it comes from the Greek
lēthargos, "forgetful." In Greek mythology,
Lethe was the name of a river that flowed in
the netherworld of Hades. The souls of the
dead were obliged to drink of its water and
so became oblivious of everything said or
done during their span on earth. One might
assume that the word **lethal,** meaning

"deadly," was of analogous origin. Not quite. "Lethal" is from the Latin *letum,* meaning death or destruction. The "h" got put in the English word in the 17th century because of confusion with the Greek *lēthe,* "oblivion." Our word, then, should be "letal," but no one would recognize it as such.

leuko- is sometimes spelled **leuco-** and is a combining form, usually a prefix, taken from the Greek *leukos,* "white," and also "light, bright, brilliant, and clear." The apostle Luke, patron saint of physicians, owes his name to the same source. **Leukemia** (+ Greek *aima,* "blood") is marked by an excess of **leukocytes** (+ Greek *kytos,* "cell") or white blood cells. The amino acid **leucine** (one of the few names wherein the "c" always appears) was so called because of its color. **Leukoplakia** (+ Greek *plakoeis,* "flat, broad") is characterized by white patches or plaques on a mucous membrane. **Leukorrhea** (+ Greek *rhoia,* "a flow") is a white vaginal discharge.

levator comes from the Latin *levare,* "to lift." There are a number of levator muscles in the body, and they all serve to lift whatever structure into which they are inserted. Muscles that lower attached structures are called **depressors,** a term derived from the Latin *depressus,* the past participle of *deprimere,* "to press down" (from *de-,* "down from," + *primum,* "above all").

levo- is a prefix or combining form taken from the Latin *laevus,* "on the left side." Purists insist it be spelled **laevo-,** and they are right insofar as the term has nothing to do with

the Latin *lĕv-* (related to "lifting") or *lēv-* (related to "smoothness"). **Levulose** was the name given by Claude Louis Berthollet (1748–1822), a French physician and chemist, to fructose (the sugar of fruits) because it caused polarized light to be rotated to the left. **Levarterenol,** also known as norepinephrine and marketed as "Levophed," is the l- (for *levo-*) isomer (and the pharmacologically active form) of the chemical mediator liberated by mammalian postganglionic adrenergic nerves.

libido is the Latin word for "desire, longing, fancy, lust, or rut." In psychoanalysis the term is applied to the motive power of the sex life; in Freudian psychology, to psychic energy in general.

lichen is a near borrowing of the Greek *leichēn,* "a tree moss." In botany, a lichen is a compound plant composed by symbiotic union of a fungus and an alga, and it grows as an excrescence on rocks or trees. The term was used by the Greeks in reference to a blight or canker on olives, and hence came to be applied, in ancient medicine, to various skin eruptions, probably most often ringworm. Now, the medical term is used almost exclusively as part of "lichen planus" (the second word is Latin for "flat"), an inflammatory skin or mucosal disease characterized by an excrescence of flat, white plaques.

lienteric refers to a type of diarrhea wherein the feces contain particles of undigested food, indicating rapid passage through the gut. The word is a combination of the Greek *leios,* "smooth," + *enteron,* "the intestine";

thus "a slippery gut." Obviously "lienteric" should be spelled "leinteric," but it isn't. And it has nothing to do with *lien,* the Latin word for "spleen."

ligament comes from the Latin *ligare,* "to bind or tie," and refers to the tough bands of connective tissue by which various structures are bound together or supported. A **ligature** is something used as a tie, especially in surgery, and to **ligate** is to tie. Oliver Wendell Holmes, the 19th-century Boston savant, wrote in his *Medical Essays,* "I would never use a long word where a short one would answer the purpose. I know there are professors in this country who 'ligate' arteries. Other surgeons only tie them, and it stops the bleeding as well." The word "obligation," in the sense of a pledge, comes from the Latin *ob,* "on account of," + *ligare,* and hence means whatever one is bound to do for a particular reason. Another related word is "religion," which can be viewed as a bond or pledge.

limbus is the Latin word for "fringe, hem, or border." Thus, the limbus of the cornea is the border where it joins the sclera. Limbo was, in ancient theology, a supposed place, not quite hell and not quite heaven, that was the abode of infants who died without baptism and of the righteous who died before the coming of Christ.

liminal is derived from the Latin *limen,* "threshold." As in "lumen" and "luminal," the second vowel of the derived adjective changes from "e" to "i." A liminal stimulus is just barely perceived by the senses, and a **subliminal** stimulus is "below the threshold" and not perceived at all.

linea is the Latin word for "line, string, or thread." To the Romans, according to Professor H. A. Skinner, the *linea alba* or "white line" was the mark made with lime or chalk across the racetrack behind which the chariots lined up for the start of a race. In anatomy, the linea alba is the longitudinal white streak of fibrous tissue between the rectus abdominis muscles.

lingual is derived from the Latin *lingua,* "tongue," and is related to the verb *lingere,* "to lick up or lap up." To pronounce the Latin word is almost to imitate licking with the tongue. For the Greeks, "to lick" was *leicho,* an imitative sound, too. "Tongue" also refers to language (the French word for "language" is *langue*), the utterance of which requires an active use of the tongue. A colloquial term for the spoken word is "lingo," recorded in English as early as 1600; it is close to the Latin. In anatomy, **lingula** (the Latin diminutive) is used as a term for anything shaped like a little tongue, as, for example, the projection from the lower portion of the upper lobe of the left lung.

liniment comes from the Latin *linere,* "to smear on or to anoint." In ancient practice, as today, a liniment was a particularly thin, liquid ointment.

lip- is a combining form taken from the Greek *lipos,* "animal fat or vegetable oil." A **lipid** is any fatty substance (although the technical definition in the U.S. is slightly different from that in the U.K.). **Lipofuscin** is a lipid-containing, granular pigment observed in various tissues and often attributed to cellular senility. It has been sometimes called "wear-and-tear pigment." The name was contrived by hybridization of the Greek *lipo-* + the Latin *fuscus,* "dark brown," because of its color. The latter Latin adjective gives a clue to the origin of "obfuscate," meaning to make murky.

liquor is Latin for anything having a fluid consistency. In anatomy and pharmacy, "liquor" is the term for various fluids or solutions used as vehicles for drugs. Thus, the "liquor amnii" is the fluid within the amniotic sac, and "liquor iodi compositus" is Lugol's solution.

litho- is a combining form derived from the Greek *lithos,* "stone." **Lithotomy** (+ Greek *tomē,* "a cutting") is the operation of "cutting for the stone" and originally referred to incision of the urinary bladder. Hippocrates, in his famous oath, required his disciples to forswear "cutting for the stone," leaving that practice to "such as are craftsmen therein," presumably meaning urologists. The condition of stones in the gallbladder is **cholelithiasis** (from the Greek *cholē,* "bile").

litmus comes from the Old Scandinavian *litmosi,* "dye moss," being a combination of *lit,* "color or dye," + *mossi,* "a moss or lichen." Litmus is a blue coloring matter obtained from certain lichens and exhibits the helpful property of turning blue in an alkaline solution ($pH > 7$) and red in an acid solution ($pH < 7$). For convenience in the laboratory, the dye usually is impregnated in paper, a slip of which is immersed in the fluid to be tested for alkalinity or acidity.

liver is the name of the largest solid organ in the body, generally acknowledged to be es-

sential to life. Its name would seem to be related to the verb "to live." Perhaps it is. Its Anglo-Saxon predecessor was *lifer.* In German, the organ is *die Leber,* and "to live" is *leben.* But scholars are not sure of the connection. It has been suggested that the Indo-European root word for the liver was *yekurt,* which became the Greek *hēpar* (from which we have hepatic, hepatitis, and similar combined forms) and the Latin *jecur.* The Latin term, oddly, has no descendant in Romance languages, being replaced by a Latin adjective, *ficatum,* "stuffed with figs." It would seem the Romans combined liver and figs in a single dish. *Ficatum* became the Italian *fegato,* the Spanish *higado,* and the French *foie.* To the ancient Babylonians, the excised liver of a sacrificial animal was an organ of divination wherefrom they read all sorts of portents. Ironically, the ancient people had not an inkling of the truly astonishing metabolic function of the liver. In fact, the liver fell into disrepute when it was found not to be the wellspring of blood and lymph, an earlier supposition. It remained for Claude Bernard (1838–1878), the renowned French physiologist, to establish the liver in its rightful place as a vital organ—"a veritable laboratory of life," as he put it. It is appropriate that "la maladie de foie" has become, in effect, the national disease of France.

livid is a derivative of the Latin *lividus,* "the color of lead," a bluish-gray. **Livedo reticularis** (from the Latin *reticulum,* "a network") is a mottled purple or dusky blue discoloration of the skin seen in hypoxic conditions. Interestingly, the Latin *lividus* also means "jealous, envious, or spiteful." Presumably this is an allusion to the complexion of persons consumed by these emotions.

lochia is the fluid that seeps from the vagina during the first week or so after childbirth. The term is derived from the Greek *locheia,* "childbirth," being related to the Greek verb *locheuō,* "I bring forth or I bear."

locus is Latin for "a place or site." The term is used in the names of various specific anatomic locations, particularly in the central nervous system. In medical practice, a **locum tenens** (from the Latin *tenere,* "to hold") is, literally, one who "holds the place," and refers to a doctor who temporarily carries on the practice of an absent colleague.

long in the tooth is an old phrase descriptive of aging. It refers to the observation that the gums tend to recede with age, thus exposing more of the teeth. The expression has been used of both horses and people.

lordosis is a borrowing of the Greek *lordos,* "bent backward." This posture results in an exaggerated anterior convexity of the lumbar spine. The term has nothing to do with a haughty or lordly bearing.

lozenge refers to the shape and not to the content or purpose of the medication so formulated. The French *losange* means "diamond-shaped." The origin probably was in the Old Gallic *lausa,* "a flat stone," + *-inga,* the Germanic suffix indicating "pertaining to." In Portuguese, *lousa* is "a tombstone." Now, in pharmacy, a lozenge is a tablet of any shape intended to be dissolved in the mouth for its topical soothing effect.

lues is the Latin word for "infection, contagion, plague, or pestilence," and may have come from the Greek *lua,* "a dissolution." To the Romans, *lues* meant any sort of virulent, contagious disease. The more specific term *lues venerea* means syphilis, a disease acquired by the act symbolizing devotion to Venus, the goddess of love.

lumbar comes from the Latin *lumbus,* "the loin," and refers to anything pertaining to the lower paraspinal region. The lumbar vertebrae are situated between the loins. **Lumbago** is an old-fashioned term for any rheumatic pain in the region of the loins.

lumbricoid comes from the Latin *lumbricus,* "a worm," and refers to whatever has the appearance of a worm. *Lumbricus* in zoology is the name of a genus of annelids, including the common earthworm. *Ascaris lumbricoides,* the scientific name of the parasitic intestinal worm, would seem to be a redundancy; the Greek *askaris* means "an intestinal worm." The **lumbrical** muscles in the hand and the foot are so called because of their wormlike shape.

lumen is Latin for "light," including the light that comes from a window or aperture. When sectioning a hollow viscus, one can see light through the opened space. Hence, "lumen" came to be a term designating that space. In the adjectival form, **luminal,** the "e" becomes an "i." Why "Luminal" was the trade name chosen for phenobarbital is uncertain; perhaps it seemed a bright idea at the time.

lunatic as a term for a person mentally disturbed comes from the Latin *luna,* "moon." Such use refers to the old belief that mental disorder was a consequence of being "moon-struck." Another derivation is the slang word "loony." The expression "crazy as a loon" refers not to the large, fish-eating diving bird but rather to the archaic *loon* that meant "a worthless or stupid fellow" and may have been derived from the Icelandic *lūinn,* "beaten." One who had been beaten senseless might well act strangely.

lung may have originated in the Sanskrit *laghu,* which meant "light" in the sense of "without weight." It is likely that the ancients were impressed by the lightness of the lungs in contrast to the density of other viscera. In almost all languages, the term for the lungs is related to the word for "lightness." For example, the Russian *legkoe,* "lung," is related to *lëgkii,* "light."

lupus is Latin for "wolf." The use of the wolf's name in the designation of various diseases reflects differing allusions. "Lupus vulgaris" (the latter word is Latin for "common") refers to tuberculosis of the skin wherein the infection appears to eat away at the skin, as by the gnawing of a wolf. "Lupus erythematosus," a skin disease wherein the malar areas become inflamed and pigmented, apparently give the patient a lupine or wolflike facies.

lutein refers to any yellow substance. The term comes from the Latin *luteus,* "mud-colored." *Lutum* is the Latin word for "mud or clay." The **corpus luteum** is the yellow body or nodule that marks the site of a mature ovarian follicle from which the ovum has been discharged.

luxation comes from the Latin luxare, "to put out of joint or to dislocate." It is akin to the Greek *loxos,* "crosswise." A **subluxation** is a less than complete dislocation. If the joint hurts and you're not sure it is really dislocated, you can gravely pronounce the injury as "subluxation."

lymph is a slightly shortened version of the Latin *lympha,* "clear water, especially that found in flowing springs." *Lympha* is a pseudoetymological formation influenced by the Greek *nymphē* (wherein the "n" was exchanged for an "l"), the word for "a bride or marriageable girl." As a proper name, Nymphē was applied to goddesses of lesser rank who presided over springs, lakes, or forests. The association seems to have been with a sense of moisture. In ancient anatomy, the lymphatic vessels were so named because, while they were thought to be veins, they were observed to carry a watery fluid rather than blood. The nodes intimately associated with these vessels were called "lymphatic glands" or, more correctly, "lymph nodes." The cells contained within the nodes were given the name **lymphocytes** by Paul Ehrlich (1854–1915), the German bacteriologist and immunologist. For the ancients, the idea of *lympha* became incorporated into the humoral system of pathology, and the supposedly cool, moist temperament became known as the phlegmatic or lymphatic type. Presumably a sluggish disposition was attributed to an overgrowth of lymphoid tissues. A person so perceived was said to be in **status lymphaticus.** Somewhat inconsistently, the Latin adjective *lymphaticus* was also used to mean "crazy or frantic."

lys- is a combining form taken from the Greek *lysis,* "a loosening or setting free." The term is used as a prefix, as in **lysozyme,** a basic protein that functions as an antibacterial enzyme; a suffix, as in **hydrolysis,** the breakdown or release of components of a substance by the addition of water (the H^+ going to one resultant part and the OH^- going to the other); or by itself, as in the **lysis** or "loosening" of adhesions.

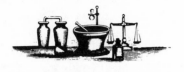

M

macerate comes from the Latin *maceratus,* the past participle of *macerare,* "to make soft or tender." The adjective *macer* means "lean or skinny" and also "thin or poor," as a depleted soil. Macerated skin is that made soft and friable by excessive moisture or oiling. A macerated fetus is one that has degenerated and disintegrated after dying in the uterus.

macro- is a prefix taken from the Greek *makros,* "long, in space or time." In medicine, the term is used only in the sense of a long distance and, more particularly, a large size. Thus, a **macrocyte** is an unusually large cell, and **macroscopic** means to be seen by the naked eye.

macula is the Latin word for "a small spot or blemish." The *-ula* ending denotes a diminutive emphasis. In dermatology, a macula is a small, flat, unraised spot or blemish in the skin (in contrast to a papule, which is a raised spot). The macula lutea (from the Latin *luteus,* "mud-colored or yellow") is the spot at the posterior pole of the retina where the keenest vision is registered.

mad as a hatter is an expression used to describe a person more than slightly daft. It usually reminds one of Lewis Carroll's Mad Hatter, an amusing character encountered in the course of *Alice's Adventures in Wonderland,* but the phrase was well known earlier. Its origin is disputed. Some say it began as "mad as an atter," the "atter" being an Anglo-Saxon word for adder, thus referring to the viper whose bite was thought to induce madness. The alternative explanation, medically more interesting, is that mercurous chloride was used in making felt for hats and that hat-makers or "hatters," inhaling the vapors, would eventually become victims of mercury poisoning. Among the symptoms of chronic mercury poisoning are tremors of the eyelids, lips, tongue, and fingers, due to cerebellar cortical atrophy.

magnesia is borrowed from the name of a town, Magnesia, that was situated in the once wealthy kingdom of Lydia, the domain of the fabulous Croesus. The area is now part of northwestern Turkey. From a small mountain near this town was obtained an ore that included what we would now call magnesium carbonate. Magnesium hydroxide is the familiar "Milk of Magnesia," commonly used as a laxative agent. Apparently there was another ore of different composition obtained from the vicinity of Magnesia that exhibited unusual properties; it was known as the Magnesian stone and led to our word "magnet."

malady is an Anglicization of the French *maladie,* "an illness." This, in turn, is derived from the Latin adverb *male,* "badly." (The Latin word is pronounced "mah-ley" and has nothing to do with "male," in the sense of the masculine gender.) This provides an opportunity to give a prime example of false etymology. The fanciful story is told that the word "marmalade" goes back to the frequent illnesses suffered by Mary, the unhappy and unfortunate queen of the Scots. When Mary complained, the cry of her French-speaking courtiers would ring through the castle, "Marie est malade!" ("Mary is sick!"). The remedy was found to be a nice dish of preserved fruit, and this took its name as an antidote for "Mary's malade." This story has not a grain of truth in it. "Marmalade" comes from the Portuguese *marmalada,* "a quince jam," and goes back to the Latin *melimelum,* "a kind of apple," and to the Greek *melimēlon,* a combination of *mel-,* "honey or a sweet," + *mēlon,* "a fruit."

malaise is a French word descended from a combination of the Old French *mal-,* "bad or ill," + *aise,* "ease"; hence "ill at ease." In medicine, "malaise" can describe any vague feeling of bodily discomfort.

malar comes from the Latin *mala,* "the cheekbone". To the Romans, this also meant the facial cheek itself, and it has been suggested that the term is related to the Latin *malum,* "an apple," presumably because of a fancied resemblance of the rosy, rounded cheek to an apple.

malaria comes from the Italian wherein *mala* means "bad" and *aria* is "air." The Italian expression used in the 18th century was *mal-'aria.* The belief was that the disease, then called "intermittent fever," was caused by *mal'aria* or noxious air emanating from marshlands. The connection with swamps was correct, but mosquitoes and not vapors carry the cause of malaria.

malignant comes from the Latin adjective *malignus,* "spiteful, mean, stingy, or malicious," this being derived from a combination of *mal-,* "bad," + [g]*nascor,* "to be born." Thus, "malignant" means, literally, "born to be bad," and this comes very close to the sense of the word as it is used in pathology. A malignant neoplasm is one that is genetically predetermined to cause trouble.

malingerer is one who feigns illness, often as a ruse to avoid an obligation. The word comes from the French adjective *malingre,* "sickly or loathsome," and is a combination of *mal-,* "bad," + the Old French *haingre,* "thin, emaciated." Presumably "to malinger" came to its present meaning from the practice of soldiers who excoriated themselves, particularly by producing ulcers on their legs, and thus appeared to have an incapacitating affliction. In modern soldiery, the self-inflicted "shot in the foot" is a supreme example of malingering.

malleus is the Latin word for "hammer or mallet." The diminutive form, *malleolus,* means "a little hammer." Inexplicably, in anatomy, the malleus, one of the tiny middle-ear ossicles that is shaped like a hammer, is considerably smaller than the **malleolus,** the bony prominence on either side of the ankle which seemed to someone to look like the protruding head of a hammer.

mamma is both the Latin and the Greek word for "the breast," especially that of the woman. The word is said to be imitative of the "ma-ma" sound uttered by mewling infants as they seek the nourishing breast. Every young mother marvels when she hears that sound: "The baby has learned my name!" Little does she know that her name came from the sound and not the other way around. Mammals are vertebrate animals that suckle their young. **Mammillation,** a word derived from the diminutive of *mamma,* refers to a small excrescence that bears a fancied resemblance to a little breast.

mandible is a transliteration of the Latin *mandibula,* "the lower jaw." The word comes from the Latin verb *mandere,* "to chew"; the suffix *-bula* indicates "the means of." The ancient anatomists used *maxilla* for both the upper and lower jaws, and only much later did the "inferior maxilla" become "the mandible."

mania is the Greek word for "madness" and is related to the verb *mainomai,* "to rage, to be furious, or to rave in anger." A **manic** disorder is one characterized by an abnormally expanded emotional state, excessive elation, and heightened verbal and motor activity.

manifest means "clearly evident," and a manifestation of disease is a readily apparent feature. "Manifest" comes from the Latin *manifestus,* which, in turn, is a combination of *manus,* "hand," + *festus,* "struck." Anything that strikes the hand or is struck by the hand is clearly evident. A palpable tumor is certainly manifest.

manometer is a word in which the "o" reveals the origin of the term. If the second vowel were "i" or "u," the first part would have to come from the Latin *manus,* "hand," but this is not the case. The "mano-" of "manometer" comes from the Greek *manos,* "scanty or sparse." The second component of the word, "-meter," comes from the Greek *metron,* "a measure." The first manometer called by that name was used early in the 18th century to record the decreasing pressure of rarefied or "scanty" air in a chamber from which the air had been extracted. Later the term was applied to any instrument capable of measuring the pressure or tension of gases or liquids.

manu- is a combining form, usually a prefix, that denotes relation to the hand. It is derived from the Latin *manus,* "the hand." The **manubrium** (+ Latin *hibrium,* from *habere,* "to hold") is the breastbone, so called because it resembles the handle of a sword. A **manual** or **handbook** is a set of instruction as to what to do with the hands in performing a given task. These terms have nothing to do with the size of such a book, in the sense of being easily held in the hand. This explains why a so-called handbook (and particularly the German *Handbuch*) can be such a ponderous volume.

marasmus is derived from the Greek *marainein,* "to quench, to extinguish" and also "to waste away, to languish." In former times, the term was used to describe the pitiable state of infants who became emaciated and wasted away from no known cause. Insofar as causes are now increasingly well defined and remedies are more available than before, "marasmus" is seldom heard nowadays. However, the adjectival forms "marantic" and "marasmic" are occasionally used.

marrow means the pith, the core, or the central substance of anything. The Latin equivalent, **medulla,** is used to refer to the pith of the kidney and brain, while the English "marrow" is used to refer to the pith of hollow bones. "Marrow" can be traced to the Anglo-Saxon *mearh* and the Sanskrit *majjan,* both of which referred alike to the marrow of bones or the pith of trees. "Spinal marrow" is an old term for the spinal cord, which was believed, incorrectly, to be the marrow of the vertebrae.

marsupial comes from the Greek *marsippos,* "a bag or pouch." Formerly, the Latin *marsupium* was applied to various anatomic pouches, such as the peritoneal cavity and the scrotum. In surgery, **marsupialization** refers to the operation whereby an external opening is provided for drainage of an internal cyst. An example would be the suturing of an opening in a pancreatic cyst to a stoma in the anterior abdominal wall, thus forming a sort of draining pouch. Such an operation is not currently favored; internal drainage by gastric or enteric anastomosis is preferred.

masochism is a distorted condition wherein self-induced pain or humiliation gives a sensation of pleasure. The term is taken from the name of Leopold von Sacher-Masoch (1836–1895), an Austrian writer who made a sufferer of this perversion the protagonist of one of his novels.

massage comes from the Greek *massein,* "I work with the hands, as in kneading dough," and probably is related to the Greek *maza,* "barley bread," and perhaps to the Hebrew *massāh,* "unleavened bread." Some patients given to colloquial speech refer to palpation, as of the abdomen, as "mashing." This is not traceable to the Greek but rather to the Middle English *mēshen,* the crushing of cereal grains in water to provide a "mash" as a food for animals or a substrate for fermentation.

masseter is the name of the jaw muscle that brings the lower teeth into contact with the upper teeth. It is so called from the Greek *masētēr,* "the chewer." The redundant "s" in the English term may have been a copyist's error.

mast cell was so named by Paul Ehrlich (1854–1915), the renowned German immunologist and bacteriologist, who first used the term *Mastzelle* in 1879. The German *mästen,* "to fatten," is related to *mast,* an old English word for food, especially as fodder for animals. This, in turn, can be traced to the Sanskrit *mēda(s),* "fat" (which, by another track, gives us "meat"). Ehrlich was impressed by the densely packed basophilic granules he observed in the cytoplasm of what he called the *Mastzelle,* at first mistaking them for particles ingested by phagocytosis. To him, the cell looked "well fed."

masticate comes from the Greek *mastazein,* "to chew or to gnash the teeth," and from this came the name *mastiche* for the resinous gum of an evergreen shrub. Yes, the ancients, too, had a "chewing gum." Though the proper Latin word for chewing is *mandere,* the Romans used *masticare* specifically for the enjoyable chewing of gum. The Greek *mastiche* also accounts for the word "mastic," a gummy substance used as a filler in masonry and as a styptic in dentistry.

mastitis is an inflammation of the breast. The first portion of the word comes from the Greek *mastos,* "the breast of a woman." An earlier Greek form was *mazos,* from which is derived "amazon," meaning literally "without a breast." According to Herodotus, the Greek historian, there was a mythical race of female warriors who lived in Scythia. To avoid impediment in drawing their bows, these formidable women were said to have deliberately cut off their right breasts. Hence, they came to be known as "Amazons." It seems that early Spanish explorers were intrigued by the notion that such warrior women abounded in the New World. Despite the fact that the immense South American river had been already named by its original discoverer the Rio Santa Maria de la Mar Dulce, another Spanish explorer, known as Orellano, in descending that river, fancied that he was engaged in battle by warrior women, and so rechristened the river "Amazonas."

mastoid refers to the smooth, rounded eminence of the temporal bone behind the ear. This was fancied to resemble a female breast. Hence, its name was taken from the Greek *mastos,* "breast," + *eidos,* "like." At one time this structure was known by the Latin term *processus mammiformis.*

materia medica is a now archaic term meaning, literally, "the stuff of medicine," and more particularly the preparation and use of drugs, now called "pharmacology." The Latin *materia* is used in the sense of "the stuff of which anything is composed." If *materia* sounds like the Latin *mater,* "mother," the resemblance is more than coincidental. In bygone times there were but two departments in the medical curriculum, that of "physic" wherein one learned of the natural course of disease, and that of "materia medica" wherein one learned how to change it.

matrix is the Latin term for any female animal kept specifically for breeding and is related to the Latin *mater* and the Greek *mētēr,* both meaning "mother" and both used in reference to the uterus as "the mother of the fetus." From this evolved the sense of matrix as a mold or enclosing mass in which anything is formed or shaped. The bony matrix is the groundwork in which bone is formed. The Latin *matrix* also was a public roll on which one's parentage was registered. Later, the diminutive *matricula* was "a little list" of the members of a university. Those named on this list could say they had "matriculated."

maxilla is the Latin word for "jawbone." It sounds like a diminutive, and it may be, but of what no one is sure. The ancients used *maxilla* for both the upper jaw and the lower jaw. Later, the lower jaw became known as the mandible, and "maxilla" was restricted to the upper jaw.

measles as the name for the familiar childhood disease always is used in the plural. The reason is that the child so afflicted is covered by many little red spots. The name originated with the Old High German *māsa*, "a spot." This was taken into Middle English as the diminutive plural *maselen*, "many little spots." There was another wholly unconnected Middle English word, *mesel*, "a wretch" and, later, "a leper." This came from the Latin *miser*, "wretched." There should be no confusion between *maselen* and *mesel*.

meatus is the Latin word for "motion or movement," but it also means "a channel" and is related to the verb *meare*, "to go or to pass." "Meatus" is used in the sense of a channel when referring to the external auditory meatus, the passage leading into the ear.

meconium is taken from the Greek *mēkōnion*, which was the dark, viscid juice obtained by pressing the poppy plant. The Greek name for the poppy is *mēkōn*. Because the bowel discharge from newborn infants was thought to resemble poppy juice, it was given the same name.

median is a borrowing of the Latin *medius*, "the middle." The median nerve extends along the middle of the forearm to the hand. In statistics, the median is the number in the exact middle of a list of numbers representing values arranged in ascending or descending order.

mediastinum sounds like a near borrowing of the Latin *mediastinus*, but to the Romans this meant "a servant or a drudge." In anatomy, the mediastinum is a partition between the bilateral pleural cavities. Despite the apparent disparity in usage of the term, there is, in a way, a connection. The word is derived from a combination of the Latin *medius*, "middle," + *stare*, "to stand." The anatomic mediastinum can be said to "stand in the middle" of the thorax, while the servant "stands in the middle" when he acts as an intermediary for his master.

medicine is taken almost directly from the Latin *medicina*, which, to the Romans, meant the same thing. This word, in turn, is related to *mederi*, "to heal." Both in ancient times and now, the same word—*medicina* or medicine—was and is used to refer both to the science of healing and to the means of healing, that is, what we also call "drugs." Although no scholarly authority makes the connection, one is tempted to think of the "medi-" in "medicine" as being related to the Latin *medius*, "middle," in the sense of "coming between," as in "mediator" and "medium." Surely the practitioner of medicine tries to intervene in a helpful way between the patient and his affliction.

medulla is the Latin word for "the marrow," in the sense of the core or central substance of anything, and is related to the Latin *medius*, "middle." Thus, the adrenal medulla is the "core" of the adrenal gland. Andreas Vesalius (1514–1564), the renowned Flemish anatomist, who taught at Padua, also used the Latin *medulla* as a name for the spinal cord, taking his cue from the Greeks, who called it *myelos rachitēs*, "the marrow of the spine," presumably because the spinal cord occupies a channel within the spinal column. In the 18th century, the term "medulla oblongata" (the latter word meaning "rather long") was limited in reference to that part of the brainstem extending from the pons to the spinal cord proper.

mega- is a combining form, usually used as a prefix, derived from the Greek *megas*, "great or big." In Latin this became *magnus*. Thus, **megacardia** refers to an enlarged heart, **hepatomegaly** refers to an enlarged liver, and a **megacyte** is an abnormally large red blood cell.

melan- is a combining form derived from the Greek *melas*, "black." The Greek verb *melainein*, "to darken or grow black," gives us **melena** as the term for blood that has become black as it traverses the gut after internal bleeding. **Melancholia** (+ Greek *cholē*, "bile") is a gloomy, depressed emotional state which, according to humoral pathology, was thought to result from an excess of "black bile." **Melanin** is the dark pigment of the skin, the hair, the choroid coat of the eye, and the substantia nigra ("black substance") of the brain. **Mela-**

nuria, a darkening of the urine, can be produced by a variety of substances, including blood, melanin, and homogentisic acid.

melitensis is the Latin adjective that means "Maltese," i.e., of or from the island of Malta. The disease now called brucellosis was formerly known as "Malta fever." The causative organism, *Bacillus melitensis*, was first isolated in 1887 by David (later Sir David) Bruce (1855–1931), an English army surgeon, from the spleens of British soldiers who died of "undulant fever" while stationed in Malta. The unfortunate soldiers had contracted the disease by drinking raw goat's-milk.

membrane comes from the Latin *membrana*, "a skin or parchment." This, in turn, has been thought to relate to the Latin *membrum*, "a member" in the sense of a part of the whole, as a limb is a "member" of the body. It was the *membrana* that covered and delineated a *membrum*. Later "membrane" was applied to any skin-like tissue.

men- is a prefix taken from the Greek *mēn*, "a month," and *mēnē*, "the moon." The cyclic changes observed in the moon provided one of the earliest measures of time, about 29½ days. Hence, a "month" is really a "moonth." In Latin, a month is *mensis* (plural, *menses*), and *menstruus* means "monthly." It early became obvious that a woman's cyclic vaginal bleeding almost coincided with the period of the lunar phases, and from this come **menstrual** and **menstruation.** Colloquially, some women still refer to their "monthlies." Because these usually occur predictably, they are often called "periods." **Menorrhagia** (+

Greek *rhēgnymi,* "to burst forth") is an excessive vaginal bleeding which occurs at regular monthly intervals. The **menopause** (+ Greek *pausis,* "cessation") signals the end of a woman's menstruation and, hence, of her fertility. Alchemists used the Medieval Latin *menstruum* to mean a solvent, and even today one occasionally hears of a solvent medium being so called, e.g., Pitkin **menstruum,** a medium for the administration of heparin. What has this to do with a woman's monthly vaginal discharge? In centuries past, the product of uterine flow or *menstrua* (in classical Latin the neuter plural was always used) was fancied as the medium by which the male and female elements (i.e., the sperm and the ovum) were united, or "dissolved," into a single being that gained form as the fetus.

meninges is the plural of the Greek *mēninx,* "a membrane," and the earliest writers used this term for membranes found anywhere in the body. Later the term was restricted and used in the plural in reference to the three membranes that envelop the brain and spinal cord. However, there is a related combining form, **myringo-,** that is familiar to otologists. In Late Latin *myringa* appeared as a term for the eardrum or tympanic membrane, probably as a corruption of the Greek *mēninx.* From a combination of *myringo-* + Greek *tomē,* "a cutting," came **myringotomy,** the operation of incising the eardrum. It is said this operation was introduced in 1760 by a Parisian quack doctor as a remedy for deafness, presumably to let the sound gain easier access to the ear. Only later did myringotomy gain respectable status as a means of providing drainage for suppurative collections in the middle ear.

meniscus is a near borrowing of the Greek *mēniskos,* "crescent-shaped." The root word, obviously, is the Greek *mēnē,* "moon." The capillary effect on fluid in a tube, such as a pipette, produces a concave or convex shape at the top of the fluid column; this is known as a "meniscus." The articulating cartilages at the proximal end of the tibia at the knee joint are crescent-shaped and, as such, were given the name "menisci."

mental really represents two words and can refer to the mind or to the chin, depending on which Latin word is considered the origin. In common and most frequent usage, "mental" refers to the mind and, as such, is derived from the Latin *mens,* "the mind or intellect." Just as properly, "mental" is derived from the Latin *mentum,* "the chin." The mental artery goes not to the brain but, as a branch of the maxillary artery, to the skin and subcutaneous tissues of the chin.

menthol is a common ingredient of liniments. It is a volatile oil and gives rise to the minty odor characteristic of athletes' training rooms. In fact, *mentha* is the Latin word for mint. This came from the Greek *mintha,* the mint plant. In Greek mythology, Minthē was the name of a nymph who caught the roving eye of Pluto. In a fit of jealousy, Proserpine, Pluto's wife, transformed the nymph into an herb that was then known by her name. The Reverend Cobham Brewer, writing a century ago, pointed out that, as Pluto was the god of the underworld, Minthē actually was saved by her transformation—presumably "from a fate worse than death"—and thus became an agent of healing.

mesmerism is so called from Franz Mesmer (1734–1815), a Viennese doctor of medicine. The newly discovered properties of magnetism had become fascinating at the time, and Mesmer evolved the theory that a similar force could exercise a profound effect on the human body. This supposed force, known as "animal magnetism," purportedly could be transferred from one person to another. The practice of summoning and exerting this force, widely promoted by Mesmer, was a form of hypnotism, and thus "to mesmerize" became a part of the language. Both Mesmer and mesmerism fell into disrepute when French authorities, commissioned to investigate the man and his method, issued an unfavorable report.

meso-, mesen- are combining forms, usually appearing as prefixes, taken from the Greek *mesos,* "middle." Thus, the **mesencephalon** (+ Greek *enkephalos,* "brain") is the midbrain. The **mesenchyme** (+ Greek *enchyma,* "instillation") is that embryologic tissue, situated in the **mesoderm** (+ Greek *derma,* "skin"), the middle germ layer between the ectoderm and the entoderm, that gives rise to connective tissue and to constituents of the vascular and musculoskeletal systems. The **mesentery,** from its derivation (+ Greek *enteron,* "intestine"), would seem to be the "middle intestine." This, of course, is not so. Rather, the Greek *enteron* originally referred to the viscera generally. The mesentery, then, is properly named as the midline membrane situated in the midst of the viscera.

meta- is a Greek preposition that can mean "among, between," or "after, above, beyond," or "by way of change." It is in these last two senses that "meta-" is incorporated in a host of scientific terms. **Metabolism** (+ Greek *ballein,* "to throw") was introduced in 1839 by Theodor Schwann (1810–1882), an eminent German anatomist and physiologist, as a term for the chemical changes whereby nutriments were converted (or "thrown into a different position") to energy and living tissues. The **metacarpal** (+ Greek *karpos,* "wrist") bones are situated in the hand "beyond" the wrist. Their counterparts in the foot are the **metatarsal** bones. The analogy may be apt, but the etymology is a bit off the mark. "Metatarsal" came into use much later than "metacarpal." The tarsal bones owe their name to the Greek *tarsos,* which means "a flat surface"; *tarsos podos* means "the flat of the foot." The metatarsal bones are "beyond" the tarsal bones, but they are not exactly beyond the flat of the foot. **Metamorphosis** (+ Greek *morphē,* "form") is a change in configuration, as from a caterpillar into a butterfly. **Metaplasia** (+ Greek *plassein,* "to shape or mold") is a process whereby a change takes place "beyond" the normal adult form, as when gastric mucosa assumes the form of intestinal mucosa in response to injury. **Metastasis** (+ Greek *stasis,* "a placing") was used by the ancient Greeks to mean "removal from one place to another." The term was introduced into Late Latin to designate the shift of disease from one part of the body to another. Now it is used almost exclusively in reference to the spread of malignant neoplasms to sites distant from their primary source. **Methemoglobin** (wherein the "t" and the "h" are pronounced separately) is a term introduced by Ernst Hoppe-Seyler (1825–1895), a German biochemist, for the change that occurs in hemoglobin when its iron has been oxidized from the ferrous to the ferric state, from which oxygen cannot be readily released.

meteorism is the condition wherein the gut is distended by excessive gas, most of which is swallowed air. The term comes from the Greek *meteōros,* "suspended in midair or raised aloft." To the patient afflicted with meteorism, his abdomen feels, indeed, as though it were a balloon. He may also feel as though he were about to take off, like a meteor.

methyl designates the radical CH$_3$, a prototype substance being **methanol** (CH$_3$OH), also called "wood alcohol." The term is attributed to Johann Jakob Berzelius (1779–1848), a Swedish chemist, who combined the Greek *methy,* "wine," + *ulē,* "wood." Chemists were well grounded in classical languages in those days.

metr- is a combining form taken from the Greek *mētra,* "uterus." Thus, the **endometrium** is the lining of the uterus, and the **myometrium** is the muscular wall of the uterus. **Metrorrhagia** (+ Greek *rhēgnymi,* "to burst forth or flow from") is bleeding from the uterus at times other than regular menstruation.

metric comes from the Greek *metron,* "a measure, rule, or standard." The metric system, as we know it today, is a product of the French Revolution. Before this momentous political upheaval, France had no uniform system of measures or weights. In 1790 the revolutionary assembly charged the Académie des Sciences with the task of devising a sensible and universally usable system. This they did, completing their work in 1799. Except for minor corrections in later years, the basic concept remains. The genius of the system is that it is designed on a base of 10, i.e., it is a "decimal system," and its derived units can be calculated merely by shifting a decimal point. The entire system is based on only two "natural" units: the meter (as a measure of length, intended to be $\frac{1}{10,000,000}$ the distance on the earth's surface from the equator to either pole) and the gram (as a measure of weight or mass, being the mass of pure water at maximum density that would fill a cube whose edges are 0.01 meter). All other units are therefrom derived. They are named in the table on page 153.

micro- is a combining form, usually used as a prefix and taken from the Greek *mikros,* "small, petty, or trivial." The number of medical terms incorporating "micro-" is not small. **Microbe** is a concoction of "micro-" + the Greek *bios,* "life," proposed in the late 19th century as a name for any minute, living organism. **Microscope** is a word invented by Johannes Faber in 1628 by combining "micro-" + the Greek *skopein,* "to view." A **microtome** (+ Greek *tomē,* "a cutting") is an instrument for cutting ultrathin sections of tissue for examination under the microscope.

midwifery refers to the performance of a **midwife,** a person who assists a woman at child-

prefix	abbreviation	derivation	power of 10	equivalent
tera-	T	Greek *teras,* "monster"	10^{12}	trillion
giga-	G	Greek *gigas,* "giant"	10^9	billion
mega-	M	Greek *megas,* "large"	10^6	million
kilo-	k	Greek *chilioi,* "thousand"	10^3	thousand
hecto-	h	Greek *hekaton,* "hundred"	10^2	hundred
deca-	da	Greek *deka,* "ten"	10^1	ten
deci-	d	Latin *decimus,* "a tenth"	10^{-1}	one-tenth
centi-	c	Latin *centum,* "a hundredth"	10^{-2}	one-hundredth
milli-	m	Latin *millesimus,* "a thousandth"	10^{-3}	one-thousandth
micro-	μ	Greek *mikros,* "small"	10^{-6}	one-millionth
nano-	n	Greek *nanos,* "dwarf"	10^{-9}	one-billionth
pico-	p	Italian *pico,* "small"	10^{-12}	one-trillionth
femto-	f	Danish *femten,* "fifteen"	10^{-15}	one-quadrillionth

birth. The name is an Anglo-Saxon combination of *mid-,* "together with," + *wif,* "a woman." A midwife, therefore, can be of either sex; it is the one who is being assisted that is the wife, not the one who is assisting. In current and common parlance, a midwife is a nurse-practitioner, specially trained in attending women at childbirth. But many years ago, in some schools, the head of the obstetrics department held the title of "professor of midwifery."

migraine is a common, severe, head pain that has long been recognized as typically occurring on only one side of the head at a time. The term began as the Latin *hemicrania,* which was derived from the Greek *hēmi,* "half," + *kranion,* "the skull." In Medieval Latin this was shortened to *migraena* and came into French as *migraine.*

miliary is often used to describe lesions that are of the size of millet seeds, e.g., those of "miliary" tuberculosis. But how many doc-

tors have ever seen a millet seed? Millet is a cereal grass cultivated through the centuries for food and fodder. Its seed is about 2 mm in diameter. The Latin word for millet is *milium,* hence the derived adjective. **Milaria** is a skin eruption characterized by numerous papules, approximately the size of millet seeds. It is caused by abnormal retention of fluid in sweat glands and is often marked by extravasation of sweat into adjacent layers of the skin, with attendant inflammatory reaction.

minim was formerly used in pharmacy and therapeutics as the term for "a small drop." It came from the Latin *minimus,* "the smallest or the least." Small doses of liquid medicines were prescribed in "minims." It became obvious that all "drops" are not of the same size, and in the mid-19th century the London College of Physicians defined a "minim" as $\frac{1}{60}$ of a dram or $\frac{1}{480}$ of a fluid ounce. Today some liquid medicines are dispensed with their own standard dropper so as to assure a proper dose.

mithridatism is the technique of inducing immunity to the effects of poison by administering at first minute amounts and then gradually increasing doses of the poisonous substance. This is somewhat akin to desensitizing an allergic person by injecting increasing amounts of the antigen to which he reacts. The term is taken from the name of Mithridates, king of Pontus, an ancient country bordering on the Black Sea. As a precaution against being poisoned, Mithridates diligently conditioned himself to the effects of some noxious substance (which one is not known). As it turned out, the experiment backfired. Mithridates was defeated in war and captured by the Roman general Pompey in 67 B.C. To evade the ignominy of his plight, Mithridates tried to commit suicide by taking poison but, of course, failed. As a last resort, he bid his slave run him through with a sword.

mitochondrium is a combination of the Greek *mitos,* "a thread," + *chondros,* "a cereal grain" or any coarsely granular substance. The term was introduced in 1902 by Karl Benda (1857–1933), a German physician, as a name for the granular structures with threadlike membranes found in the cytoplasm of cells.

mitosis was suggested in 1882 as a term for cell division by Walther Flemming (1843–1905), a German cytologist. The term was taken from the Greek *mitos,* "thread," the allusion being to the threadlike formation of the nuclear chromatin as it becomes conspicuous in a cell preparing to divide.

mitral as a descriptive term for the bicuspid valve between the left atrium and ventricle of the heart is so used because the two cusps of the valve resemble a bishop's miter or headdress. The Latin *mitra* referred to a turban; the Greek *mitra* referred to a cloth band that could be worn either as a girdle, or as a snood or headband. These terms perhaps are related to the Greek *mitos,* "the thread of the warp," as in woven cloth.

mnemonic comes from the Greek *mnēme,* "memory." Mnemonics is the art of improving the memory, and mnemonic devices are those that aid recollection. Medical students through the ages have been among the cleverest users of mnemonic devices. One that comes to mind: "Never lower Tillie's pants; Grandmother might come home!" The initial letter of each word in this admonition is also the initial letter of the names of the carpal bones, conveniently listed in their proper order: *n*avicular, *l*unate, *t*riangular, *p*isiform, greater *m*ultangular, lesser *m*ultangular, *c*apitate, *h*amate. The problem is, of course, that sometimes one remembers the mnemonic device but forgets what it stands for.

moiety comes by way of the French *moitié* from the Latin *medietas,* "the middle or mean." Originally, "moiety" meant "half," but now it can refer to any designated portion, e.g., the carbohydrate moiety of a glycoprotein.

molar is the name for a tooth that grinds. It comes from the Latin *mola,* "a millstone." Thus, the molar teeth are distinguished from the incisor teeth, which are designed for a different purpose. Ask anyone whose

154

molar teeth have been extracted how well he can chew with only his front teeth.

mole can mean a number of things: a dark spot on the skin, a uterine mass, a chemical mass, a breakwater or pier, or a small burrowing animal. The mole of the skin comes from the Gothic *mail,* "a wrinkle or blemish." The mole that is a fleshy mass forming in the uterus as a result of degeneration or abortive development of an embedded ovum comes from the Latin *moles,* "a mass or pile." From this same Latin source comes the word for the mole that is the massive pile of stone forming a breakwater or pier, and also for the mole that is the mass in grams of a chemical compound equivalent to its molecular weight. This latter mole is a convenient abbreviation of **molecule,** which itself is a diminutive of the Latin *moles,* i.e., "a little mass." Thus, we have the odd sequence of a standard term converted to its diminutive, then back again to its standard form.

molluscum as in "molluscum contagiosum" comes from the Latin *mollis,* "soft or spongy." Originally the Latin *molluscum* referred to a soft fungus growing on trees, and also to a sort of nut with a soft shell. The phylum Mollusca includes snails, squids, and octopuses. "To mollycoddle" means to pamper or make soft. Somehow, the image of mollycoddling an octopus does not readily come to mind. In pathology, "molluscum contagiosum" is a spongy excrescence of the skin caused by a transmissible virus.

moniliasis is an exudative inflammation of the skin or mucous membranes consequent to infection by the fungus *Candida albicans* (and, in some quarters, is better known as "candidiasis"). The genus in which the fungus is classified was known formerly as *Monilia,* this name being taken from the Latin *monile,* "a necklace." Under the microscope, the organism appears arrayed as a string of beads. The speckled white exudate, especially as it occurs in the mouth or throat, has long been commonly referred to as **thrush.** Possibly this may be an allusion to the speckled throat and breast of a familiar songbird, the thrush. The disease known as **sprue** gets that name from the Dutch *spruw* or *sprouw,* as the monilia-induced thrush is called in Holland. The connection is that patients afflicted with sprue can become severely debilitated and, hence, liable to infection by the monilial fungus.

mono- is a prefix derived from the Greek *monos,* "single," and denotes a reference to only one thing or part. Thus, a **monomania** (+ Greek *mania,* "madness") is a psychosis limited to a single delusion. A **mononuclear** cell contains but a single nuclear clump. Occasionally one hears "mono" as a nickname for infectious mononucleosis.

monster is sometimes construed as being related to "huge," but its use in reference to size reflects only a subsidiary meaning. In mythology, a monster is a fabled creature that hideously combines animal and human forms. In pathology, a monster is an infant born with a grotesque anomaly, such as an absence or excess of limbs, or other misshapen form. Whatever its use, "monster" comes from the Latin *monstrum,* "a divine omen, portent, or warning," this being related to the verb *monere,* "to warn." Fortunately, the belief has long dissipated that the delivery of a deformed infant is a sign of divine wrath.

mons veneris is the rounded prominence covering the pubic arch just above the female external genitalia. *Mons* is Latin for "hill or mountain"; *veneris* refers to Venus, the Roman goddess of love.

morbid is an adjective derived from the Latin *morbus,* "sickness or disease." What we now call "pathology" formerly was known as "morbid anatomy."

morgue is the French name for a place where the bodies of persons recently dead can be viewed and identified. The term comes from the Old French verb *morguer,* "to regard solemnly." Knowing the derivation of "morgue" can remind us of the proper demeanor when attending a necropsy.

moribund is a near borrowing of the Latin *moribundus,* "at the point of death." The Latin word is equivalent to the verb *mori,* "to die," + *bundus,* an adjectival suffix.

moron is a term codified about 1905 by two Frenchmen, Alfred Binet and Theodore Simon (a physiologist and a physician, respectively), who were charged by the authorities responsible for the care of the feebleminded with the task of devising tests to determine the levels of mental retardation. According to the Binet-Simon scale, the mental ages of retarded adults are: one to two years, "idiot"; three to seven years, "imbecile"; and eight to twelve years, "moron." Perhaps Binet and Simon were inspired in their choice of the last term by their compatriot, the 17th-century French playwright Molière, who gave the name

Moron to the fool in one of his plays. In any event, the name can be traced to the Greek *moros,* "dull, sluggish, slow in wit."

morphology combines the Greek *morphē,* "form, shape, or appearance," + *logos,* "a discourse." In biology, "morphology" properly refers to a study or treatise on the form or structure of an organism or its parts, as contrasted with a study of its function. The Greek *morphē* appears in the name of Morpheus, the mythological god of dreams who, in the parlance of show business, "created, designed, and produced" those nocturnal fantasies. Perhaps thus inspired, a German apothecary, Adolf Sertürner (1783–1841), gave the name **morphine** in 1805 to the principal psychotropic alkaloid of opium.

mountebank is an epithet for a quack doctor and comes from the Italian *montambanco,* a combination of *montare,* "to mount," + *banco,* "bench," literally "one who mounts a bench" to proclaim his nostrums. If what a mountebank had to say carried the weight of truth, he wouldn't have to make such a fuss about it.

mucus is the Latin word for "a semifluid, slimy discharge from the nose." The Greek *muktēr* is "the nose or snout." Incidentally, the colloquial, vulgar term "snot" comes from "snout," literally. In current usage, "mucus" designates a clear, viscid fluid expressed from any epithelial surface. **Mucosa** is a convenient shortening of the Latin *membrana mucosa,* which refers to any membrane or surface that is slimy. Some people who are slipshod in their spelling tend to confuse "mucus" (the noun) and "mucous" (the adjective).

multi- is a combining form, usually a prefix, that comes from the Latin adjective *multus,* "many or abundant." The medical terms so formed are, indeed, multiple. One example is **multipara** (+ Latin *parere,* "to give birth to"), the term for a fecund woman who has spawned many children.

mumps probably is related to the Icelandic *mumpa,* "to eat greedily, to fill the mouth too full." The person afflicted with marked swelling of the parotid glands has the appearance of one with a large mouthful. A related word is "mumble," meaning to speak indistinctly, as if one's mouth were full of marbles. However, "mumps" also has been attributed to the Old English verb "to mump," which meant to appear sulky or sullen. This, too, could describe the countenance of a patient afflicted by mumps.

Munchausen syndrome was so named by Dr. Richard Asher (*Lancet* 1:339, 1951), an exceptionally perceptive and articulate English physician, to describe the startling and often bizarre presentation by arch-malingerers who feign catastrophic illness. Baron Karl Friedrich Hieronymus Munchausen was the protagonist in a pseudo-autobiographical narrative of impossible adventures, written in English, in 1785, by the German Rudolf Eric Raspe. In 1850 the word "Munchausenism," meaning exaggerated tales, was applied to the writings of Herodotus.

murmur is a Latin as well as an English word and has the same meaning in the two languages. To the Romans, *murmur* could also mean "growling, rumbling, or roaring." A related word is the Sanskrit *marmaras,* "noisy, as the rustling wind." The onomatopoeic quality of the word is enhanced by its reduplication. When the French clinicians in the early 19th century described what they heard from the heart, all sounds were called by the French word **bruit.** It was Joseph Skoda (1805–1881), an Austrian physician, who clearly distinguished normal heart tones from adventitious murmurs.

muscarinic refers to the parasympathomimetic action of certain cholinergic agonists. The origin of the term is in the Latin *musca,* "a fly." The prototype is muscarine, a natural alkaloid isolated in 1869 from a species of poisonous mushroom called *Amanita muscaria. Amanita* is an ancient Greek name for a kind of fungus; *muscaria* refers to its hairy appearance. The Latin *muscarium* means, literally, "pertaining to flies," but to the Romans a *muscarium* was specifically a sort of flyswatter made up of hairs from a horse's tail. If a horse can get rid of flies with a flick of his tail, the Romans could follow suit. So, the hairy mushroom that looked a little like a flyswatter was found to contain a poisonous alkaloid that was given the name of the flyswatter.

muscle comes from the Latin *musculus,* the diminutive of *mus,* "a mouse," hence, literally, "a little mouse." The use of *musculus* for "muscle," and this is what it meant to the Romans, usually is explained by the allusion to the movement of muscles under the skin to the scurrying of little mice. Or perhaps it was fancied that the shape of dissected muscles resembled that of small rodents. This may seem farfetched, but the fact is that pre-Galenic anatomists had little knowledge of the function of muscles. Indeed, Plato and Aristotle, among other ancient authorities, conceived of muscular tissue as simply another form of flesh serving as a cover for the body. This brings us to two Greek words: *mys* means both "mouse" and "a muscle of the body," while *myō,* a different word, means "I close," especially the lips and eyes, thus implying a muscular function. To either of these Greek words, the combining form **myo-** may be owed. The prefix can define a structure (as in "myocardium" or "myometrium") or tell the origin of a substance (as in "myoglobin"). **Myotonia** (+ Greek *tonos,* "tension") is a spastic condition of skeletal muscle. **Myopia,** or nearsightedness, however, is a special case. This clearly is a combination of the Greek *myō* + *ōps* (the "ps" being the Greek letter psi), which means "the eye." This adds up, literally, to "shut eye." Observe the nearsighted person as he tries, without glasses, to look at a distant object. He squints. It is the squint or closing of the lids that suggested the term "myopia."

mutation is derived from the Latin *mutare,* "to move, shift, change, or alter." In biology, a **mutant** is an offspring whose **phenotype** ("pheno-" comes from the Greek *phainein,* "to show"), or outward expression of its heredity, differs from that normally expected of its **genotype** ("geno-" comes from the Greek *gennaō,* "I produce"), or genetic disposition of its parents. The genetic theory of mutation was advanced in 1886 by Hugo de Vries (1848–1935), a Dutch botanist. Previous to de Vries's ex-

planation, such aberrant individuals were recognized but poorly understood and were called **sports.** "Sport" is a contraction of the Middle English disporter, "to amuse oneself, as from being removed from labor." This, in turn, is derived from the Latin *dis-,* "away," + *portare,* "to carry." This accounts for "sport" as an amusing game and for "sport" as a mutant; in both there is a sense of being "carried away."

mycelium comes from the Greek *mykēs,* "fungus," + *hēlos,* "an ornamental nail or stud." Presumably, the array of fungal filaments or "mycelia" was thought to resemble a collection of decorative nails. The combining prefixes **myc-, myco-,** and **mycet-** appear in a number of biological terms and denote a relationship to fungus.

mydriasis is a Latin term meaning an unnatural dilatation of the pupil of the eye. Such a dilatation can be induced by an anticholinergic drug, such as atropine, or by an intense, endogenous, adrenergic (sympathomimetic) stimulus. The latter phenomenon could explain the origin of the term in the Greek *mydros,* "a red-hot mass." The Greek phrase *mydrous airein cheroin* can be translated as "to grasp masses of red-hot iron," as an ordeal. Surely under such trying circumstances, the pupils of the eyes would be dilated. In contrast, **miosis** is an excessive contraction of the pupil of the eye, the term being a near borrowing of the Greek *meiōsis,* "a lessening." This is in no way related or connected to "myopia" or nearsightedness.

myelo- is a combining form taken from the Greek *myelos,* "the marrow or inmost core." In medicine, this can refer either to the marrow of bone or to the "marrow" of the central nervous system, viz., the brain, the peripheral nerves, and especially the spinal cord. It is easy to conceive of bone marrow as the core of a hollow bone. But the application of the term to the central nervous system is more difficult to appreciate unless one looks at these structures through the eyes of ancient observers. Then, the spinal cord might appear to be the "marrow" of the spinal canal, and the brain the "marrow" of the skull. By tradition, then, **myelitis** can be either an inflammation of the spinal cord or an inflammation of bone (though the latter usually is qualified as an **osteomyelitis**). **Myeloma,** on the other hand, is restricted as a designation for a tumor related to bone marrow or its constituents, not to nervous tissue. But sometimes tradition persists despite logic. What we call **myelin** is actually the substance of a fatty

sheath covering nerve fibers and clearly not the core of nerve tracts.

mylohyoid is a muscle whose name tells us that it extends from the lower jaw to the hyoid bone. The first part, "mylo-," comes from the Greek *mylē,* "a mill" (the lower jaw is part of a mill wherein the teeth are grinders). "Hyoid" is a Greek way of saying "U-shaped," and that describes the **hyoid** bone.

myxedema is contrived by a combination of the Greek *myxa,* "mucus," originally used in reference to the discharge from the nose, + *oidēma,* "a swelling up." It was Sir William Gull (1816–1890), an English physician, who first described in 1873 the peculiar swelling of the subcutaneous tissue associated with thyroid insufficiency, as observed in a "cretinoid state" in adults. In 1877 William Ord (1834–1902), an English surgeon, proposed the term "myxoedema" (the British spelling) for this "mucoid dropsy."

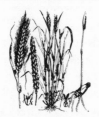

N

nape has served since the Middle Ages as a term for the back of the neck. It might be related to the Old German *noppe,* "to pluck," insofar as the back of the neck is a convenient place to grab and hold a man or animal. In this way, too, we may refer to the "scruff of the neck." "Scruff" is related to the Gothic *skruft,* "hair of the head." "Nape" may be related to the Old Frisian *hals-knap,* "the bump on the neck," and the Anglo-Saxon *cnaep,* "top of the hill" (from which also comes "knob"). Whether "nape" originally meant the external occipital protuberance at the posterior base of the skull or the protuberant spine of the seventh cervical vertebra is uncertain. The anatomic adjective **nuchal** is derived from the Arabic *nukha',* "the back of the neck."

narcissism is taken from the name of the mythological Narcissus, son of Cephisus, the river god, and the nymph Liriope. Narcissus was a handsome but heedless youth who attracted, then shunned, the woodland nymphs. One such forsaken nymph prayed that Narcissus would himself learn how it felt to be spurned. And so he did. One day, kneeling by a sylvan pond, Narcissus saw his own reflection mirrored in the water. Not recognizing the image as his own but thinking it to be a gorgeous inhabitant of the pond, he reached out to embrace the reflection. With the water thus disturbed, the image disappeared, only to return when the water was still. The more he looked, the more Narcissus became enamored of his own visage; the more often the figure eluded his grasp, the more frustrated he became. And thus Narcissus languished and died, shunned by his own image. His place at the edge of the pond was taken by the lovely white flower that is still known by his name. Psychiatrists refer to narcissism as a warped sexual attraction to oneself.

narcosis comes from the Greek *narkē,* "numbness or torpor." A **narcotic** drug is one that numbs or induces torpor. **Narcolepsy,** contrived by combining "narco-" + the Greek *lēpsis,* "a seizure," is the term used for a condition marked by sudden, uncontrollable compulsion to sleep.

nasal is an adjectival formation taken from the Latin *nasus,* "the nose." To the Romans, *nasus* always meant the external nose or snout, but now "nasal" refers to whatever pertains to the nose, inner as well as outer.

nausea is an almost direct borrowing of the Greek *nausia,* "seasickness." Quite logically this comes from the Greek *naus,* "ship," as does our word "nautical." Only later did "nausea" acquire the broader meaning of that disagreeably queasy feeling that often precedes vomiting.

navel is an ancient word, traceable in various forms through all Teutonic languages, with the same meaning as now. The Anglo-Saxon *nafe* was the center or hub of a wheel where the axle was inserted; its diminutive, *nafela,* was the name given to the belly button, probably because it looked like a "little hub" and was situated in the center of the abdomen. ("Nave" as the central part of a church is derived from the Latin *navis,* "a ship.") To the Greeks, the navel was *omphalos* (from which we take our combining form **omphalo-,** "pertaining to the navel") and to the Romans **umbilicus** (the anatomic term we use as a noun today).

navicular is taken from the diminutive of the Latin *navis,* "a ship," hence "a little ship." Early anatomists used "navicular" for any structure they fancied to have a ship-like shape. The navicular bone in the wrist was so named. But some classically minded anatomists preferred the Greek, so they called it the **scaphoid** bone (from *skaphē,* "a light boat or skiff," + *eidos,* "like").

necrosis is an almost direct borrowing of the Greek *nekrosis,* "becoming dead," from *nekros,* "a dead body or corpse." In pathology, "necrosis" refers to the lethal degeneration of cells or tissues rather than to the death of the entire organism. **Necropsy** ("necr-" + Greek *opsis,* "a viewing"; hence, literally, "a viewing of the corpse") is the proper term for postmortem examination and should be used as such rather than "autopsy." The Greeks did not have a word like "necropsy," but they would have understood the term. The Germans rendered it *Leichenbeschauung,* "a corpse-beholding or corpse-showing."

neck comes by way of the Middle English *nekke* from the Anglo-Saxon *hnecca,* originally "the nape of the neck." Whereas we now think of the neck as the entire structure interposed between the head and the torso, the original term referred to the back or nape of the neck. The Teutonic *hnakkon* conveyed the sense of a projection, as in the Gaelic *cnoc,* "hill."

nematoda is concocted from a combination of the Greek *nēma,* "a thread," + *eidos,* "like," hence "threadlike." The Nematoidea is a multitudinous order of intestinal worms characterized, in most species, by an intricate, threadlike alimentary tract. The reference, then, is not to the shape of the worm but to the worm's own innards.

neo- is a combining form, usually a prefix, taken from the Greek *neos,* "new, young, fresh, or recent." The prefix serves a variety of medical terms. In neuroanatomy, it designates those structures that are considered to represent more recent, advanced evolution, e.g., the neopallium and the neothalamus. **Neoplasm** (+ Greek *plasma,* "that which is formed") refers to tumors in the sense that the abnormal proliferation is among cells that have reverted to a primordial or "young" configuration; the implication is not that the tumor or growth itself is recent. "Neo-" is sometimes added to the trade names of drugs to convey the idea that something new (and presumably better) is being purveyed. Examples are Neo-Synephrine®, Neo-Cortef®, Neogesic®, Neoloid®, Neosporin®, and Neomycin.

nephro- denotes that which pertains to the kidney and is taken from *nephros,* the Greek word for that organ. While the Greek term is used as a combining form, the Latin *renes* is the source of the adjective **"renal."** We still use the Greek word **nephritis,** though to the Greeks this would have been any kidney condition, while we have restricted the term to denote an inflammatory disease. **Nephrosis** to the Greeks would have meant simply "pertaining to the kidney," while to us it means any noninflammatory, non-neoplastic disease. **Nephrolithiasis** (+ Greek *lithos,* "stone") means a condition of concrements in the kidney, and **nephrosclerosis** (+ Greek *skleros,* "hard") means a degenerative process, usually of vascular origin, that is marked by pervasive scarring or "harden-

ing" of the kidney. The surgical excision of the kidney is **nephrectomy** (+ Greek *tomē,* "a cutting").

nerve is descended from the Greek *neuron* and the Latin *nervus,* both of which have physical and metaphysical meanings. The Greek and Latin terms, in a physical sense, mean "a sinew, a tendon, a thong, a string, or a wire." But, in the metaphysical sense, the terms also mean a sort of "strength, force, or energy." Our word "nerve" is used in a dual sense, too. There is a big difference when we say, "He has nerves" (an unlikely, superfluous remark, inasmuch as we all possess these structures) and when we say, "He has nerve!" or "He is nervous." In ancient anatomy, the Greek *neuron* was used as a name for any white, cord-like structure; thus, tendons and nerves were confused (and this confusion persists in what we still call an "aponeurosis"). Aristotle and Galen were among the first to restrict *neuron* to the nerves. The Greek word gives us both our noun **neuron** and **neuro-,** a combining form that designates anything pertaining to nerves.

neutrophil combines the Latin *neuter,* "neither," + the Greek *philos,* "fondness." This hybrid term, meaning literally "fond of neither," was given by Paul Ehrlich (1854–1915), the renowned German bacteriologist, to those blood corpuscles that appeared to be attracted neither to the acidic stains (as were the oxyphils or eosinophils) nor to the basic stains (as were the basophils). The neutrophils were fancied to have a "fondness for neither." If Ehrlich had been as good a linguist as he was a cytologist, the "neutrophil" could have been called "neutramor."

nevus is a near borrowing of the Latin *naevus,* "a body mole, especially a birthmark." It has been suggested that the word is related to the Latin *nativus,* "inborn or congenital." Certain moles or blemishes, particularly the striking vascular lesions, are clearly evident at birth, and it is logical they would be so named.

nightmare is readily understood in its first part, "night," but what about "mare"? This has nothing to do with a female horse, but rather comes from the Anglo-Saxon *maere,* an imaginary demon or evil spirit said to descend on sleeping persons. More specifically, a *maere* was conceived as a male demon intent on having sexual intercourse with a sleeping woman. The Romans, too, had a word for a nightmare, and it was *incubus,* from the Latin verb *incubare,* "to lie upon." *Incubus* also came to be the name of the male demon who made the nocturnal visitation to sleeping women. A female demon of similar proclivity was known as *Succuba,* her name being taken, appropriately, from the Latin *succubare,* "to lie under."

nigra is the feminine adjectival derivative of the Latin *niger,* "black, dark, or swarthy." Thus, the "substantia nigra" is a layer of dark, pigmented substance separating the tegmentum from the cerebral peduncles in the brain. **Nigricans,** as in the skin disease known as "acanthosis nigricans," means "of a dark hue, almost black."

nihilism is derived from the Latin *nihilum,* "nothing, not a bit of," this being a combination of *ni,* "not," + *hilum,* "a trifle." The term refers to an attitude of despair, assumed by almost all doctors at one time or another when no remedy seems available. This is "therapeutic nihilism." On occasion such an approach can be of benefit to the patient when he is thus spared the possibly adverse effects of nostrums. Writing at a time when the dangerous use of nostrums prevailed, Oliver Wendell Holmes (1809–1894), the noted Boston physician and savant, put it well: "I firmly believe that if the whole materia medica, as now used, could be sunk to the bottom of the sea, it would be better for mankind—and all the worse for the fishes." Happily, we now practice our art in a more enlightened era when, for most conditions, safe and effective therapy is at hand. But even now, on occasion, a little therapeutic nihilism can serve us well.

nipple is the derived diminutive of the Anglo-Saxon *neb* or *nib,* "a beak or nose"; hence, literally, "a little beak." It is not farfetched to imagine the pigmented projection from the female breast as "a little beak." The word "nibble," meaning to peck away at, comes from the same source.

nitrogen can be traced through the French *nitre* to the Latin *nitrum,* the Greek *nitron,* and the Hebrew *nether,* all of these being related to the Latin *natron* and the Arabic *natrun.* In ancient times *nitrum* and *natron* were sometimes used interchangeably for any sort of chemical salt that was used as a cleanser. The actual chemical constituents of these salts were unknown in those days. Probably *natron* was often a crude sodium carbonate, while *nitron* was likely to have been saltpeter (potassium nitrate). It was not until the 18th century that the distinction between sodium and potassium became clear. The name "natron" was then assigned to sodium carbonate, and "nitron" to the nitrate. Meanwhile, the gas we know as nitrogen was identified as a constituent of air in 1772 by Daniel Rutherford (1749–1819), a Scottish physician, who called it "mephitic [noxious] air." To Joseph Priestley (1733–1804), the noted English clergyman, author, and chemist, the residue after removing oxygen from air was "dephlogisticated air" ("phlogiston" being a supposed substance released during combustion but now known to be nonexistent). To early French chemists, this residue was known as *azote* (from the Greek *a-*, "not," + *zoein*, "to live") because it was found not to support life. They had observed that when a mouse and a lighted candle were both placed in a sealed glass jar, and the oxygen was consumed in the flame of the candle, the candle was extinguished, and the mouse expired. From *azote* comes the medical term **azotemia,** meaning an accumulation of nitrogen in the blood. Finally, Henry Cavendish (1731–1810) found that the same gas as *azote* could be produced from *nitre* (potassium nitrate); hence, it was given the name "nitrogen," concocted from *nitro-* + the Greek *genos,* "a descendant."

node is a near borrowing of the Latin *nodus,* "a knot or a knob," this being probably related to the Sanskrit *gandh,* "to grasp" (from which "handle" descends). Surely a subcutaneous bump, be it bone, scar, or lymph gland, could be taken to feel like a knotted rope or the knot in the wood of a tree. If the bump was small, it was called by the diminutive **nodule** or "little knot."

nomenclature is taken from the Latin *nomenclator,* "a name caller," this being a combination of *nomen,* "name," + *clamare,* "to proclaim." In Roman times, a *nomenclator* (the poet Martial used a variant spelling, *nomenculator*) was a servant or slave who accompanied his master and identified those whom they met, especially during a political campaign. It is hoped this small volume can serve the reader as well by helping to identify the words encountered in the study and practice of medicine.

nondisease is a term introduced in 1965 by C. K. Meador of the University of Alabama in a delightful essay, "The Art and Science of Nondisease" (*New Eng J Med* 272:92–95, 1965). The author cited numerous circumstances wherein symptoms appeared to be present, but the disease they were thought to represent was not. Dr. Meador concluded by admonishing, "The treatment of nondisease is never the treatment indicated for the corresponding disease entity." In this statement lies the ultimate value of the science of nondisease.

normal comes from the Latin *norma,* "a carpenter's square" or, figuratively, "a rule or standard." In medicine, "normal" is defined as that which conforms to the common or established type. Whatever deviates from this standard is called **abnormal** (from the Latin *abnormis,* "irregular or unorthodox," this being a combination of the Latin *ab-,* "away from," + *norma,* "the standard"). In statistical usage, "normal" often is considered to be the average or mean, give or take two standard deviations. On a Gaussian or bell-shaped curve, this accounts for approximately 95% of presumably normal subjects. For example, this is the way the "normal" range is established for values of various blood-chemistry determinations in print-outs issuing from multichannel analyzers.

nose is a modern version of the Anglo-Saxon *nosu* and is related to the Latin *nasus,* both meaning "the nose." This term and its antecedents refer to the external, midline projection from the face. Each of its two openings is called a **nostril,** and this term, as unlikely as it may seem, is related to our common word "thrill." The Middle English *thrillen* originally meant "to pierce." To be thrilled was to be "pierced with emotion." "Nostril" used to be spelled "nosethirl" and meant, literally, "a hole pierced in the nose."

nosology is not the province of one who deals with noses; it is the proper term for the science of disease, especially its classification. The term has been contrived by combining the Greek *nosos,* "disease," + *logos,* "a study or discourse." The prefix **noso-** has come to be attached to a variety of medical terms and indicates a reference to disease. A **nosocomial** infection is one acquired in a hospital, the adjective being derived from a combination of *noso-* + the Greek *komeō,* "I take care of." The patient is said to have acquired his disease while being taken care of.

nostrum means a worthless remedy and comes directly from the Latin as the neuter form of the adjective *noster,* meaning "our own." The explanation is that a proprietary concoction whose secret formulation was closely guarded as "our own" probably has little actual efficacy. Many of the so-called patent medicines flamboyantly purveyed in years past were eventually recognized as nostrums.

noxious is a near borrowing of the Latin *noxius,* "harmful or injurious." The Indo-European root word probably was *nek,* "death," but the sense became softened a bit as the word descended to later tongues.

nucleus began as the Latin word for "a little nut or kernel," this being a diminutive of *nux, nucis,* "nut or nut tree." To the Romans, *nucleus* usually referred to the kernel or pit of a fruit, hence the hard core or central body of a mass. That there was a central spot in the blood corpuscles of fish had been noted by Antonj van Leeuwenhoek (1632–1723), the pioneer Dutch microscopist. But it was not until the early 19th century that "nucleus" appeared in English writings as a name for the "kernel" of a cell. When finer structural details became apparent, the nucleus was found to contain a still smaller body, and the term **nucleolus** was coined (there being no such ancient Latin word). Thus, in "nucleolus" we have a diminutive of a diminutive.

nullipara is contrived as a combination of the Latin *nullus,* "not at all," + *parere,* "to give birth." The term is used in obstetrics and gynecology to designate a woman who has never borne a viable child.

numbers derived from classical sources are often incorporated in medical terms. The following list of combining forms used as prefixes, including a few that pertain to relative quantity, can be helpful in identification.

English	Latin	Greek
1	uni-	mono-
2	bi-	di-
3	ter-	tri-
4	quadri-	tetra-
5	quinque-	penta-
6	sex-	hexa-
7	septi-	hepta-
8	octo-	octo-
9	novem-	ennea-
10	decem-	deka-
11	undecim-	endeka-
12	duodecem-	dodeka-
100	cent-	hecto-
1000	milli-	kilo-
half	semi-	hemi-
one and one-half times	sesqui-	
whole	omni-	holo-
equal	equi-	homo-
many	multi-	poly-
more	super-	hyper-
less	sub-	hypo-

nurse is derived from the Latin *nutrix,* "a nurse." In the plural *nutrices* this meant "the female breasts." The Latin verb *nutrire* means "to suckle or nourish an infant" but also, by extension, "to bring up or to take care of." Originally, a "nurse" was a woman hired to suckle a baby—what we would call today a "wet-nurse." Later the name was given to an attendant who cared for any sick or helpless person. The Latin term became the French *nourrice* and the Middle English *nurice.*

nutrition apparently is related to the Sanskrit *snauti,* "drips," which implies flowing or wetness. From this descended, by various paths, the Latin *nutrire,* "to suckle" (from which we get nourish, nurse, nursery, and nurture); the Anglo-Saxon *gesnott* (from which comes snoot, snooty, snot, and snotty); and the Old High German *snūzen* (later corrupted as schnozzle). To the Romans, the idea of nourishment as a means of promoting growth was expressed as *nutrimentum.* To them this meant both food and, by extension, support in general. Today, we still use "nourish" in both a literal and a figurative sense. We nourish our bodies by the assimilation of food, but we can also nourish an idea or a thought. But we restrict "nutrition" to the sense of providing food, in one form or another, by mouth or parenterally.

nyctalopia is a contrived combination of the Greek *nycto-,* "night," + *alaos,* "obscure or blind," + *opsis,* "vision." The term refers to impaired vision in dim light or at night. It is symptomatic of a deficiency of vitamin A.

nymphomania first appeared in the English medical literature about 1800 as a term for a morbid, uncontrollable sexual desire by women. It is not related to an actual Greek word but was concocted by combining the Greek *nymphē,* "a bride or maiden," + *mania,* "madness." Among the more attractive creatures of Greek mythology, the nymphs were lovely maidens who combined certain divine and human features. The

Greeks were fond of believing that there were nymphs abounding in the woods (the Dryads) and in the hills (the Oreads), cavorting about springs and streams (the Naiads), and abiding in the sea (the Nereids). Nymphs were playful and sexually seductive. In a more down-to-earth sense, a Greek *nymphē* was any marriageable maiden. Early anatomists applied the Latinized *nympha* as a term for the clitoris and, in the plural, *nymphae* to the labia minora.

nystagmus comes from the Greek *nystakēs,* "nodding or drowsy." The meaning has changed from that of a drooping of the head or eyes as a sign of sleepiness to that of a repetitive, involuntary movement of the eyeball in a horizontal, vertical, or rotatory direction. It was Johannes Purkinje (1787–1869), the Bohemian physiologist, who first associated nystagmus with vertigo. Later, nystagmus was recognized as a sign of vestibular disease by Robert Bárány (1876–1936), a Viennese otologist who was awarded the Nobel prize in 1914 for his studies on the physiology and pathology of the vestibular apparatus.

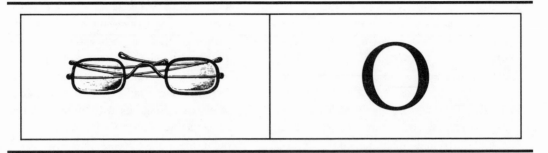

obese is from the Latin adjective *obesus,* meaning "fat, plump, swollen, or coarse." This, in turn, is the past participle of *obedere,* "to eat upon." The ancients, in their wisdom, knew that whoever was fat probably had "eaten upon" to excess.

obstetrics is a near borrowing of the Latin *obstetrix,* "a midwife." Note the feminine ending *-trix* (as in aviatrix or executrix). The term comes from the Latin *obstare* (*ob-,* "in front of," + *stare,* "to stand"). Thus, the *obstetrix* was a woman who stood in front of the mother-to-be and assisted in the delivery of the baby.

obtunded refers to a dulled mentality. It comes from the Latin verb *obtundere,* "to beat upon or to stun." Anyone who has been beaten upon, as by the ravages of disease, is likely to be mentally dull or insensible.

obturator comes from the Latin *obturare,* "to block up or to plug." The obturator of a needle or a catheter is the insertable shaft that plugs the lumen. The obturator foramen in the pelvis is the large opening in the innominate bone that is almost occluded by a tough, fibrous membrane.

occiput is a direct borrowing of the Latin term for the back of the head. The word is a combination of *ob-* (which here becomes *oc-*) + *caput,* "head." The Latin *ob-* has all sorts of prepositional meanings, among which are "in front of" but also "against" in the sense of opposite to or other than. Thus, the occiput is the side of the head opposite to the front.

occult is from the Latin *occultus,* the past participle of *occulere,* "to cover up or to hide." Occult blood, as in feces, is present but hidden from view and can be discerned only by chemical tests.

ochronosis is a sign of a rare metabolic disorder now known as "alkaptonuria" (sometimes spelled with a "c"). The disease is characterized by the deposition, mainly in cartilage, of a yellow-brown pigment (a homogentisic acid polymer). Thus, ochronosis is "the yellow disease," the name being contrived from the Greek *ōchros,* "yellow," + *nosos,* "disease." But be careful. The pigmented cartilage showing through the skin, as in the pinna of the ear, often appears blue or slate-gray. So, if you see blue, think of "the yellow disease."

ocular refers to the eye, the Latin word for which is *oculus.* It is interesting to note that we use the English noun "eye," but for an adjectival form we resort to the Latin derivative "ocular." Professor H. A. Skinner explains this by pointing out that in Old English there were few adjectives. When one was needed, the noun was used, as in "eyeball" or "eyelid." This sufficed in common usage, but scientists insisted on something more highfalutin. One could say "eyenerve," but somehow "ocular nerve" sounds better. Most "eye doctors" prefer to be called "oculists." Other examples cited by Professor Skinner of Old English nouns for which classical adjectives have been adopted are: mouth *(oral),* nose *(nasal),* mind *(mental),* moon *(lunar),* and star *(stellar).*

odontoid describes anything fancied to be in the shape of a tooth and is derived from the Greek *odous (odont-),* "tooth," + *eidos,* "like." The odontoid process is a toothlike projection from the body of the axis, the second cervical vertebra.

odyno- is a combining form taken from the Greek *odynē,* "pain." **Odynophagia** (+ Greek *phagein,* "to eat") is pain on swallowing. An **anodyne** (Greek *a[n]-,* "without") is an old word for a drug that relieves pain.

oenophile is derived from the Greek *oinos,* "wine," + *philos,* "affinity or love," and refers to a person not only fond of wine but generally regarded as a connoisseur of the grape. An oenophile does not become of professional concern to physicians unless or until he becomes an **oenomaniac,** that is, one who is overly wild about wine.

-oid is a suffix taken from the Greek *eidos,* "that which is seen, the form or shape of something, the sort or kind." It has been hooked on to numerous classical terms to form adjectives or nouns, thereby conveying either of two senses: *(a)* having the appearance of, as in **scaphoid** (like the hull of a boat); or *(b)* almost, but not quite, like, as in **carcinoid** (a tumor resembling, but not really, a carcinoma).

ointment can be traced to the Latin *ungere,* "to anoint or to apply oil." The Old French *oignement* was "an anointing" but also could designate the substance thereby applied. This was taken into Middle English as *oinement.* Later, a "t" was interposed between the syllables, either to facilitate pronunciation or to make the word sound more like "anoint." In pharmacology, an ointment, having an oleaginous base, is usually distinguished from a cream, which has a water-soluble base.

olecranon is an almost direct borrowing of the Greek *ōlekranon,* "the point of the elbow." This combines *ōlenē,* "the arm from the elbow to the wrist" (from which comes the Latin *ulna*), + *kranos,* "helmet." Apparently, someone thought that the proximal end of the larger bone in the forearm looked a little like a helmet.

oleum is the Latin word for "oil," being related to the Greek *elaion*. Originally, the Greek and Latin terms referred specifically to olive oil. Later, the term was used for any natural oil.

olfactory comes from the Latin *olfactare*, "to sniff at," this being related to the transitive verb *olfacere*, "to smell." In the Latin *olere*, "to smell of," as in the English "to smell," the verb can function as both transitive and intransitive. The combination of *olere* + *facere* (Latin, "to make") intensifies the transitive sense of the verb.

oligo- is a combining form, usually a prefix, taken from the Greek *oligos*, "few or scanty." **Oligodontia** (+ Greek *odous*, "tooth") is an insufficiency in the number of teeth owing to a developmental failure of dental eruption. **Oligodendroglia** (+ Greek *dendron*, "tree," + Greek *glia*, "glue") are ectodermal, non-neural cells that form part of the adventitial structure of the nervous system. Linear projections of the cells suggest the branches of a tree. If the cells become neoplastic, a fourth Greek component is added to form **oligodendroglioma**. **Oligohydramnios** (+ Greek *hydōr*, "water," + "*amnion*") refers to a paucity of amniotic fluid surrounding the fetus, usually taken to be less than 300 ml. **Oligomenorrhea** (+ Greek *mēn*, "month," + Greek *rhoia*, "a flowing") is abnormally infrequent or scanty menstruation. **Oliguria** (+ Greek *ouron*, "urine") is diminished formation or excretion of urine.

-oma is taken from the inseparable Greek suffix *-ōma*, which, as explained by Professor H. A. Skinner, was used in the back formation of nouns from verbs. An example of the Greek sequence would be *adēn*, "a gland"; *adenoō*, "I form a gland"; *adenōma*, "a gland formation." In its early medical application, "-oma" could refer to any swelling or tumor. Later it became restricted to neoplasms.

omentum is the Latin word that Celsus used for the fatty caul or cap that covers most of the abdominal viscera. The origin of the term is obscure. Some authors relate it to the Latin *operimentum*, "a lid or cover," assuming "omentum" to be a contraction thereof.

omphalos is the Greek word for "the navel." In a figurative sense, *omphalos* meant "the center of anything." Thus, the word referred to the boss or decorative knob at the center of a warrior's shield or to the knob in the middle of a yoke. In medicine, the word is not used alone but only as a combining form, as in **omphalocele** (+ Greek *kēlē*, "tumor or hernia"), a protrusion of the intestine, enclosed in a thin-walled sac, through a defect in the umbilicus.

onanism refers to the practice of "coitus interruptus" (wherein the penis is withdrawn from the vagina before ejaculation) and also to masturbation. The term immortalizes the name of a man whose fate is told in the Old Testament, Genesis 38:7–10, as follows:

And Er, Judah's firstborn, was wicked in the sight of the Lord; and the Lord slew him. And Judah said unto Onan, Go in unto thy brother's wife and marry her, and raise up seed to thy brother. And Onan knew that the seed should not be his; and it came to pass, when he went in unto his brother's wife, that he spilled it [his semen] on the ground, lest that he should give seed to his brother. And the thing which he did displeased the Lord; wherefore he slew him also.

oncology is derived from the Greek *o[n]gkos,* "a bulk or mass" and, later, "a tumor." By custom, the Greek "g" (gamma), when preceding "k" (kappa), becomes "n" as a word moves from the classical to a modern vocabulary. Also, the Greek "k" becomes the English "c." Hence, the scientific combining form is **onco-.** An **oncologist** is one who specializes in the science of tumors, specifically neoplasia.

ontogeny refers to the sequential development of an individual organism. The word is a combination of the Greek *on* (genitive *ontos*), "that which actually exists, a being," + *genos,* "descent," in the sense of origin. This is in contrast to **phylogeny,** the development of a whole kind or type of organisms. The Greek *phylon* means "a race, stock, or tribe."

oö- is a combining form taken from the Greek *ōon,* "egg," and denotes a relationship to an ovum. The diaeresis (¨) placed over the second "o" indicates it is to be pronounced distinctly from the first "o" and that "oö" is not a diphthong. An **oöcyst** (+ Greek *kystis,* "bladder") is the encapsulated fertilized form of the malaria parasite in the stomach of a mosquito, just waiting for its chance to infect a man. **Oöphoro-** is a combining form contrived by putting together the Greek *ōon,* "egg," + *phora,* "a bearing or producing," and thus is an apt reference

to the ovary. **Oöphoritis** is an inflammation in the ovary, and **oöphorectomy** (+ Greek *tomē,* "a cutting") is the surgical removal of the ovary.

operculum is a direct borrowing of the Latin word for "a lid or cover." In anatomy various structures are called "opercula" because they cover something. For example, the dental operculum is the hood of gingival tissue overlying the crown of an erupting tooth.

ophthalmo- is a combining form taken from the Greek *ophthalmos,* "the eye." A common error in spelling is to omit the first "h." To avoid this lapse it helps to remember that the "-phth-" represents the Greek letters Φ and Θ (phi and theta). **Ophthalmia** can refer to any disease of the eye, but usually it is restricted to an inflammatory condition ("ophthalmitis" is seldom used by ophthalmologists). The suffix *-ia* was used by ancient medical writers to denote any morbid condition of a structure. Another example is "pneumonia."

opisthotonus is a posture of recumbent, rigid hyperextension wherein the head and legs are bent backward and the trunk is bowed forward. This is the position of tetanic muscular spasm observed in severe meningitis and in tetanus. Obviously, all muscles are spastic, but the stronger extensors predominate over the flexors. The term combines the Greek *opisthe,* "backward," + *tonos,* "stretching."

opium originated in the Greek *opos,* "the juice, sap, resin, or gum of trees or plants." Opium, the juice of the poppy plant, was known to the ancients as a drug. Homer

171

described it as "the healing draught that drowns all pain and sorrow."

opsonin is an antibody which renders bacteria or other cells particularly susceptible to phagocytosis. The term was proposed in 1903 by Sir Almroth Wright (1861–1947), an eminent English pathologist, who cleverly took it from the Greek *opsōnion,* "victuals." The Greek *opsōnein* means "to buy provisions." Thus, Sir Almroth fancied that opsonin rendered bacteria available to satisfy hungry phagocytes.

optic is derived from the Greek *optikos,* "pertaining to sight," which originated in *opsis,* "a sight, view, or vision." An optometrist (+ Greek *metron,* "a rule or measure") is one who measures eyesight (and usually purveys a corrective lens).

orbit comes from the Latin *orbita,* "the track or rut made by a wheel." The Latin *orbis* could be applied to almost anything circular, including a wheel. In the Middle Ages *orbita* came to be used as a name for the eye socket. **Orbicularis** is a diminutive of *orbis,* hence "a small disk." This name applies to the flat muscles (not sphincters) that surround certain apertures, such as the mouth or eye.

orchid is recognized by everyone as a highly prized and much admired flower, but its name means "like a testicle" and comes from the Greek *orchis,* "testicle." Pliny the Elder, the Roman author and naturalist, pointed out 2,000 years ago that the bulbous double roots of the plant resemble the testicles. We do not call testicles "orchids," but we use **"orchi-"** as a combining form in "orchitis" and "orchidectomy."

organ is a derivative of the Greek *organon* and the Latin *organum,* both meaning "an instrument or an implement." The Greek word was derived from *ergein,* "to do work." In biology, the etymologic sense of "organ," then, is of function rather than structure. The concept is not of what an organ is but of what it does.

orgasm comes from the Greek *orgainein,* "to swell," which, in the case of fruit, means to swell until it ripens, or, in the case of animals, to swell with lust or to be at heat. In English the word was first used to describe any turgid fit of anger or passion. Later it was applied specifically to the climax of coitus.

ornithosis is a viral disease of birds that is transmissible to man. The origin of the term is in the Greek *ornis,* "a bird." If a parrot transmits the disease, it is **psittacosis,** from the Greek *psittakos,* "a parrot."

orphan is derived from the Greek *orphanos,* "the state of being left without parents" and, by extension, "bereft or destitute." "Orphan diseases" are those bereft of needed attention by researchers, not for lack of interest but because such diseases are so rare that funding agencies, particularly those of government, decline to provide the support required for research. Drugs that are postulated or proved to be effective in the treatment of these rare diseases are called "orphan drugs," because pharmaceutical manufacturers are, in some cases, loath to produce medications on which there will be only a negligible commercial return.

ortho- is a combining form originating in the Greek *orthos,* "straight or erect." *Orthop-*

noia (+ Greek *pnoia,* "breath"), usually spelled in American English as **orthopnea,** was used by Hippocrates to describe the plight of patients who could breathe easily only when in an upright posture. **Orthodontics** (+ Greek *odous,* "tooth") is the practice of straightening misaligned teeth. **Orthopaedics** (+ Greek *paes* or *pais,* "child") is, literally, the practice of "child straightening." Now, by spelling this term with "ae" rather than with just "e," a bag of worms has burst. Some people might look upon "orthopaedics" as archaic pedantry, but it is not. To spell it "orthopedics" would relate the term to the Latin *pes, pedis,* "foot." This is incorrect on two counts: *(a)* the practice was never intended to be restricted to "foot straightening"; and *(b)* to link the Greek *ortho-* and the Latin *pedis* would create a mongrel word. Those who might still want to argue are referred to an exhaustive discussion in the journal *Medical Communications* 9:93–99, 1981.

os is the Latin word for both "mouth" and "bone." The Latin genitive *oris* means "of or pertaining to the mouth," and from this we have "oral." In anatomy, the classical noun is occasionally used, as in "the cervical os," meaning the mouth of the uterine cervix. The Latin *os,* meaning "bone," is related to the Greek *osteon,* and it is the Greek that provides the combining form **osteo-** in terms such as osteitis, osteoblast, osteoclast, and osteomyelitis. **Osteomalacia** (+ Greek *malakia,* "softness," especially in the sense of weakness consequent to depletion) is a degenerative softening or weakening of bones, particularly that due to depletion of calcium. **Osteopathy** (+ Greek *pathos,* "suffering or disease") could mean any disease of bones, but it doesn't. It is now usually taken to be the name of a system of therapy founded in 1874 by Andrew Still (1828–1917), an American medical practitioner. It is based on the supposition that most diseases are caused by a bony deformation and can be cured by manipulation of the skeletal structure.

-osis is a suffix of Greek origin that denotes "a condition of," as in "nephrosis" (thus providing a distinction from inflammation, as in "nephritis"), and also "an increase in," as in "leukocytosis." It is comparable to the Latin *-osus,* "abounding in or having the quality of," from which is derived the English suffix "-ous," as in "cancerous" or "poisonous."

osmosis is derived from the Greek *ōsmos,* "a push or impulse," this being related to *ōtheō,* "I thrust, push, or shove." Osmosis is the passage (or "shoving", if you will) of a solvent through a semipermeable membrane from a solution of a lesser to a greater concentration. The term was introduced in 1854 by Thomas Graham (1805–1869), an English chemist.

oto- is a combining form taken from the Greek *ōtos,* genitive of *ous,* "the ear." An example of its use is **otosclerosis** (+ Greek *sklēros,* "hard or tough"), an abnormal formation of new bone around the oval window of the ear, immobilizing the stapes and resulting in a progressive loss of auditory acuity.

ovary is a near borrowing of the Late Latin *ovarium,* meaning "a receptacle of eggs." Ancient writers did not use this term but rather referred to "the female testis or gonad." The term "ovary" became generally adopted after the writings, in 1672, of Reijnier de Graaf (1641–1673), the Dutch anatomist. The Greek *ōon,* "an egg" (which became the Latin *ovum*), led to *oophoros* (+ Greek *pherein,* "to carry"), literally "an egg bearer." Classically, this term referred, in general, to animals that bear eggs. From *oophoros* was derived the combining form **oöphor-,** since used specifically to refer to the ovary and incorporated in such terms as oöphoritis and oöphorectomy.

oxygen is a word introduced as a result of the seminal discoveries by Antoine Laurent Lavoisier (1743–1794), the celebrated French chemist. Curiously, the word signifies a mistaken concept in that it was contrived from a combination of the Greek *oxys,* "sharp, as an acid," + *gennaō,* "I produce." Originally it was thought that the newly discovered "vital air" conferred the property of an acid when it was combined with another radical and, thus, was an "acid producer." It was not until sixty years later,

in 1837, that Justus von Liebig (1803–1873), the renowned German chemist, showed that the essential component of acids was actually hydrogen (which, if anything, more aptly deserves the name of "acid producer"). **Oxyntic** comes from the Greek *oxynō,* "I make sour," and was applied, in the 1880s, by an English physiologist, John Langley (1852–1925), to the acid-producing (or parietal) cells of the gastric mucosa. **Oxalic** is a chemical designation that has nothing to do with oxygen but comes from the Greek *oxalis,* "the sorrel plant," from whose succulent leaves a sour or acid juice was obtained.

oxytocic was contrived by a combination of the Greek *oxys,* "sharp or quick," + *tokos,* "a bringing forth, a birth, a time of delivery." Hence, an oxytocic is any agent that hastens childbirth.

oxyuriasis is a fancy name for pinworm infection. The pinworm, *Enterobius vermicularis,* is a member of the family Oxyuridae, so called from the Greek *oxys,* "sharp or pointed," + *oura,* "tail."

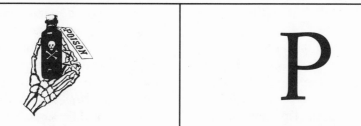

P

pagophagia is a perverted craving for the eating of ice. The term incorporates the Greek *pagos,* "anything stiffened or hardened, such as frozen water," + *phagein,* "to eat." Pagophagia is a form of pica and is symptomatic of iron deficiency.

pain comes through the French *peine* from the Latin *poena,* "a penalty or punishment." Sadly, the origin of "pain" reflects the old belief that suffering was divinely decreed as penance for sinful acts. This idea still lurks in the minds of some benighted patients who bewail their fate by asking, "What have I done to deserve this?"

palate is the name of the arched partition that separates the oral and nasal cavities. The term is derived from the Latin *palatum,* which means the same thing but was extended, figuratively, to "taste" in the sense of discrimination, as in what is palatable and what is unpalatable. Scholars debate the origin of the Latin term for the roof of the mouth, but probably it is related to the Latin *pala,* "a shovel or spade," in part because of its shape and in part because it helps convey food into the gullet.

palindromic is used in medicine to describe a recurring disease or symptom, particularly one marked by complete remissions. The word is a near borrowing of the Greek *palindromos,* "a running back again." Palindromic rheumatism is a recurring polyarthritis that results in no permanent joint deformity or functional impairment. More intriguing are the palindromes that are words, phrases, or sentences that read the same backward as forward. Among the best known (and, one might guess, probably the first) is "Madam, I'm Adam," said to be Adam's manner of introducing himself to Eve. Another is "Dennis sinned." The award for the perfect palindrome goes to the

San Diego Zoological Society for the title of its journal, *ZOONOOZ.* It reads the same upside down, too.

palliate is derived from the Latin *pallium,* "a coverlet or cloak." More specifically, this was a garb worn by scholars in ancient times. It consisted of a rectangular woolen cloak draped over the left shoulder, thus partly covering the body. When we palliate a disease, we do not provide a complete remedy or cure but rather treat it partially and insofar as possible, so that its manifestations are not fully evident.

pallid is a near borrowing of the Latin *pallidus,* "pale or sallow," said to be related to the Greek *polios,* "gray-white, particularly of the hair as a sign of aging." The globus pallidus is a pale, gray portion of the corpus striatum in the brain. Persons who become anemic also become pallid or pale because the normally rich red blood coursing in the capillaries no longer shows through the skin. To be appalled by some shocking circumstance means to grow pale. The shock stimulates a reaction in the sympathetic nervous system that entails constriction of the cutaneous arterioles.

palpate comes from the Latin *palpare,* "to stroke or to pat." The sense of the Latin word is to touch or feel lightly, and this is precisely the manner in which palpation, as a part of the physical examination of a patient, should be undertaken. The related Latin intransitive verb *palpitare* means "to throb or to quiver," and from this come **palpitation,** a consciousness by the patient of his own heart throbbing, and **palpebral,**

meaning whatever refers to the eyelid, a structure given to quivering.

palsy is an old, almost archaic term for **paralysis.** Indeed, it is an Anglicized contraction of the French *paralysie.* For some reason, its use persists in the designation "Bell's palsy," a peripheral facial paralysis caused by a lesion of the seventh cranial nerve. The eponym is owed to Sir Charles Bell (1774–1842), a Scottish anatomist and neurologist who described the condition in 1830.

pan- is a prefix taken from the Greek *pan,* this being the neuter form of *pas,* "all, the whole of." A **panangiitis** (+ Greek *a*[*n*]*ggeion,* "a vessel") is an inflammation affecting all coats of a blood vessel; more specifically, a **panarteritis** (+ Greek *artēria,* "a conduit") indicates inflammation involving all coats of an artery. In these designations, it is important to point out that "pan-" refers to the whole of the individual vessel involved and not to all the vessels throughout the body. A **panhysterectomy** (+ Greek *hystera,* "the uterus," + *tomē,* "a cutting") is extirpation of the whole uterus, including its cervix.

panacea comes from Panaceia, the name of one of the daughters of Asklēpios, the Greek god of healing. Another daughter was Hygieia. Both daughters followed their father's calling, but their paths took different turns. Panaceia became the patroness of clinical medicine or what today we might call "critical-care medicine." She advocated the use of specific remedies as indicated by the occurrence of particular needs. Hygieia was concerned rather with preserving health or what might be called "preventive medicine." As it turned out, the goddesses competed more often than they cooperated. "Panacea" is taken to mean "a universal remedy," of which no example exists in modern medicine. To the ancient Greeks, *panakeia* (a combination of *pan-*, "all," + *akos,* "remedy") was an "all-healing" herb.

pancreas is a near borrowing of the Greek *pa[n]gkreas.* Remember that the Greeks pronounced their letter "g" (gamma) as "n" in "ng" when it preceded palatals. The term is a combination of *pan,* "all," + *kreas,* "flesh," and was used by Herophilus to describe the "all meaty" structure of the gland. The pancreas is, indeed, a thoroughly fleshy gland, though of rather firm consistency.

panniculus is the diminutive of the Latin *pannus,* "a patch of cloth or a rag." Originally, in anatomy, "panniculus" was applied to a variety of membranes. Currently, its use is usually restricted to the layer of fatty subcutaneous tissue. When we refer to an obese person as having a "heavy panniculus" we mean that he is well padded. To use "heavy" in the same breath as a diminutive of a term seems odd, but oddities abound in medical parlance.

pannus is a direct borrowing of the Latin word for "a piece of cloth." In pathology, "pannus" has come to mean either *(a)* a superficial vascularization of the cornea accompanied by a granulomatous infiltrate; or *(b)* an inflammatory exudate overlying the synovial membrane of a joint. In both instances, the allusion is to a piece of cloth covering the affected structure.

papaverine is an alkaloid having the property of relaxing smooth muscle generally. Although originally (in 1848) isolated from opium, it possesses none of the analgesic or soporific properties of other opioid alkaloids. Its name indicates that it is a derivative of the poppy plant *Papaver somniferum. Papaver* is the Latin name for the poppy plant.

papilla is the Latin word for "nipple or teat," being related to the Latin verb *pappare,* "to eat pap [baby food] in the manner of an infant." In early treatises on anatomy, "papilla" was restricted to designate the nipple of the breast, but later the term was applied to various structures fancied to have a nipple-like appearance. Thus, among others, were so called the small projections on the surface of the tongue that bear taste buds, the projections of the renal medulla into the pelvis of the kidney, and the mucosal projections from the luminal surface of the duodenum that serve as exits for the biliary and pancreatic ducts.

papule is a near borrowing of the Latin *papula,* "a pimple." Dermatologists use "papule" to designate any small, circumscribed, solid elevation on the skin surface, as distinct from a vesicle, which contains a fluid substance, and a macule, which is flat and even with the skin surface. **Pimple** seems to have descended, as a diminutive and by a devious route, from the Greek *pomphos,* "a bubble or a blister."

para- is a combining form, usually a prefix, taken from the Greek preposition *para,* "along the side of, in comparison with, or during." The list of Greek words and their derivatives to which "para-" has become affixed is almost endless. Mention has been made of how Paracelsus took his name (see **laudanum**). **Paracentesis** (+ Greek *kentēsis*, "puncture") is the tapping of a body cavity, usually the abdomen, to relieve an abnormal accumulation of fluid. **Paralysis** (+ Greek *lysis*, "a loosening") originated as the Greek word *paralytikos*, meaning, literally, one whose side was lax, this being the typical condition of a person afflicted with apoplexy. Later, "paralysis" was extended to designate a loss of motor function in any part. **Paraplegia**, as the Greek *paraplēgia* (+ *plēgē*, "a stroke"), also originally meant "a stroke on one side," but the medical meaning has now shifted to designate a paralysis of both legs and the lower portion of the body consequent to a lesion of the spinal cord. **Paranoia** is a direct borrowing of the Greek word for "madness or mental derangement," the Greek *noein* meaning "to think." Probably the idea is akin to the figurative sense of one beset or "beside himself." A **parasite** (+ Greek *sitos*, "food") is an organism that feeds along with its host. The original Greek *parasitos* meant "eating at the table of another," but later the sense changed to that of a poor friend or relation who boarded at the expense of another. "Parasite" was introduced into English as a biologic term in the early 18th century. **Parenchyma** (+ Greek *encheō*, "I pour in") refers to the essential, functional elements contained within an organ, as distinct from its capsule or supporting structures. Incidentally, the "y" in "parenchyma" is always

pronounced as a short "ĭ," not as "eye." **Paregoric,** when prepared according to the specifications of the *United States Pharmacopoeia,* is a tincture of opium (equivalent to 0.04% anhydrous morphine) in which there is also benzoic acid, camphor, and anise oil. Though now paregoric is administered usually to suppress diarrhea, formerly its principal use was as a sedative and analgesic agent. The name comes from the Greek *parēgorikos,* "soothing." This, in turn, is derived from the verb *parēgoreō,* meaning "I address in a consoling or soothing manner." In *parēgoreō* we see the prefix *para-* together with a derivative of *agora,* "a place of assembly for commercial or political purposes." Such a place could be a scene of raucous confusion, and anyone who could temper the tumult by a soothing speech would be highly regarded. Hence, paregoric, as a drug, was seen to address a paroxysm of pain in a soothing manner. And it can quell the uproarious bowel, too. **Parotid** (+ Greek *ōtos,* "the ear") is the large salivary gland situated beside (actually in front of) the ear. A **paroxysm** is a sudden recurrence or exacerbation of a symptom. The term combines *para-,* in the sense of "during," + Greek *oxus,* "sharp or acute." Thus, one can have a cough or a fever, but a paroxysm is an acute, recurring attack of that symptom.

paresis is a direct borrowing of the Greek word for "a slackening" or, by extension, "a loss of strength." In modern medicine, the term is used in two ways: *(a)* as another name for dementia paralytica, the chronic and inexorable condition due to degeneration of the central nervous system consequent to syphilis; and *(b)* for a partial loss of motor function in a part, short of total paralysis. The latter is the more frequent use.

parietal is a derivative of the Latin *parietalis,* "belonging to a wall," this being related to *paries,* "a wall that encircles" or "goes around." Ancient writers used *parietalis* to designate the wall of a body cavity. Thus, the parietal peritoneum lines the wall of the abdominal cavity, while the visceral peritoneum covers the abdominal organs.

parturition is another word for the process of giving birth to a baby. It comes from the Latin *parturire,* "to be ready to bear young." The Latin *partus* is the past participle of *parere,* "to produce."

Pascal's wager has been cited to support the position of a doctor who knowingly (or unknowingly) invokes a "hanging-of-the-crepe" strategy when dealing with the plight of a critically ill patient. By this strategy, the doctor intimates—or, in effect, wagers—that the patient is sure to die. If, then, the patient dies, the doctor is credited with an accurate prediction. If the patient is treated and miraculously survives, the doctor appears to have wrought a seemingly impossible victory over insurmountable odds. By "hanging the crepe," the doctor may feel he has set up an "all gain, no loss" condition. But has he? Blaise Pascal (1623–1662), the French philosopher of nature and religion, thought he had achieved a similar condition when he stated: "Let us weigh the gain and loss in wagering that God is. Let us estimate the two chances. If you gain, you gain all; if you lose, you lose nothing. Wager, then,

without hesitation that He is." But, for a number of reasons explored in a perceptive essay by Dr. Mark Siegler (*New Eng J Med* 293:853, 1975), neither Pascal's wager nor the "hanging-of-the-crepe" strategy is unassailable.

patella is the Latin word for "a small pan, dish, or plate," this being related to the verb *patere,* "to stand open or to be accessible to." The small bone in the front of the knee came to be called the patella, though its shape is hardly suggestive of a saucer. "Kneecap" seems a better name.

patho-, -pathy are combining forms taken from the Greek *pathos,* "suffering or disease." **Pathogenesis** (+ Greek *gennaō,* "I bring forth") refers to the manner in which a diseased state or lesion evolves; it may include, but is not limited to, a consideration of initial cause. **Pathology** (+ Greek *logos,* "a treatise") is properly a discourse or study of disease. Commonly, "pathology" is deplorably used by medical speakers and writers as a pseudo-esoteric synonym for a given disease or a lesion itself. To say, "There's no 'pathology' there" (when what one means is that no lesion exists) is ridiculous unless, of course, one is referring to a school of medicine whose curriculum does not include a study of disease. **Pathognomonic** is a near borrowing of the Greek *pathognōmonikos,* "skilled in judging diseases." The Greek *gnōmōn* designated both "one who knows" and "the indicator pin on a sundial." A pathognomonic symptom or sign is one so characteristic that it clearly indicates, not merely suggests, a given disease.

patient is derived from the Latin verb *patior,* which means "to suffer," both in the sense of feeling pain and of forbearance. Therefore, the two English uses of "patient"—one as a noun, a person who suffers, and the other as an adjective, to bear with fortitude —are of common origin. The identity of the adjective and the noun can lead to awkward, if not impossible, constructions: persons who suffer may lack forbearance, but to call them "impatient patients" sounds odd, if not nonsensical.

pectinate is derived from the Latin *pecten* or the Greek *pektēn,* both meaning "a comb." The Indo-European root *pek* meant "to pluck wool or hair." The pectinate line is the sinuous border marking the junction at the anus between the squamous epithelium of skin and the columnar epithelium of the rectum. It vaguely resembles the teeth of a comb. Pectinate is not to be confused with "pectin" (from the Greek *pēktos,* "congealed or curdled"), a carbohydrate substance used to produce a gel.

pectoral refers to the anterior chest and comes from the Latus *pectus,* "the breast." One can reflect on the Greek *pēktis,* an ancient sort of harp, and on *pēkte,* a cage to catch birds, and conjure up an allusion to the appearance of the bony thorax. **Pectoriloquy** (+ Latin *loqui,* "to speak") is a term invented by René Théophile Hyacinthe Laënnec (1781–1826), who also invented the stethoscope, to describe the sound of the patient's voice as transmitted by cavities in the lung, as detected by auscultation.

pediatrics used to be spelled (and is still so spelled by the British) "paediatrics," which, though it looks stilted that way, serves to remind us that the prefix of "pediatrics" comes from the Greek *pais, paidos,* "a child," and not from the Latin *pes, pedis,* "a foot," or from the Latin *pedis,* "a louse." The "-iatrics" is of Greek derivation and means "treatment of disease." **Pederasty,** meaning a perverted sexual relationship with children, especially with young boys, comes from *pais* + the Greek *erastēs,* "a lover."

pedicle is taken from the Latin *pediculus,* the diminutive of *pes, pedis,* hence "a little foot." Pediculus was adopted in the 16th century as a name for the footstalk of a fruit or flower and, soon after, as a term for the point of attachment for various organs of the body, e.g., the pedicle of the kidney. In Late Latin, *peduncle* was contrived as a variant of *pediculus,* mainly because the latter term also was used as a name for the louse (because of its many little legs). Incidentally, **pedigree** is an English way of pronouncing and spelling the French *pied de grue,* literally, "the foot of a crane." Apparently the graphic tracing of a family lineage reminded someone of the imprint of a crane's foot.

pellagra is a disease characterized by "the four D's": dermatitis, diarrhea, dementia, and death. The Italians were impressed mainly by the cutaneous and nervous manifestations of the disease, and the name "pellagra" was proposed by Francesco Frapolli in 1771, apparently combining the Latin *pellis,* "skin or hide," + the Greek *agra,* "a seizing." Frapolli also was probably aware of another term, *pellarella,* perhaps used for a similar condition, that had appeared in the register of the Milan hospital as early as the 16th century. The solution to the ancient mystery of the cause of pellagra is a fascinating story (see *Hospital Practice,* March 1978, pp. 136–164). Its protagonist is a U.S. Public Health Service doctor, Joseph Goldberger (1874–1929), who found, by his determined research in the early 1900s, that the disease resulted from a lack of dietary niacin and could be cured by assuring an adequate intake of that vitamin.

pellucidum combines the equivalent of the Latin *per-,* "through," + *lucere,* "to shine." The septum pellucidum is the translucent membrane that separates the anterior horns of the lateral ventricles of the brain.

pelvis is the Latin word for "a basin or bucket," and is related to the Greek *pyelos,* "a tub or trough." Thus, "pelvis" aptly describes the basin-like structure at the bottom of the torso that is bounded by the pubis anteriorly, the hip bones laterally, and the sacrum posteriorly. The pelvis of the kidney is really the funnel-shaped expansion of the uppermost ureter and is more accurately an "infundibulum." But to save syllables, everyone calls it a "pelvis."

pemphigus is a generic term for a group of severe, sometimes fatal, skin diseases characterized by crops of blisters that, after they subside, leave pigmented spots in the skin. The term is taken from the Greek *pemphix,* "a blister." **Pemphigoid** (+ Greek *eidos,* "like") is the name given to a vesicular eruption in the skin that looks like pemphigus but is clearly distinguished as being relatively benign.

-penia is a neo-Latin combining form taken from the Greek *penēs,* "poverty stricken." The word "penury," meaning a state of utter destitution, comes from the same source. In pathology, "-penia" refers to a lack or deficiency of something. **Leukopenia** is a deficiency of white blood cells, **neutropenia** being specifically a deficiency of neutrophils and **lymphopenia** specifically a deficiency of lymphocytes (not of lymph). **Osteopenia** is a deficiency in bony substance that can include both **osteoporosis** (an impaired maintenance of the bony matrix) and **osteomalacia** (a demineralization of bone).

penicillin immediately suggests the name of an antibiotic agent, but there was a *penicillium* long before the celebrated discovery in 1928 by Alexander Fleming (1881–1955), an English bacteriologist, that staphylococci failed to grow in a culture medium contaminated by the fungus *Penicillium notatum.* The name is taken from the Latin *penicillum,* "a painter's brush," to which the fronds of the fungus bear a resemblance.

penis originally in Latin meant "a tail." The Romans showed a proclivity, apparently common through the ages, for having numerous names for the male reproductive organ. Among these, in addition to *penis,* Professor H. A. Skinner lists *clava* ("club"), *gladius* ("sword"), *radix* ("root"), *ramus* ("branch"), and *vomer* ("plow"). "Penis" became so closely associated with the male organ that the Romans enlisted *cauda* for an actual tail. The Latin *penis* is related to the verb *pendere,* "to hang down."

pep is a sprightly little word for "spirited animation and vigor" (a quality many patients complain they lack). It is actually a contraction of "pepper." The allusion to the pungent spice is obvious. "Pepper" is a name of ancient lineage and, with minor changes in spelling, goes back to Sanskrit. Common pepper is made from the berries of the plant *Piper nigrum,* which probably was known to the earliest people who inhabited the globe.

pepsin comes from the Greek *pepsis,* "a cooking," this being related to the Greek verbs *peptō* and *pessō,* "I soften, ripen, cook, or digest." Pepsin is a proteolytic enzyme, and one might think the term should end in "-ase." It should, and the correct name is "protease." But pepsin was named before the suffix denoting enzymes became customary. The "-in" at the end means simply that pepsin has something to do with digestion.

per- is a combining form taken from the Latin preposition *per,* "through, throughout, or by means of," also used as an intensive. **Percussion** (Latin *percutere,* "to strike," from *per* + *quatere,* "to cause to vibrate") is a method of physical examination whereby a resonant part, usually the chest, is tapped so as to elicit a sound that varies according to the underlying consistency. The diagnostic implications of percussion were first recognized about 1754 by Leopold Auenbrugger (1722–1809), chief physician at the Hospital of the Holy Trinity, in Vienna, and published by him in 1761. But not until the publications in French by Jean Nicolas Corvisart (1808) and René Laënnec (1816) did the method become widely applied. **Perforate** (+ Latin *forare,* "to bore") is the making of a hole into or through something.

Perlèche is a French word combining *per-,* in the sense of excessive, + *lecher,* "to lick." In French, the connotation is one of "over-polishing." The term describes a thickening and cracking of the lips, particularly at the corners of the mouth, consequent to drooling and excessive licking of the lips. The condition is similar to **cheilosis** (Greek *cheilos,* "lip"). "Perlèche" has been applied specifically to the result of frequent licking of the lips as a symptom of oral moniliasis in children. **Pernicious** is an almost direct borrowing of the Latin *perniciosus,* "ruinous," derived in turn from the noun *pernicies,* "death-dealing disaster or calamity" and also "a pestilence or curse." The Latin word combines *per-* + *nex, necis,* "death." In lay language, "pernicious" has been softened to "hurtful." But in medicine, before a remedy was found in liver extract and later in vitamin B-12, "pernicious anemia" was a fatal disease. **Pertussis** is a term wherein the *per-* indicates intensity and is coupled with the Latin *tussis,* "a cough"; hence "a violent cough." "Pertussis" was introduced into English by Thomas Sydenham (1624–1689), the celebrated English physician, and thereafter became identified with the disease of children commonly known as whooping cough, the "whoop" describing the strident cough typical of the disease.

peri- is a prefix meaning "around or about" and is a direct borrowing of the Greek preposition of the same meaning, equivalent to the Latin *circum.* "Peri-" has been attached to numerous words to make up a host of medical terms. **Pericardium** (+ Greek *kardia,* "heart") is the membrane forming the sac that surrounds the heart. **Periosteum** (+ Greek *osteon,* "bone") is the tough fibrous covering of a bone. **Peristalsis** (+ Greek *stalsis,* from *stellein,* "to set up, bring together, or contract") is literally "a contracting around," as in the muscular activity of the intestine. **Peritoneum** (+ Greek *tonos,* "a stretching") is the membrane that is stretched around the abdominal viscera and the inner surface of the cavity containing them. It is essential to distinguish between "peri-" and "para-," the latter being the Greek for "beside." Thus, there is a significant difference between *peri*umbilical, "around the umbilicus," and *para*umbilical, "beside the umbilicus," when, for example, referring to the site of abdominal pain. Also, there is an important difference between *peri*neal and *pero*neal. **Perineum,** a near borrowing of the Greek *perinaion,* refers to the area between the anus and the scrotum or vulva. The first part of the Greek word is clearly *peri-,* but the origin of the last part is obscure. It may have been the Greek *naios,* "a dwelling," or *neos,* "new," or the word may be related to *perineō,* "I pile around," but none of these seems wholly satisfactory.

peroneal refers to the fibula or to the anterior, lateral aspect of the lower part of the leg, and to the muscles, blood vessels, and nerves serving that region. The adjective comes from the Greek *peronē,* meaning "anything pointed for piercing," especially the tongue of a buckle or brooch. This refers to the shape of the *fibula,* which is the Latin word for "clasp or pin."

pes is the Latin word for "foot." It is incorporated in pes anserinus (Latin *anser,* "goose"), the parotid branches of the facial (seventh cranial) nerve, said to resemble a goose's webbed foot. Pes planus (Latin *planus,* "flat") is literally "flat foot," while pes cavus (Latin *cavus,* "hollow or vaulted") is a foot with an abnormally high arch.

pessary comes through the Latin *pessarium* from the Greek *pessos,* the name given to an oval stone used by the Greeks in playing a game similar to our checkers. The same term was used for a round plug of lint that the Greeks used as a sort of vaginal tampon. According to Professor H. A. Skinner, Hippocrates advised the insertion of half a pomegranate in the treatment of prolapsed uterus. The prototype of the ring-shaped pessary used in more modern times was devised by Rodericus à Castro (1546–1627), a Portuguese physician who practiced in Hamburg, Germany.

pestle is a small, club-shaped instrument, now almost obsolete, once used in pharmacies to convert friable solids into powders. The term is derived from the Latin *pistillum,* "a pounder," this being related to the Latin verb *pinsere,* "to pound." The pounding was done in a dish called a "mortar," also the name of the mixture of calcined clay and crushed limestone used as an adhesive between stones or bricks in building. More often, mortar was mixed on a flat palette. The traditional academic headdress that American students don only at graduation ceremonies resembles such a palette and is called a "mortarboard."

petechia is a near borrowing of the Italian *petechio,* "a fleabite." The minute, flat, red spots that indicate focal bleeding in the skin are seen in various blood and vascular disorders. They resemble the punctate bites of fleas.

petit mal is a French term meaning, literally, "a little illness." The term is used in medicine to designate a minor form of epilepsy, typically occurring in young children and characterized by sudden, brief lapses in consciousness. In contrast, **grand mal** designates the major tonic and clonic seizures of epilepsy.

petrous is an adjective derived from the Latin *petra,* "rock." The petrous portion of the temporal bone, wedged in at the base of the skull between the sphenoid and occipital bones, is composed of an unusually dense form of bone. The petrosal nerves and the petrous ganglion are so named because they are situated in or near the petrous portion of the temporal bone.

pH is the symbol signifying the logarithm of the reciprocal of the hydrogen ion concentration of a given solution in gram atoms per liter. The pH of various body fluids, such as blood, is a critical factor in determining health or disease. The "p" can be thought of as standing either for "potential," i.e., the hydrogen potential, or for "para," in the sense of "another expression for"; the "H," of course, stands for "hydrogen."

phage is a sort of nickname for **bacteriophage,** a group of viruses that infect bacteria and cause their dissolution. The term "bacteriophage" was concocted from the Greek *phagein,* "to devour." A **phagedenic** ulcer is one which spreads rapidly, seeming to devour all surrounding tissue.

phagocytosis is the process whereby certain scavenger cells of the body ingest and destroy dead or foreign material such as bacteria. The concept and its name were introduced in 1884 by Elie Metchnikoff (1845–1916), the celebrated Russian pathologist. The term was contrived by combining the Greek *phagein,* "to eat," + *kytos,* "cell."

phalanges is the plural of the Greek *phala[n]gx,* the name given by Aristotle to the bones of the fingers (later extended to the bones of the toes) because they are arranged in ranks and rows suggesting the military formation favored by Greek warriors in battle.

phallus is derived from the Greek *phallos,* which is primly defined in Greek lexicons as the *membrum virile* ("the manly member"). Apparently lexicographers figure that if you are old enough to translate Greek, you are old enough to know this means the penis. An effigy of the *phallos* was borne in solemn procession in the Bacchic orgies as a symbol of the generative power of nature. In embryology, the phallus is the primordium of the penis or the clitoris.

pharmacy comes from the Greek *pharmakon,* "a drug." The Greek term was used to designate remedies, particularly those applied externally as salves or ointments, and also charms or poisons. Pharmacology (+ Greek *logos,* "treatise") is the study of drugs, their sources, and their properties. **Pharmacopoeia** (+ Greek *poiein,* "to make") is an authoritative or official listing of drugs and their components. The first U. S. Pharmacopoeia was published in 1820. It was printed in both English and Latin, and it listed 217 drugs that were considered worthy of mention.

pheno- is a combining form only slightly modified from the Greek *phainō,* "I bring to light, I show." This is best exemplified by **phenotype,** the visibly evident expression of the hereditary constitution of an organism. A **phenomenon** today is almost exactly what *phainomenon* was to the Greeks, "a thing observed or brought to light." The use of "pheno-" in the designation of numerous organic chemical compounds is owed to the naming in 1840 of the prototype **phenol** (+ Latin *oleum,* "oil"), literally "the shining oil" because of its derivation from coal oil, which was used in lamps.

pheochromocytoma is a catecholamine-producing tumor arising from cells related to the sympathetic nervous system, especially those in the adrenal medulla. The name can be dissected according to its contrived derivation: Greek *phaios,* "dark or dusky," + *chroma,* "color," + *kytos,* "cell," + *-oma,* "tumor." The explanation is that unfixed sections of such a tumor, when exposed to chromium salts, take on a dusky brown color. This is because they are composed of **chromaffin** cells.

-phil is a combining form taken from the Greek *philos,* "loved." In some instances it denotes possession in the absence of affection. In scientific usage, "-phil-" has the sense of "affinity." An example, in addition to many others cited in this volume, is **drosophila** as the name for the fruit fly, commonly used in the study of heredity. The drosophila was so named because, in addition to its fondness for fruit, it also has an affinity for frolicking in the dew (Greek *drosos,* "dew"). Both the Greeks and the Romans had their love charms or love potions, known in the singular as *philtron* and *philtrum,* in their respective languages. Why the median vertical groove in the upper lip is called the **philtrum** is unknown.

phimosis is a condition wherein the foreskin of the penis (or clitoris) is so tight it cannot be drawn back over the glans. The term originated in the Greek *phimos,* "a muzzle," such as used to keep an animal's mouth shut, and also for the noseband on a horse's bridle.

phlebo- is a combining form taken from the Greek *phleps* (genitive *phlebos*), "vein," which could also mean a vein of ore or a spring of water. The Greek root verb was *phlein,* "to gush or overflow." Hippocratic writers used *phleps* for blood vessels generally, including both arteries and veins. Probably it was the gushing of blood from a severed vessel that first suggested a name related to *phleō.* When the arteries were later distinguished as such (under the mistaken impression they conveyed air), *phleps* was restricted to veins. **Phlebotomy** (+ Greek *tomē,* "a cutting") is an incision into a vein to permit the outpouring of blood. **Phlebotomus** is a genus of pesky flies that bite hard and suck blood, thereby transmitting "sandfly fever," kala-azar, and probably other diseases.

phlegm comes from the Greek *phlegma,* "a flame or heat." Ancient writers used the term in reference to inflammation generally. Even today, **phlegmon** designates an infiltrating inflammation leading to abscess and ulceration. The Greek *phlegma* was incorporated into the archaic "humoral pathology," but, oddly, the term was assigned to the cold, moist "humor." From this came the custom of referring to the mucous secretion of the respiratory tract as "phlegm." Echoing the idea of cold and moist is the use of phlegmatic to describe a person of a sluggish or indifferent temperament, also known as "a cold fish" or "a wet blanket."

phobia   is a near borrowing of the Greek *phobos,* "fear." Psychologists cite all sorts of morbid phobias or aversions, ranging from **acrophobia** (Greek *akron,* "peak"), a fear of high places, to **zoophobia** (Greek *zōon,* "a living creature"), a fear of animals. A few other phobias are:

agoraphobia (Greek *agora,* "market place"), a fear of venturing into any crowded place

ailurophobia (Greek *ailouros,* "a cat")

anemophobia (Greek *anemos,* "wind"), a fear of hurricanes

bromidrosiphobia (Greek *brōmos,* "stench," + *idrōs,* "sweat"), a dread of body odors, real or imaginary

claustrophobia (Latin *claustrum,* "a barrier or fence")

noctiphobia (Latin *nox, noctis,* "night")

pantophobia (Greek *pantos*, "all"), a fear of everything

photophobia (Greek *phōs,* "light"), a painful sensitivity to light

stenophobia (Greek *stenos,* "narrow [place]"), a fear of caves

taphophobia (Greek *taphos,* "a grave"), a fear of cemeteries or a fear of being buried alive

topophobia (Greek *topos,* "place"), a fear of being in a particular place, as in "stage fright"

triskaidekaphobia (Greek *treis-kai-deka,* "thirteen"), a superstitious aversion to thirteen of anything

tropophobia (Greek *tropos,* "a turning"), a fear of making decisions or changes

and finally,

xenophobia (Greek *xenos,* "a stranger")

phrenic is an adjective derived from the Greek word which in the singular, *phrēn,* means "the mind or the seat of reason and of passion" and from which come such turbulent words as frenetic, frantic, and frenzy. The plural, *phrenes,* means "the muscular diaphragm" (perhaps because that structure lies so close to the heart and spleen). Actually, the Greeks also had a much more recognizable term, *diaphragma* ("a partition"), for the muscle that separates the chest from the abdomen. In any case, "phrenic" now is used for whatever pertains to the diaphragm. **Phrenology** was a pseudoscience of the 19th century. It was based on the belief that a person's character could be determined by closely observing the shape of his head, particularly noting any bumps. The term was taken, obviously, from the Greek *phrēn* and *logos.* The 19th-century concept of "phrenology" was so absurd that the sensible Greeks would have been appalled by this abasement of their language.

Phrygian cap   is the name given to an anatomic variant of the gallbladder wherein the fundus appears, in oral cholecystograms, to fold over on itself. The name comes from the floppy, conical headdress worn by liberated slaves, as a sign of their freedom, in Phrygia, an ancient country in Asia Minor. This sort of cap, often hoisted on a pole, was displayed by the proletariat in the French Revolution. The Phrygian cap of a gallbladder usually has no clinical significance.

phthisis is an archaic name for tuberculosis and was used when, because of its devastating effect, tuberculosis was commonly known as "the consumption." The Greek *phthisis* means "a dwindling or wasting away."

physician is a designation for a practitioner of the healing arts and is used only in English-speaking countries. Everywhere else in the world such a practitioner is known, in one form or another, as "a healer." To the Greeks, whatever pertained to nature or its laws was known as *physikos,* and *physikoi* were philosophers who pondered the origin and existence of material things rather than abstract or moral issues. The Greek *physikos* when taken into English provided two words: **physic** and "physics." The latter is that branch of science that deals with matter and energy, and its practitioners are known as "physicists." The former word is a now almost forgotten term for the practice of medicine, once used presumably because doctors were supposed to know the nature of things. At Harvard University there still is a Hersey Professor of the Theory and Practice of Physic. In addition, there was another use of "physic," and that was as a colloquial term for a cathartic, probably because cathartics were among the few effective drugs that practitioners of "physic" at one time used. In a cathartic vein, it has been said that the ancient Egyptian equivalent of a physician was called *swnw* (pronounced "soo-noo") or "shepherd of the anus." In the pathophysiology of that time long ago, the anus was considered the repository for the various bodily humors, including a product of putrefaction called *okhedu.* The physician was charged with removing this deleterious residue by administering enemas to both the living and the dead.

physiology is an almost direct borrowing of the Greek *physiologia,* "an inquiry into the nature of things," this combining *physis,* "nature," + *logos,* "a treatise, discourse, or study." Through the centuries, *physiologia* covered all that was known of natural science. As various specialized studies established purviews of their own, "physiology" became restricted to that department of natural science that deals with the functions of living organisms and their parts.

physostigmine is an alkaloid whose principal property is inhibition of cholinesterase activity; thereby it exerts a cholinergic effect. It is derived from the calabar bean, a product of the plant *Physostigma venenosum.* The botanical name is a combination of the Greek *physa,* "a bellows," + *stigma,* used here to refer to that part of the pistil which receives the pollen. This describes the shape of the flower. The Latin *venenosum* means it is poisonous.

pia mater is a delicate membrane, the innermost of the three meninges that cover the brain and spinal cord. *Pia* is the feminine of the Latin *pius,* in this sense "tender," the feminine form being required to agree with *mater,* which is used here in the Arabic sense of "covering or protecting" (even though the Latin *mater* ordinarily means "mother").

pica is the Latin word for "magpie," a bird noted for its indiscriminate gleaning of all sorts of objects for inclusion in its nest. Medically, pica is an inordinate craving for bizarre foods or the eating of substances not ordinarily considered as foods. The commonest cravings are for ice, clay, chalk, or cornstarch, and such craving is now recognized as a sign of iron deficiency.

Pickwickian syndrome was so named by Dr. C. S. Burwell and his coauthors (*Amer J Med* 21:811, 1956) as a whimsical allusion to the sleepy, red-faced, fat boy of Charles Dickens's *Pickwick Papers.* The syndrome of obesity, plethoric facies, and reduced vital capacity was first described twenty years earlier by Dr. W. J. Kerr and Dr. J. B. Lagen (*Ann Int Med* 10:569, 1936).

pill is a shortened, Anglicized version of the French *pilule,* which is taken from the Latin *pilula,* the diminutive of *pila,* "a ball." Thus, "a little ball" comes close to describing a medicinal pill. The Latin *pila* is related to the Greek *pilos,* "wool, or hair made into a sort of felt." The balls used in play by the Romans were made of felt.

pineal is a shortening of the Latin *pinealis,* "pertaining to the pine [tree]," or more specifically, "the pinecone." The small, cone-shaped structure, an outgrowth of the epithalamus in the brain, is called the "pineal body" because of its fancied resemblance to a little pinecone. While the pineal body was known and described by ancient anatomists, its function remains uncertain to this day. It has been found to harbor a remarkable variety of neurotransmitter substances, and some say the pineal body is implicated in the regulation of circadian rhythms, as a sort of internal "clock."

pinna is the Latin word for "feather or wing" and, by allusion, could easily be applied as a name for the winglike external ear that projects from either side of the head. It is so applied.

pinocytosis is the process whereby certain cells can imbibe fluids from their environment. They do this by forming invaginations in their cell walls, thus engulfing droplets of surrounding fluid. The term was contrived by combining the Greek *pinein,* "to drink," + *kytos,* "a cell."

piriform comes from a combination of the Latin *pirum,* "a pear," + *forma,* "shape." The term has been used to describe various pear-shaped structures and lesions. An example is the piriform fossa or sinus in the lateral wall of the laryngeal pharynx. Inexplicably, the term sometimes is misspelled "pyriform," thus utterly destroying its meaning. "Pyri-" would suggest a relation to the Greek *pyr,* "fire."

pisiform is derived from a combination of the Latin *pisum,* "a pea," + *forma,* "shape." The pisiform, as one of the carpal bones is called, might be said to resemble a large pea in shape and size.

pituitary comes from the Latin *pituita,* "phlegm," this being related to the Greek *ptuō,* "I spit." The Greek word, obviously, is vividly imitative and is the forerunner of the expletives "Ptooey!" and "Phooey!" The ancients entertained the notion that the brain secreted a mucoid substance which was discharged through the nose. Aristotle, no less, suggested that this was a cooling process, designed to allay an unduly hot temper. Indeed, Vesalius used the Latin *infundibulum,* "funnel," to describe the attachment of the pituitary gland to the brain. The idea that the pituitary gland elaborated a sort of spit was discarded in the 17th century, but the name stuck. A much less interesting name for the gland is **hypophysis** (Greek *hypo,* "below," + *physis,* "a growth"), which simply tells us that the structure grows underneath the brain.

pityriasis is a word that Hippocrates and Dioscorides used to describe a scurfy excrescence on the skin. The scurf or dandruff resembled the husks of cereal grain, known in Greek as *pityron.* We still use "pityriasis," much as did the ancient writers, for a group of scaly diseases of the skin, though we usually designate specific types of modifying terms.

placebo is the first person singular of the future tense of the Latin *placere* and is literally translated "I will please." In medicine, a placebo is any relatively inert substance given, in a form that resembles a medicament, merely for the purpose of pleasing or gratifying the patient (or, sometimes, the doctor who gives it). In that strict sense, placebos are rarely, if ever, knowingly prescribed, except in the conduct of controlled therapeutic trials wherein a drug of purported effect is to be compared with an inactive dummy.

placenta is the Latin word for "a cake" and is related to the Greek *plakous,* "a flat cake." This is descriptive of the shape of the placenta in the gravid uterus, where it serves as a communication, by way of the umbilical cord, between the fetus and its mother. To the ancient Greeks the placenta was known as *ta deutera,* and to the Romans as *secundae,* both terms meaning "the second thing" expelled after childbirth. A **placenta praevia** (Latin *praevia* being the feminine of *praevius,* "leading the way") is a placenta that develops in the lower part of the uterus at or near its outlet and, at the time of delivery, tends to precede the fetus. **Abruptio placentae** (Latin *abruptio,* "breaking off") is premature detachment of the placenta from the uterine lining.

plague is a derivative of the Greek *plēgē,* "a blow or stroke." The Latin *plangere* means "to beat or to strike" and also "to bewail or lament." In reference to devastating pestilence, the image is both that of a divine stroke of retribution and of the lamentation that this evokes. Originally the term was applied to any destructive epidemic disease, particularly that marked by fever. The "black plague" of the 14th century was so called because the extensive subcutaneous hemorrhages of its victims gave their bodies a dark-blue hue. In some areas, the pestilence was known as the **bubonic** plague (Greek *boubōniaō,* "I suffer from swollen groins") because of the characteristic inguinal adenopathy or "buboes." This disease, which still occurs sporadically in various parts of the world, is now known to be the result of infection by *Pasteurella pestis,* a microorganism transmitted to man from rodents by fleas. The "Great Plague" that devastated London in 1665 probably was typhus.

plane comes from the Latin adjective *planus,* "flat," and has been used in English anatomy since the 16th century to designate various flat surfaces, real and imagined, in reference to the body. Among the most widely used of the imagined anatomic planes, referable to the body as a whole or any part thereof, are the **transverse** plane (Latin *transversus,* "lying crosswise"), the **frontal** plane (Latin *frons, frontis,* "facade"), and the **sagittal** plane (Latin *sagitta,* "arrow"). The last is so called because it is the plane within which would lie an arrow if it penetrated the body squarely from front to back.

plasma is a direct borrowing of the Greek word for "anything formed," this being related to the Greek verb *plassein,* "to form or to mold." As noted by Professor H. A. Skinner, the ancients "believed that the vital principle or spirit of the body was a diffuse principle able to pervade any structure or tissue and adapt itself to any condition." It was in the 19th century that "plasma" was given as a name for the fluid content of blood (as opposed to its cellular elements). This was a logical extension of the idea that this "plastic" fluid substance pervaded all tissues of the body and, in a way, took their form.

platelets are, as the diminutive ending suggests, "little plates," and this seems an apt name for the smallest of the formed elements in blood. When first identified in the mid-19th century, they were called "globulins" because they were thought to resemble little globes or spheres. However, this conflicted with the use of the same name, given about the same time, to the proteinaceous substance thought to be a product of the "globules" or cells of the blood. Later, the minute formed elements in blood were called, in German, *Blutplättchen,* and this was translated literally into English as "blood platelets," thus solving the problem.

platy- is a combining form taken from the Greek *platys,* "flat, wide, or broad." The **platysma** is a thin, flat muscle that lies just beneath the skin of the anterior neck and inserts in the lower jaw and the tissues around the mouth. **Platyhelminthes** (+ Greek *helmins,* "worm") is a phylum of flatworms. Several of these, such as the trematodes or flukes and the cestodes or tapeworms, are parasitic in man.

pleo- is a combining form taken from the Greek *pleiōn,* "more." In some words this is spelled "pleio-," as in **pleiotropy** (+ Greek *tropos,* "a turning"), which, in genetics, means the capacity of a gene to manifest itself in different ways. Whatever is **pleomorphic** (+ Greek *morphē,* "form") appears in more differing shapes than are normal. An example would be the varying configuration of parenchymal cells in certain liver diseases.

plethoric describes the florid countenance of a person whose skin, particularly that of the face and neck, is suffused with an excess of blood. "Plethora" offers an example of a disease having been demoted, through the ages, to the status of a symptom. To ancient Greek physicians, *plēthōrē* meant an excess of "humors," notably blood. The Greek term was related to the verb *plēthyō,* "I am full." In modern medicine, there is a disease characterized by an overabundance of blood, and it does confer a plethoric countenance on the patient, but it is called "polycythemia." Today, "plethoric" is used to describe anyone who is red-faced for any reason.

pleura is the plural of the Greek word for "the rib" and also refers to the side or body wall containing the ribs. Even ancient writers began to limit the term to the lining of the chest cavity. **Pleurodynia** (+ Greek *odynē,* "pain") is pain in the chest wall, especially that aggravated by breathing. **Pleuritis** was used by the ancient Greeks to denote disease in the chest wall; now the word refers specifically to inflammation and has been Anglicized, through the French, to **pleurisy.** The combining form, "pleuro-," refers to whatever is related to the membrane lining the chest cavity or that covering the external surface of the lungs.

plexus originated in the Indo-European *plēk,* "to weave together," which gave rise to the Latin *plexus,* "plaited or braided." This is also related to the Greek verb *plekō,* "I twist or I weave," and to the Greek *diploō,* "I bend double." In Anglo-Saxon, the root word gave rise to *fleax,* which became "flax" as a name for the plant yielding a fiber that can be woven into cloth, specifically linen. A related Anglo-Saxon word, *fealden,* has become "to fold." In anatomy,

a plexus is an intricate network of fine nerve fibers or vascular channels. An example is the **solar plexus** (more properly designated the "celiac plexus"), the largest of the three sympathetic nerve plexuses situated in front of the lumbar vertebrae, so called because its ramifications radiate like the rays of the sun (Latin *sol,* "sun").

plumbism is lead poisoning. The Latin for lead is *plumbum,* whence comes the symbol "Pb." The Romans used this malleable metal to construct water pipes. Two causes related to lead water pipes have been postulated for the decline and fall of the Roman Empire. One is that Roman plumbers pauperized the populace by their ever-increasing charges for fixing the pipes, and the other is that the citizens of Rome became afflicted with lead poisoning, a common symptom of which is mental impairment.

pneumo- is a combining form taken from the Greek *pneuma,* "wind, air, or breath." The Greek *pneumōn* is "the lung," and **pneumonia** is both a Greek and an English word for "disease of the lungs"; to us it means specifically an inflammatory, usually infectious, disease. The list of medical terms incorporating "pneumo-" in reference to the lung, breathing, or air is lengthy. Among these terms are **pneumoconiosis** (+ Greek *konis,* "dust"), any one of a number of diseases resulting from the inhalation of irritant particles, and **pneumococcus,** a species of bacteria that often causes pneumonia. When the combining form is **"pneumat-,"** the reference usually is to gas or air, as in **pneumaturia** (+ Greek *ouron,* "urine"), the urinating of air, a startling symptom pathognomonic of a fistula between the bowel and the bladder.

podagra is a direct borrowing of the Greek word that originally denoted "a trap or snare for the feet." Later it came to mean "a seizure of pain in the foot," such as one might experience if one's foot were caught in a trap. The term is a combination of the Greek *podos,* "foot," + *agra,* "a seizure." Early on, podagra was identified with gout. Today, it refers to gouty arthritis as it specifically affects the big toe.

podiatry is an invented combination of the Greek *pous, podos,* "foot," + *iatreia,* "a healing." A podiatrist is a nonmedical practitioner who specializes in alleviating various ailments of the foot. Formerly such practitioners were known as "chiropodists," but **chiropody** was a confusing term, combining as it does the Greek *cheir,* "hand," + *podos,* "foot" (the idea having been that the hand is used to manipulate the foot). What had been known as the National Association of Chiropodists officially changed its name, in 1958, to the American Podiatry Association. **Podalic version** (Latin *vertere,* "to turn") is an obstetrical maneuver wherein the about-to-be-born fetus is turned so that the feet present first.

poison came originally from the Latin *potio,* "a drink," from which we also derive **potion.** To the Romans, *potio* also meant a magical draught. In early French the word became *puison,* and in Medieval English it was *poysoun.*

poliomyelitis is an acute viral disease characterized by inflammation of the central nervous system, particularly the anterior horn cells of the spinal cord and brainstem. Inasmuch as these are the cells having to do with motor function, the aftermath of the disease can be a disabling paralysis. Because youngsters are particularly susceptible, the disease was once called "infantile paralysis." Older clinicians still remember the devastating onslaught of poliomyelitis in the summer and early autumn of each year. Among the true triumphs of modern medicine has been the virtual obliteration of the disease by the universal use of effective vaccines. "Poliomyelitis" is a combination of the Greek *polios,* "gray," + *myelos,* "marrow," referring to the focus of the disease in the gray matter of the spinal cord.

pollex is the Latin name for the thumb and the big toe. In anatomy the reference is restricted to the thumb. The name is derived from the Latin *pollere,* "to be strong." In a contest of strength, the thumb wins over the other digits.

poly- is a combining form, usually a prefix, taken from the Greek *polys,* "many." When used in medical terms, "poly-" usually means "too many" or "more than normal." All medical terms incorporating "poly-" are too many to list, and only a few are cited here. **Polydactyly** (+ Greek *dactylos,* "finger") means having more than the normal allotment of fingers or toes. **Polydipsia** (+ Greek *dipsia,* "thirst") is excessive craving for water, while **polyuria** (+ Greek *ouron,* "urine") is the passage of an excessive volume of urine (both being symptoms of diabetes). **Polycythemia** (+ Greek *kytos,* "cell," + *haima,* "blood") is having too many red blood cells. This condition often is secondary to the hypoxia of chronic pulmonary disease, but when it occurs as a primary manifestation of myeloproliferative disease it is called "polycythemia **vera**" (the feminine of the Latin *verus,* "true"). **Polyp** is a strange word, coming as it does from a combination of the Greek *polys* + *pous,* "foot." This was Latinized as *polypus,* then shortened to "polyp." The allusion to many feet presumably relates to an observation that globular excrescences from the skin or mucous membranes can have an irregular, rootlike attachment. Actually, most such excrescences have a single, well-defined pedicle, but nevertheless the name "polyp" has become firmly attached. Another point: "polyp" often carries the connotation of a benign growth. This is not always true. A polyp can be cancerous, and not all benign growths are polypoid. "Polyp" should be used only as a descriptive term; it does not represent a diagnosis.

pons is the Latin word for "a bridge." The anatomic pons is that portion of the central nervous system "bridging" the mesencephalon and the medulla oblongata beneath the cerebellum.

popliteal comes from the Latin *poples,* "the hollow of the knee," and refers to the concavity at the back of the knee. It has been suggested that *poples,* in turn, may have originated in a combination of the Latin *post,* "behind," + *plicare,* "to fold"; thus the "fold behind" the knee.

pore can be traced to the Greek *poros,* "a way through." Although the ancients could examine the skin only with the eye, aided at best by means of a most primitive lens, they clearly recognized the presence of pores or passageways through which sweat was excreted.

porphyria designates a group of metabolic diseases, some of them hereditary, characterized clinically by neurologic and cutaneous manifestations and chemically by an excessive production of **porphyrins,** pyrrole derivatives that are ubiquitous in protoplasm. The terms are taken from the Greek *porphyra,* "purple," because of the color assumed by these compounds in certain chemical reactions.

porta is the Latin word for "gate" and is related to the verb *portare,* "to carry." The porta hepatis is the fissure on the underside of the liver, a "gateway" into which enter the **portal** vein and hepatic artery and from which departs the bile duct.

post- is a combining form taken from the Latin preposition and adverb *post,* "behind, backward, later, or afterward." It has been attached as a prefix to a host of medical terms to indicate a subsequent or following relation in space or time. Often the prefix is separated by a hyphen from the word it is intended to modify, but in recent usage the hyphen tends to be omitted. Thus, **postmortem** (+ Latin *mors, mortis,* "death") and **postpartum** (+ Latin *partus,* "born") now usually appear as single words. **Postprandial** is an oddly mixed-up word wherein *post-* is hooked onto the Latin *prandium,* "a late breakfast or lunch," which itself is derived from a combination of the Greek *pro-,* "before," + *endios,* "midday." Literally, then, "postprandial" translates as "after the time before midday." Nowadays "postprandial" refers to the time after any meal. The initials **p.c.,** for the Latin *post cibum* (the latter part coming from the Latin *cibus,* "food"), are used on prescriptions to instruct the patient to take his medication after meals. The word **posthumous,** incidentally, is the result of a mistake. The original classical Latin *postumus* means "last or coming after." Some now-forgotten scribe must have thought the "-umus" stood for the Latin *humus,* "ground or soil," and that he would amend the spelling to look more like "after burial."

post hoc ergo propter hoc is a succinct statement of a well known but often ignored fallacy of reasoning. It translates literally as "after that, therefore because of that," but it sounds more forceful in the original Latin. The fallacy is pertinent to medicine, and its pitfall is to be carefully avoided by doctor and patient alike. The truth, as everyone knows but does not always remember, is that simply because two events occur in sequence it does not necessarily mean the first is the cause and the second is the result. If a patient is given a dose of penicillin for a bad cold on Tuesday and then reports that he feels better on Wednesday, one cannot rightly assume that penicillin cured the cold. Medical practice is replete with similar examples of fallacious reasoning wherein *post* is confused with *propter.*

poultice comes through the French from the Latin *pulta* and the Greek *poltos,* both meaning "porridge." Originally, the idea was that of exerting heat on a part by applying a warm, moist cloth on which had been smeared a boiled mixture of bread, cake, or herbs. Later, mildly irritating substances were so applied. Some may recall the mustard plaster of bygone days. The concept was that supposed "bad humors" would be thus "drawn out" from the affected part. This was a mistaken idea, yet the effect of a counterirritant was probably to allay a more deep-seated ache or pain. Countless jars and tubes of mentholated products are still sold today for this purpose and, what's more, they often work. Incidentally, "poultice" bears no relation to "poultry," which comes from the Latin *pullus,* "a chicken."

pox is a variant spelling of the plural of "pock." The term seldom occurs in the singular except as in "pockmark." "Pock" seems to have come from the Norman French *poque,* "pouch," and its diminutive, *poquet.* A pock, then, was "a little pocket" in the skin. In bygone times, a great variety of pustular eruptions in both man and beast were called "pox." The **smallpox** was so called not only because the pustules, though many, were small, but also because the disease, as bad as it was, seemed the lesser of two evils. The "great pox" was syphilis.

pre- is a slightly shortened version of the Latin *prae,* "before, in front of, by reason of." "Pre-" usually appears as a prefix (+ Latin *figere,* "to fasten"). The number of medical terms incorporating "pre-" is almost endless. Some are derivatives of actual Latin words, such as **precipitate,** which is a borrowing of the Latin *praecipitare,* "to throw down," this being a combination of *prae + caput,* "head," in the sense of "headlong" or "headfirst." Some are obviously concoctions, though perfectly serviceable, such as "precancerous." **Predilection** often is misspelled and mispronounced as if it were "predelection." This error is avoided if one remembers the word comes from a combination of *pre* + Latin *dilectus,* "selection." A disease that has a predilection for certain persons is one that tends to preselect its victims. **Pregnant** (+ Latin [g]*natus,* "birth") carries a little different meaning from **prenatal,** even though the two words share the same origin. **Prepuce** comes from the Latin *praeputium,* "the foreskin [of the penis]," but this is a hybrid combination of the Latin *prae-* + the Greek *posthē,* "penis." A medicinal **preparation** owes its name to the Latin *praeparatus,* "to be ready in advance," this being a combination of *prae-* + *paratus,* "ready." A **prescription** is something written beforehand, i.e., preceding the actual treatment. The Latin *praescriptus* combines *prae-* + *scribere,* "to write." In his *Devil's Dictionary,* Ambrose Bierce defines "prescription" a bit differently: "A physician's guess at what will best prolong the situation with least harm to the patient." The **prevalence** of a disease is the number of cases existing at a given time in a given place. The term relates to the Latin *praevalere,* "to be stronger, to exert the greater influence," this being a combination of *prae-* + *valere,* "to be strong."

precarious can describe the condition of a patient who may well be in need of prayer. The Latin *precarius* means "obtained by prayer" or "dependent on another's will," hence uncertain or risky. The adjective is derived from the Latin verb *precari,* "to pray for." The sense of uncertainty was epitomized by the phrase, popular during World War II, that described a crippled airplane as "coming in on a wing and a prayer."

presbyopia is a condition of faltering vision, especially for near objects, in the elderly. The term combines the Greek *presbys,* "an elder", + *ōps,* "the eye."

priapism is a persistent, abnormal erection of the penis, such as occurs in the absence of sexual desire. It can be the consequence of certain spinal cord injuries or can be associated with a bladder calculus or sickle-cell anemia. Priapus was the mythologic god of procreation whose nude statues made abundantly evident his chief attribute. It is said that statues of Priapus were placed in vineyards or cultivated fields as scarecrows.

primum non nocere is a time-honored maxim essential to sound medical practice. Literally translated from the Latin it means "first of all do no harm." The principle dates back to Hippocrates, who is quoted as saying, "As to disease, make a habit of two things: to help, or at least to do no harm." The author vividly recalls his own introduction to this fundamental precept. It came as our instructor's concluding remark in his final lecture on dermatology. Our professor was an earnest, diminutive, bald-pated Viennese. For eight weeks he had been catechizing us on the various salves and ointments for what to me, as a junior medical student, was a bewildering array of rashes and eruptions. His final admonition, as he carefully lifted his pince-nez, was, "Boyce [which is Viennese for "boys"]! Whatever you do, for God's sake, don't make it any worse!"

pro- is a combining form, usually a prefix, borrowed from the *pro* of both Greek and Latin, a preposition meaning "before, in front of, in behalf of, in place of, or the same as." The initials **p.r.n.** stand for the Latin *pro re nata,* "according as the circumstances arise." In anatomy, a **process** is a projection of a structure, the term being derived from the Latin *processus,* "a going forward," which combines *pro- + cedere,* "to go." A **procedure** is an action that must "go before" a desired result. **Procaine** was given as a name for a substance used in local anesthesia "in place of" cocaine (with the misconception that "-caine" denoted an anesthetic property). **Procidentia** refers to a prolapse of the uterus; this Latin word combines *pro- + cadere,* "to fall," and therefore means "a falling forward." A **prodrome** (+ Greek *dromos,* "a running") is an early stage of a disease that "runs before" the period when the characteristic symptoms are fully evident. **Progeria** (+ Greek *geraios,* "old") is a rare condition of premature degeneration wherein young children acquire the appearance of wizened age. **Progestin** is a concocted name for a hormone that prepares the endometrium to receive the fertilized ovum; it combines *pro- +* the Latin *gestare,* "to bear." **Prognathism** (+ Greek *gnathos,* "the lower jaw") is an abnormal protrusion of the mandible in relation to the maxilla. **Prognosis** is a direct borrowing of the Greek word for "perceiving beforehand." The word was used by Hippocrates, as we use it now, to mean a foretelling of the course of a disease. The word combines *pro- +* the Greek *gnō-*

sis, "a knowing." **Prolapse** is taken from the Latin *prolapsus sum,* "to slip forward." **Prophylaxis** is a borrowing of the Greek word for "an advance guard" and an apt term for whatever measure can be taken to fend off a disease. "Pro" is a nickname for "prophylactic" and was commonly used before the advent of penicillin therapy to denote the method of genital lavage once promulgated as a measure to prevent venereal disease. In the early days of World War II, military authorities established "pro stations" at convenient locations in large cities where errant soldiers and sailors could repair for succor of sorts following a night of dalliance. The naming of the **prostate** gland followed a somewhat tortuous path. A Greek *prostatēs* (+ *histēmi,* "to stand") was "one who stands before, as a leader of the first rank, a president." To the Greek anatomist Herophilus, the *prostatai adēnoeidēs* was "that which stands before the glands," the "glands" being the testicles.

probe comes from the Latin *probare,* "to test or to try." As surgical instruments in the form of slender, malleable rods with blunt ends, probes were used by the ancients, as they are now, to explore wounds, ducts, fistulas, and cavities.

procto- is taken from the Greek *prōktos,* "the anus or hinder parts," but is used only as a combining form. For nouns, we rely on the Latin-derived "anus" and "rectum." **Proctology** (+ Greek *logos,* "a treatise") is the art and science of dealing with anorectal problems. A **proctoscope** (+ Greek *skopein,* "to view") is an instrument by which the inner recesses of the rectum can be inspected. **Proctalgia** (+ Greek *algos,* "pain") is, in the vernacular, "a pain in the arse." **Proctalgia fugax** (Latin *fugax,* "swiftly passing") is a fleeting anorectal pain that, strangely, strikes mainly during the night.

Proprioceptive is a concoction of the Latin *proprius,* "one's own," + *capere,* "to take," and was introduced in 1906 by Sir Charles Sherrington (1857–1952), a renowned English physiologist, to describe the capacity of an organism to sense stimuli arising in its own body. By the faculty of proprioception we can tell whether our legs are crossed or outstretched, even with our eyes closed.

prosthesis is a direct borrowing of the Greek word for "an addition." Today we use the term more in the sense of a substitution whereby parts lost to disease or injury are replaced by artificial devices, particularly for the purpose of restoring function. A set of false teeth is a dental prosthesis. Probably the ultimate prosthesis was the "Six Million Dollar Man," the protagonist of a recent television series. **Enthesis,** a concoction of the Greek *en-,* "in," + *thesis,* "a placing or an arranging," refers to the insertion or "putting in" of nonliving material in the repair of a defect or deformity of the body. Placing a metal plate so as to fill a hole in the skull is an example of an enthesis.

protean is always pronounced in three syllables and describes the capacity to assume different appearances. A protean symptom is one that can appear in various guises characteristic of different diseases. Fever is an example of a protean symptom, appearing in diseases as diverse as a common cold

and acute leukemia. The word comes from Proteus, the name of a Greek sea god who had the peculiar ability to change his shape or appearance at will.

proto- is a combining form taken from the Greek *prōtos,* "first, foremost, or earliest." The term **protein** was introduced in 1838 by a Dutch chemist, Gerard Johann Mulder (1802–1880), to designate what he thought to be the essential constituent of all organic bodies. He took the term from the Greek *prōteios,* "the chief rank or first place." **Protamine** is a term contrived in the late 19th century to designate certain elemental protein substances of low molecular weight. **Protocol** is occasionally used in medical practice to designate a particular scheme for diagnosis or treatment. For example, an endoscopic protocol is an orderly outline of the procedure used and the observations made when a patient is examined by means of an endoscope. A protocol for chemotherapy is an agreed-upon schedule, in orderly sequence, of the drugs and their dosages used in treating patients requiring such chemical agents. The word comes from the Late Greek *protokollon,* which was the first page or front leaf attached to a manuscript and which contained an outline of its contents. *Protokollon* combines *protos,* "first," + *kolla,* "glue"; hence "something stuck on at the beginning." **Protoplasm** (+ Greek *plasma,* "the thing formed") was introduced in 1839 by Johannes Evangelista Purkinje (1787–1869), a Czech anatomist from Breslau, as a term for the formative substance of embryos. Shortly thereafter the term was extended by Hugo von Mohl

(1805–1872), a professor of botany at Tübingen, in Germany, to describe the mucilaginous substance contained within the cell membranes of plants and animals. Previously, this substance had been known by the prosaic German *Schleim.* **Protozoa** (+ Greek *zōon,* "a living animal") is a term introduced in the early 19th century to more properly designate the single-celled, presumably primordial "animalcules" that had been described by van Leeuwenhoek in 1675.

proximal is taken from the Latin adjective *proximus,* "nearest, next following, adjoining." With reference to position, proximal is opposed to **distal,** which is taken from the Latin verb *distare,* "to stand apart, to be distant from." Whenever such relative terms are used, there must be a point of reference. In most cases this is obvious. Everyone understands that in a finger a proximal phalanx is the bone nearest the hand; a distal phalanx is the bone at the end of a finger. But in some other cases, the relation is not always clear unless stated. For example, the upper part of the rectum is proximal with reference to the colon but distal with reference to the anus. In whatever situation there may be ambiguity, the point of reference should be made clear.

pruritus is from the Latin *prurire,* "to itch." The term has nothing to do with inflammation, and its ending must be spelled "-itus," never "-itis." A prurient thought occurs in a mind itching with lewd or lascivious ideas.

psammoma is a combination of the Greek *psammos,* "sand," + *-oma,* designating a tumor. Psammoma bodies are minute foci of calcification sometimes seen in various neoplasms, particularly those of the prostate gland.

pseudo- is a combining form taken from the Greek *pseudēs,* "false." When incorporated in medical terms, "pseudo-" is used in the sense of "mistaken" or "not of the true type." **Pseudocyesis** (+ Greek *kyēsis,* "conception") is a delusion of pregnancy. A **pseudocyst** (+ Greek *kystis,* "a bag or bladder") is real enough, but it does not contain in its wall all the histologic components of its parent structure. A **pseudomembrane** is something that looks like a membrane, such as a sheet of exudate, but really isn't. "Pseudo-" has been affixed to the names of a number of diseases to indicate a condition that can mimic the prototype or, sometimes, simply differ from it. For example, "pseudohypoparathyroidism" is a condition that resembles hypoparathyroidism except that the defect is a failure of response to the parathyroid hormone rather than a deficiency in its secretion. Now, we also have "pseudopseudohypoparathyroidism" which resembles the one-pseudo condition except that the serum levels of calcium and phosphorus are in the normal range. Can "pseudopseudopseudohypoparathyroidism" be far behind?

psoas comes from the Greek *psoa,* usually used in the plural, *hai psoai,* "the loins." The psoas muscles are those of the loins.

psoriasis is a direct borrowing of the Greek word denoting "an itchy or scaly condition" and is related to *psora,* "a cutaneous disease, particularly the itch or the mange." Ancient writers applied the term to a variety of pruritic, scaly diseases. By the end of the 18th century these diseases were more or less sorted out, and "psoriasis" was restricted to the chronically recurring, papulosquamous dermatosis we recognize today.

psyche is our word for the human faculty for thought, judgment, and emotion. To the Greeks, *psychē* was "the spirit or soul of man" and also "the seat of the will, desires, and passions." The concept is felicitously defined in the Greek myth concerning Psyche, a mortal maid who aroused the jealousy and ire of Venus, not only because of her surpassing beauty but also because she was beloved by Venus' handsome son, Cupid. Seeking rapprochement with Venus, Psyche was required to perform three nearly impossible tasks, in which she almost failed because of her human character, being saved only by the intervention of kindly gods. Eventually, Psyche was taken into the celestial realm by a benevolent Jove and reunited with her husband, Cupid. The allegory is that of the human soul gaining immortality. The Greek name for the butterfly also is *psychē,* the allusion being to the transformation of the plodding caterpillar into the transcendent glory of the butterfly. **Psychiatry** (+ Greek *iatreia,* "healing") is that branch of medicine that deals with the diagnosis and treatment of mental disorders. **Psychology** (+ Greek *logos,* "a treatise") is that branch of science dealing with mental sensation and behavior. In medicine, there is a curious distinction between "psychosis" and "psychoneurosis." A **psychosis** is a more profound mental aberration whereby the afflicted person has lost all touch with reality, while a **psychoneurosis** is a behavioral disorder suggesting a functional nervous disturbance of mental origin. **Psychosomatic** (+ Greek *sōma,* "the body") describes whatever has an integral mind-body relationship. **Psychedelic,** a word of more recent currency, incorporates the Greek *dēloō,* "to make visible or known." A psychedelic drug is one that purportedly makes mental perceptions, particularly those that delight but sometimes those that depress, clearly evident.

pterygoid combines the Greek *pteryx,* "wing," + *eidos,* "like," and describes whatever resembles a wing. The pterygoid processes are paired, winglike extensions of the sphenoid bone at the base of the skull. A **pterygium** is a sort of winglike, triangular membrane that sometimes emerges as an abnormal extension of the conjunctiva from the inner canthus of the eye. The usual cause is prolonged exposure of the eye to wind and weather.

ptomaine is now an almost obsolete word, but until comparatively recently any acute illness thought to be due to the ingestion of spoiled food was often called "ptomaine poisoning." An Italian chemist, Francesco Selmi (1817–1881), is said to have invented the word *ptomana,* "from a corpse" (using the Greek *ptōma,* "corpse"), to describe certain poisonous substances that he had extracted from cadavers. "Ptomaine" later was used to refer to various products of organic decomposition.

ptosis is a direct borrowing of the Greek word for "a falling," and is related to the verb *piptein,* "to fall." While not used as a medical term by ancient writers, "ptosis" later was applied to drooping of the eyelid consequent to impairment of the third cranial (oculomotor) nerve. About the turn of the present century it was fashionable to attribute various obscure abdominal complaints to a downward displacement of the viscera. There ensued a flurry of high-sounding but meaningless diagnoses, such as "gastroptosis," "nephroptosis," or—if one wasn't quite sure just which organ drooped—"visceroptosis." Fortunately, the organs were as difficult to pin down as was the diagnosis, so little harm was done.

ptyalin comes from the Greek *ptyalon,* "saliva," this being related to the imitative verb *ptyein,* "to spit." Ptyalin, an enzyme occurring in saliva, converts starch into maltose and dextrose. The longer one chews a morsel of bread, the sweeter it tastes because of the action of ptyalin.

pubis is taken from the Latin *pubes,* which as an adjective means "grown-up, adult," and as a noun designates the growth of hair that comes to adorn the genital area of adults. In anatomy the term shifted in meaning from the hair-covered area to the underlying bone. The Latin *pubertas,* "coming to the age of manhood," led to **puberty.**

pudenda are what the Victorians primly called "the private parts," i.e., the external genital structures, especially those of a woman. The word comes from the Latin *pudere,* "to be ashamed." The more familiar word "impudent" means "brazen or lacking in shame."

puerperal is but a slight shortening of the Latin *puerperalis,* "pertaining to childbirth." The word is derived by a combination of *puer,* "a child," + *parere,* "to bear or to bring forth." Puerperal fever, an often fatal illness afflicting the mother shortly after delivery (and commonly known all too well as "childbed fever"), was recognized by Hippocrates. In 1660 the condition was described and named *febris puerperarum* by Thomas Willis (1621–1675), the famous English physician and anatomist. But it was not until 1843 that Oliver Wendell Holmes (1809–1894), a proper Bostonian physician, and 1847 that Ignaz Semmelweiss (1818–1865), a Viennese obstetrician, proclaimed their conviction that puerperal fever was, indeed, an infectious disease spread by untidy, unwashed doctors. Needless to say, this was an affront to the profession and aroused bitter controversy on both sides of the Atlantic. When doctors and midwives were finally persuaded to employ antiseptic procedures as they attended women in labor, the malady became nearly extinct.

puke is a venerable English word for the act of vomiting. In *As You Like It,* Shakespeare describes the infant "mewling and puking in the nurse's arms." Probably it is an imitative word, akin to "spit."

pulmonary comes from the Latin *pulmo* (genitive *pulmonis*), "the lung." Some authorities hold that this is derived, by a transposition of letters, from the Greek *pleumōn,* a variant of *pneumōn,* "the lung." In any case, the pulmonary vessels puzzled ancient anatomists. Lacking knowledge of the circulation of the blood, they were perplexed by the structure of the vessels connecting the lung to the right and left sides of the heart. Thus, the pulmonary artery and vein were once known, respectively, as "the vein-like artery" and "the artery-like vein."

pulse comes from the Latin *pulsus,* "a pushing, beating, or striking," this being related to the verb *pello, pellere, pepuli, pulsum* of similar meaning. The ancients connected the pulsation in peripheral arteries with the beating of the heart and came within a whisker of discovering the circulation of the blood. It was an ignorance of the capillary connection between arteries and veins that stumped them.

punctate comes from the Latin *punctum,* "a point or spot," this being related to the verb *pingere,* "to prick, sting, or stab." The punctum lacrimale is the pinpoint opening at the inner canthus of the eye which leads to the tear duct that drains into the nasal cavity. A **puncture** is the result of pricking or stabbing and may be more specifically designated as, for example, a **venepuncture.** A "pungent" odor is sharp or biting.

pupil referring to the aperture of the iris in the eye is derived from the Latin *pupa,* "a doll." Presumably this came from the early observation that when one peered closely into the eye of another, one saw a minute image of himself. The Greeks, in similar fashion, used the word *korē* for "maiden or doll" and also for "the pupil of the eye." From the Greek word we obtain **anisocoria** (Greek *a-,* "not," + *iso,* "equal"), a condition wherein the pupils are of different diameters.

purgative is taken from the Latin *purgatio,* "a cleansing," this being related to the verb *purgare,* "to clear away, to cleanse, to purify." The idea of cleansing the body by the use of enemas or cathartics is as old as time itself. Incidentally, to "expurgate" a piece of literature is to remove from it whatever may be considered offensive or objectionable.

purpura is the Latin word for "purple" and may be related, in turn, to the Greek *porphyra,* the name of a mollusk or shellfish from which a purple dye was extracted. In medieval times, patients afflicted with febrile illnesses marked by extensive subcutaneous hemorrhages were said to suffer from "purple fever." Later it was recognized that similar hemorrhages occurred in the absence of fever, and such conditions were referred to simply as "purpura." Purpura is distinguished from petechiae by the confluence of hemorrhagic spots and by their being observed at a stage when fresh red blood has been degraded to a purple color. An ecchymosis usually is a larger focal extravasation of blood in the skin.

pus comes from the Greek *pyon,* "corrupt matter, specifically that which exudes from sores." The Sanskrit root *pu-* meant "fetid or stinking." From this came the Latin *puter,* "rotten," and our word "putrid." Can it be that the colloquial exclamation "pee-yew!" represents a legacy from the Vedas of India bequeathed two-and-a-half millennia ago? **Putrefaction** (Latin *putris,* "rotten," + *facere,* "to make") is an enzymatic decomposition, especially of proteins and usually by bacteria, resulting in fetid products, such as hydrogen sulfide, mercaptans, and ammonia. The diminutive **pustule** (Latin *pustula,* "blister") is a little, pussy pimple. **Pyemia** is a contrived term combining the Greek *pyon* + *haima,* "blood," and is used to denote pus in the blood. In modern medicine, this has been superseded by the more precise "leukocytosis" (an excess of white blood cells), "septicemia" (bacterial toxins in the blood), and "bacteremia" (bacteria in the blood). **Pyorrhea** (+ Greek *rhoia,* "a flowing") is, literally, "a flow of pus," but currently the term tends to be restricted to purulent exudate from infected tooth sockets.

putamen is the Latin word for "whatever falls off with paring, such as a shell or husk." The related Latin verb is *putare,* "to trim or to prune." In anatomy, the putamen is the outer part of the lenticular nucleus of the brain, so called because of its fancied resemblance to a husk or shell. The original sense of the Latin *putare* was "to make clean, as by pruning or trimming." Later, *putare* was extended to the sense of "making clear," hence "to think or reckon." From this sense we have derived a number of commonly used words, such as putative, compute, impute, and repute.

pyelo- is a combining form taken from the Greek *pyelos,* "a pan or basin," to which the Latin *pelvis* is related. In modern anatomy, "pyelo-" has been limited to the pelvis of the kidney and has been incorporated in numerous terms pertaining thereto, e.g., **pyelography** (+ Greek *graphein,* "to write"), **pyelonephritis** (+ Greek *nephros,* "kidney"), and **pyelolithotomy** (+ Greek *lithos,* "stone," + *tomē,* "a cutting"). It is neces-

sary to distinguish "pyelo-" from "pyle-"; the latter refers to the portal vein.

pyknic is taken from the Greek *pyknos,* "close, compact, solid, or dense." A person of a pyknic habitus has a short, stocky build. A **pyknotic** nucleus of a cell is contracted by condensation of its chromatin into a dense clump, usually as a sign of impending mitosis or of degeneration.

pylorus is a near borrowing of the Greek word for "gatekeeper," this being related to *pylē,* "gateway." The Greeks used *pylōros* to designate the lower end of the stomach, while Latin authors tended to restrict the term to the narrow opening into the duodenum, as we do now. From the Greek *pylē* also comes the combining form **pyle-,** which designates whatever pertains to the portal vein. Thus, **pylethrombosis** (+ Greek *thrombos,* "a clot") refers to the formation of a blood clot in the portal vein. **Pylephlebitis** (+ Greek *phleps,* "vein") is an inflammation of the portal vein.

pyrexia is taken from the Greek *pyrēxis,* "feverishness," related to *pyr,* "fire." **Pyretic** denotes whatever pertains to fever. An **antipyretic** is whatever quells fever. **Pyrogenic** (+ Greek *gennaō,* "I produce") refers to whatever may stimulate or cause fever. **Pyrosis** is derived from the Greek and is now restricted to a retrosternal burning sensation that most sensible people would call "heartburn." It is not a febrile condition.

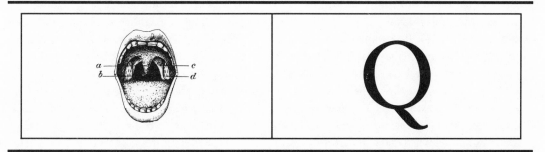

Q

Q fever is the only disease whose name is a single letter. It is a self-limited, acute, febrile disease with constitutional manifestations, but its symptoms tend to focus on the respiratory tract. It occurs throughout most of the world but seems more prevalent where cattle are raised. Its odd name is shrouded in obscurity. Most writers interpret the "Q" as standing for "Query" because the cause of the disease was for so long unknown. It is now recognized as an infection by *Coxiella burnetti,* a rickettsial organism.

quack is a pejorative name for an unqualified practitioner of medicine and owes its origin to the sound of the word (and, perhaps, to that of a duck). "Croak" in Dutch is *kwakken,* which means "a loud, boisterous sound" or "a trifling utterance." According to one explanation, this form was long ago combined in Dutch as *kwakzalver,* meaning one who purveyed all sorts of salves and other remedies, all generously laced with humbug. This became "quacksalver" in English, later shortened simply to "quack."

quadrant is a near borrowing of the Latin *quadrans,* "a fourth part, a quarter." Thus, in surface anatomy, the right upper abdominal quadrant, for example, is that area extending from the midline laterally to the right flank, bounded above by the right costal margin and below by the level of the umbilicus. **Quadrate** (Latin *quadratus,* "squared") describes whatever is shaped like a square, as is, more or less, the quadrate lobe of the liver.

quarantine is a period of isolation decreed to control the spread of contagious diseases. The duration might vary according to the known incubation period of the given disease or other circumstances. In the old days the period was a flat forty days, hence the derivation of the term from the Latin *quadraginta,* "forty." Why forty? Probably because it was known empirically that the in-

203

cubation period of most infectious diseases was less than forty days.

quinine comes from a Peruvian Indian word, *kina,* "bark of a tree," that was Latinized to *quina.* A particular bark came from what the Andean Indians called "the fever tree," now properly classified as *Cinchona calisaya.* The active principle in the extract from this bark was isolated and named "quinine" in 1820. When 18-year-old William (later Sir William) Perkin, an English chemist, unwittingly founded the coal-tar dye industry in 1856, he was actually seeking a synthetic source of quinine so as to relieve Europe of dependence on the cinchona bark, then available only in faraway South America and the East Indies. Perkin failed to form quinine, but he reaped the rewards of serendipity on a grand scale. **Quinidine,** an alkaloid of cinchona with quite different properties, was recognized in 1833 and so named because of its isomeric relation to quinine (a sort of quin*oid*ine).

quinsy is an almost archaic term for a peritonsillar abscess. It originated as the Greek *kyna*[*n*]*gchē,* "a bad sore throat," this being a combination of *kyōn,* "a dog," + *a*[*n*]*g-chōne,* "a choking or throttling" (whence "anguish"). The allusion might have been either to the pain and soreness one would suffer were a dog to chew on one's neck or, perhaps, to a sore throat "as mean as a dog." From *kyna*[*n*]*gchē* a shift in spelling led to the Medieval Latin *quinancia,* to the Middle English *quinesye,* and finally to "quinsy."

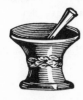

R

rabies is the Latin word for "rage or madness." This disease of warmblooded animals, incidentally transmitted to man by a bite or other contact with an infected beast, was known to the ancients. Its dramatic neurologic manifestations led to its being called "rabies." In medieval times the disease was known as **hydrophobia** (Greek *hydōr,* "water," + *phobos,* "fear") because its victims eschewed water on account of the painful throat spasm induced by attempting to drink. In the 17th century the term "rabies" was revived, and the victims of the disease, both human and animal, were described as being rabid.

racemose is taken from the Latin *racemus,* "a cluster or bunch, especially of grapes." In anatomy, the term is applied to whatever has the appearance of a bunch of grapes on a stalk, such as a cluster of glands attached to a ductal system.

radical is used in science, particularly in mathematics and chemistry, to denote something essential or fundamental on which other forms can be constructed. The term also can be spelled "radicle." Thus, sulfate (SO_4) is a simple chemical radical from which more complex chemical compounds can be formed. This scientific usage is much closer to the origin of the word, which is in the Latin *radix,* "root," than the present-day vernacular use of "radical" would suggest, but there is a connection. In 18th-century England, certain political reformers came to be known as "radicals" because they insisted on getting to the root of matter and advocated revamping the social structure from the ground up. The political conservatives were content with little or no change at all. In anatomy, **radicle,** as a diminutive derivative of *radix,* is "a little root" and thus is applied to the smallest extension of a nerve or vessel.

radiology had to be contrived by hybridizing the Latin *radius,* "a ray," + the Greek *logos,* "a treatise," to come up with a name for the new science emanating from the discovery of X-rays in 1895 by Wilhelm Konrad Röntgen (1845–1923), a German physicist. As a tribute to the discoverer, who was awarded a Nobel prize in 1901, the science also has been known as **roentgenology. A roentgen** (usually symbolized by "r") is an international unit of gamma (γ) radiation. **Radiation** comes from the Latin *radius* (related to the Greek *rhabdos,* "a rod"), which was first a stick or wand, then the spoke of a wheel, and, by allusion, a ray of light. **Radium** is the name given to a metallic elemental source of X-irradiation that was discovered in 1898 by Pierre and Marie Curie, husband-and-wife French physicists. Their surname is commemorated in the **curie,** a term for the quantity of radionuclide in which the number of disintegrations is 3.7×10^{10} per second. **Radon** is a gaseous radioactive element with a short half-life that has been used in implantable capsules as a source of radiotherapy.

radius is the name of the smaller bone in the forearm and was so called because it was thought to resemble the spoke of a wheel. At least that is what it looked like to Celsus, the 1st-century Roman writer who introduced the term to anatomy. The spoke of a wheel, in Latin, is *radius.* The **radial** nerve is so called because of its proximity to the radius, not because of its shape or distribution.

râle is taken from the French verb *râler,* "to have a rattle in one's throat, or to grumble." In medicine, "râle" was first used as a term for the "death rattle" of mucus accumulating in the throat of a dying person. Laënnec, the French physician who invented the stethoscope in 1816, applied the term to certain adventitious crackling sounds he heard when he applied his new device to the chests of patients with various congestive cardiopulmonary diseases.

ramus is Latin for "a branch or bough." In anatomy, a ramus is a small structure emanating like a branch from a larger structure, be it bone, nerve, or vessel. If there are many such branches, they are **rami** (the Latin plural).

ranula is the diminutive of the Latin *rana,* "a frog," and has been given as the name of a cystic tumor, actually a mucocele, that can occur beneath the tongue when the submaxillary or sublingual salivary glands are obstructed. There are three possible explanations for the use of the term: *(a)* "ranine" is an archaic adjective referring to the tip of the tongue as "the frog of the mouth"; *(b)* a swelling in the floor of the mouth may be fancied to resemble the throat of a croaking frog; or *(c)* such a swelling may cause hoarseness, i.e., "a frog in the throat."

raphe is a borrowing of the Greek *rhaphē,* "a seam," as sewn with a needle. The median line extending from the anus to the pudenda is known as the "perineal raphe." The Greek term is synonymous with the Latin *sutura.*

rash comes from the Latin verb *rado, radere, rasi,* "to scrape or to scratch." An erythematous eruption in the skin has the appearance of having been scraped or scratched. Also, some rashes itch and, therefore, prompt scratching. "Rash" came into English from the French *raser,* meaning "to shave or slice thin." A "rasher" of bacon is a thin slice, and the connection with "razor" is obvious.

reagin designates an antibody or whatever behaves like an antibody in complement fixation reactions. The term is modeled on **reagent** and is derived by combining the Latin *re-,* "back," + *agere,* "to drive, act, or perform."

receptor comes from the Latin *recipere,* "to receive." A receptor nerve ending is the sensory terminal that receives and registers stimuli from its environment. Paul Ehrlich (1854–1915), the pioneer German immunologist, postulated the presence in cell membranes of special receptor sites where substances might attach and gain entrance. The basic validity of Ehrlich's side-chain, or receptor, theory has been borne out in modern immunology.

recrudescence comes from the Latin *recrudescere,* "to become raw or sore again." To the Romans this referred to the reopening of a wound which had appeared to heal. Later the meaning was extended to the recurrence of any symptom or disease, and now we may speak of the recrudescence of a rash or even of a fever.

rectum is derived from the Latin *rectus,* "straight." Aristotle referred to the most distal segment of the bowel as "the straight passage" from the lower colon to the anus. The reference puzzles most students of anatomy because they find the lumen of the rectum to be anything but straight. A possible explanation for the early and persistent use of the term is that the ancients derived most of what they learned of anatomy from the dissection of lower animals, and the most distal segment of the bowel is more nearly straight in many quadrupeds than in humans.

recuperate comes from the Latin *recuperare,* "to regain, to get back, or to recover." The Reverend W. W. Skeat, in his 19th-century etymological dictionary, explains that *recuperare* may have originally meant "to make good again," from the Sabine *cuprus,* "good," as related to the Latin verb *cupere,* "to desire." Another explanation is that *recuperare* might be a transliterated combination of *re-,* "again," + *capere,* "to grasp or to gain."

recurrent comes from the Latin *recurrere,* "to run back or to return." The recurrent laryngeal nerve is a branch of the vagus (tenth cranial) nerve that runs down the neck, then turns back up to invest the larynx. In medicine, as generally, "recurrent" is used to describe anything that "comes back again."

reflex is derived from the Latin *reflectere,* "to bend back or to turn around," from which, obviously, we obtain "reflection." René Descartes (1596–1650), the celebrated French savant, may have been the first to perceive reflex actions wherein mental impressions generated impulses, conducted automatically along nerve pathways, that were then "thrown back" to call forth movement.

reflux is derived from the Latin *refluere,* "to flow back." Fluid flowing in a retrograde manner from the stomach into the esophagus is an example of reflux, as is the motion of fluid and electrolytes from the internal environment into the gut lumen and back again, through the epithelial cells. A term of related meaning is **regurgitation,** from a combination of the Latin *re-,* "back," + *gurgitare,* "to flood," This implies a somewhat more forceful action than "reflux." The retrograde flooding of blood from the left ventricle of the heart, during systole, through an incompetent bicuspid valve into the left atrium, whence it came, is known as "mitral regurgitation."

refraction comes from the Latin *refractus,* the past participle of *refringere,* "to break down (or up)." The original scientific application of the term was to describe the "breaking up," by a crystal, of a beam of white light into its component colors of different wavelengths. In clinical medicine, a refractory condition is one that is so "broken down" that it resists treatment. In this vein, a patient or a symptom that defies treatment is said to be **recalcitrant.** This term is taken from the Latin *recalcitrare,* "to kick back." This relates to *calcaneum,* the Latin word for "the heel."

regimen is often confused with "regime," and vice versa. Both have their origin in the Indo-European *reg,* whose dual meanings, "to move in a straight line" and "to rule," gave rise to the Latin *regio* and *rex, regis,* respectively. A regime is a mode or system of government. A regimen, in medicine, is a regulated course of diet, exercise, or therapy designed to attain a favorable result.

relapse is a near borrowing of the Latin *relapsus,* the past participle of *relabi,* "to slide back or to sink down." In medicine, a re-

lapse is marked by a return of symptoms or signs of disease that had appeared to subside. A **remission** (Latin *remissio,* "a release or abatement") is the period during which a disease appears to subside. The implication is one of uncertainty. A remission may lead to a cure or to a relapse.

remedy designates anything that is known to cure or palliate a disease. The word comes from the Latin *remedium,* "that which heals again." The prefix *re-* is essential to the meaning in that a true remedy has been proved to work, again and again. An experimental, unproved method of treatment can hardly be called a "remedy."

renal is a adjective derived from the Latin *renes,* "the kidneys." We do not use a Latin-derived noun in modern English for this pair of organs, though *reins* (among other spellings) is an archaic English and Old French word for the kidneys or the lower back. None of this has anything to do with the "reins" by which a horse is controlled; this comes from the Latin *retinere,* "to hold back."

research is obviously a compound of "re-" + "search" and is related to the French *recherche,* "search, quest, or pursuit." If research is essentially an inquiry or a quest, why the "re-"? Why not just "search"? This explanation is found in translating the prefix "re-" as "back." We have to "search back" to find something new. We think of researchers as looking ahead, and they do. But they are sitting on the shoulders of the giants of the past. As the Roman Didacus Stella put it, "Pigmaei gigantum humeris impositi plusquam ipsi gigantes vident" ("A dwarf sitting on the shoulders of a giant may see farther than the giant himself").

resection is a near borrowing of the Latin *resectio,* "a trimming or a pruning." In surgery, the meaning of "resection" has been extended to that of "cutting away" for the purpose of removal. Gastric resection is the surgical removal of all or part of the stomach. A related term is **extirpation** (Latin *ex-,* "out," + *stirpes,* "stem or stalk") and another is **eradication** (Latin *e*(*x*)-, "out," + *radix,* "root"). These terms are aptly applied to the thorough surgical removal of lesions by their stalks or their roots.

respiration comes from the Latin *respirare,* "to breathe." The Latin *spirare* also is "to breathe," among more figurative meanings. Why the "re-"? The Romans used *respirare* especially as "to catch one's breath" or "to breathe forcefully, as after combat or other exertion," i.e., "to breathe again." Also, "respiration" conveys the sense of breathing repetitively, which, experience teaches, is a good way to breathe. In biomedical usage, "internal respiration" denotes the exchange of gaseous constituents between a cell and its environment.

retching means an involuntary and unproductive effort to vomit. It comes from the Anglo-Saxon *hraecan,* "to clear one's throat," whence we have also "to hawk up [phlegm]."

rete is Latin for "a net." The term *rete mirabile* ("marvelous network") has been given to an elaborate vascular plexus found at the base of the brain in some animals and formerly believed to exist in man. At the base of the human brain there is a remarkable interconnection of arteries known as the circle of Willis (named after Thomas Willis, a 17th-century English anatomist and physician), but this is not really a counterpart. If one defines *rete mirabile* as a capillary plexus interposed in an arterial channel, then the only example in man is the capillary tuft within the renal glomerulus. The *rete testis* is the network of seminiferous tubules leading from the testis into the vas deferens.

reticulum is the diminutive of the Latin *rete,* "a net," hence "a little net." The term is used in histology to describe a fine network of connective or supporting tissues. A **reticulocyte** is an immature erythrocyte, so called because its cytoplasm, when vitally stained, is seen to contain a fine, basophilic network.

retina is a Latinized term, but no such word exists in classical Latin. Probably it comes from the Latin *rete,* "net," but this cannot be firmly established. Obviously the innermost tunic of the eyeball bears no resemblance to a net. According to Professor H. A. Skinner, Galen described the retina using the Greek *amphiblēstron,* which meant "anything put on or thrown around," as a tunic, though the same word was also used for a fishnet. Galen used the term in the former sense when he described the eye, but translators read the term in the latter sense and took it to be equivalent to the Latin *rete.* "Retina," although of confused origin, still serves adequately in modern anatomy.

retinaculum is the singular of the Latin neuter noun *retinacula,* used in the plural to mean "cable, rope, or tether." This relates to the

Latin verb *retinere,* "to hold back." In anatomy, a retinaculum can be a restraining ligament or a fibrous cord that restrains tendons. In surgery, a retinaculum is a clawed instrument that is used to hold or pull back tissue from the field of operation, as a sort of small retractor.

retractor is related to the Latin adjective *retractus,* "withdrawn," from the verb *retrahere,* "to draw back." The ancients used the term, as we do, to refer to an instrument for holding back structures that would obscure an operative field. Of interest is that the Latin *retrahere* also means "to bring to light again," and this is what a retractor does in the hands of the surgeon.

retro- is a combining form borrowed from the Latin adverb *retro,* "backward, behind, or in the past." In anatomy, "retro-" refers to space, as in **retrobulbar** (+ Latin *bulbus,* "onion"), meaning the space behind the eyeball, which resembles, in shape, a medium-sized onion. In clinical investigation, **retrospective** (+ Latin *spectare,* "to observe") studies are those that evaluate previous experiences; **prospective** (Latin *pro-,* "in front of") studies are those that are planned in advance so as to evaluate forthcoming experiences according to an antecedent protocol.

rhabdo- is a combining form taken from the Greek *rhabdos,* "a stick, rod, or wand," or from the Greek *rhabdōtos,* "striped." There is an obscure genus of rod-shaped microorganisms called **Rhabdomonas** (+ Greek *monas,* "a unit"). More often, in medicine, "rhabdo-" is combined with "myo-" to designate a reference to striated (striped) voluntary muscle, as opposed to "leiomyo-" (+ Greek *leios,* "smooth"), which refers to smooth or involuntary muscle. Thus, a **rhabdomyoma** is a tumor of striated muscle origin, while a **leiomyoma** is a tumor of smooth muscle origin.

rhagades is the plural of the Greek *rhagas,* "a rent or chink," this being related to the Greek verb *rhēgnymi,* "to break open or to burst forth." Originally, "rhagades" was used by the ancients to refer to chapping or excoriations in the skin of the scrotum, pudenda, or anus. Later, the term was extended to cracks or fissures occurring around any bodily orifice subject to movement, including the mouth.

rheumatism is derived from the Greek *rheuma,* "that which flows, as a stream or river." In ancient medical writings, *rheuma* was used to describe any thin or watery discharge from a body surface or orifice. We still refer to a person with watery eyes as being "rheumy-eyed." In the 17th century, "rheumatismos" was applied to an affection of the joints, presumably because various forms of arthritis are marked by effusion into the joint spaces. In modern medicine, an odd circumstance pertains. There is no recognized disease known as **rheumatism,** though lay persons often use the term to describe any sort of stiffness or soreness in the joints. Nevertheless, physicians skilled in musculoskeletal diseases and disorders have dubbed their specialty **rheumatology** (+ Greek *logos,* "a treatise") and style themselves as "rheumatologists." There is, of course, **rheumatic** fever, an acute febrile disease marked by polyarthritis and various immunopathic manifestations related to group-A streptococcal infection. And there is **rheumatoid** (+ Greek *eidos,* "like") arthritis, a term introduced in 1858 by Sir Alfred Garrod (1819–1907), a London physician, to distinguish the condition from acute rheumatic fever and gouty arthritis.

rhexis is a term, now seldom used, that denotes "a rupture." The word is a direct borrowing of the Greek term for a rent or a cleft and is related to the Greek *rhēgnymi,* "to break forth." **Angiorhexis** (+ Greek *a*[*n*]*ggeion,* "a vessel") is rupture of a blood vessel.

Rh factor refers to one of the phenotypic blood groupings. "Rh" stands for "Rhesus," the factor having been first recognized in the red blood cells of rhesus monkeys. It was later found that antibody to the "rhesus factor" agglutinated the erythrocytes of certain persons, who were then identified as being "Rh-positive." The initial letter of "Rh" when referring to the blood factor is customarily capitalized though the name of the monkey is not. The rhesus monkey is a macaque native to India. Presumably, the name was taken from that of Rhesus, the mythical king of ancient Thrace, a realm northeast of Greece whose boundaries were indefinite and may have been thought to extend as far as the home of the monkey.

rhino- is a combining form taken from *rhinos,* the genitive of the Greek *rhis,* "the nose." The **rhinencephalon** (+ Greek *enkephalos,* "the brain") is that part of the cerebral cortex associated with the sense of smell. **Rhinophyma** (+ Greek *phyma,* "a swelling or tumor") is a form of rosacea characterized by a grotesque, nodular enlargement of the nose. **Rhinoplasty** (+ Greek *plassein,* "to form or mold") is a cosmetic operation performed to improve the appearance of the nose. In the vernacular, this is known as a "nose job." **Rhinorrhea** (+ Greek *rhoia,* "a flowing") is a fancy way of characterizing a runny nose.

rhizotomy is the surgical interruption of the sensory or posterior roots of spinal nerves and is performed for the relief of otherwise intractable pain. The term combines the Greek *rhiza,* "a root," + *tomē,* "a cutting." The ancient Greeks had a rhizotomist who practiced *rhizotomos,* but he was not a surgeon. He was a vagrant gatherer of roots and herbs for the preparation of agents used in medicine or in witchcraft (or, perhaps, both at the same time).

rhodopsin is the "visual purple," i.e., the purple-red protein substance in retinal rods that is bleached to "visual yellow" by light, thereby stimulating the sensory nerve endings in the retina. The term combines the Greek *rhodon,* "the rose," + *opsis,* "vision."

rhomboid means "like a rhombus." The Greek *rhombos* was a sort of toy that could be spun around to make a whirring noise. The word also means a figure shaped in such a way that all sides are equal but only the opposite angles are equal: ⬭ "Rhomboid" extends that definition to include an oblique angled, four-sided figure wherein opposite sides and opposite angles are equal: ▱. The rhomboid muscles, major and minor, of the back (originating along the spinous processes and inserting on the scapula) were so named because of their shape.

rhonchus is a near borrowing of the Greek *rho*[*n*]*gchos,* "a snore," this being derived from *rhe*[*n*]*gchō,* "I snore or I snort" (a sort of imitative word). In physical diagnosis, the term denotes the crackling or gurgling sounds emanating from the respiratory tract in which excess mucus or pus has accumulated. Rhonchi are louder and coarser than râles.

rib is probably derived from an obscure Teutonic root word for "strip, spar, lath, or rib." Most Teutonic languages have similar words with these meanings. The classical Latin word for "rib" is *costa.* This yields "coast" as the name for a strip of land that borders the sea.

ribose is a carbohydrate (an aldopentose) that characterizes the nucleic acid found in yeast. The term is derived from **arabinose**, also known as "gum sugar," a similar carbohydrate obtained by acid hydrolysis of certain vegetable gums, such as "gum arabic" (obviously a reference to its origin in Araby). A derivative of ribose is **riboflavin** (+ Latin *flavus,* "yellow"), a vitamin. When this factor was discovered in the 1930s, confusion arose by its being designated vitamin G in the U.S. and vitamine B_2 in Europe. It is now properly known by its name rather than by a letter.

rickets is a disease of children (somewhat similar to osteomalacia in adults) wherein a dysplasia of the developing bone and cartilage results in spinal deformity with twisting and bending of the upper spine and long bones and distortion of the skull. The disease was recognized long before its cause—a dietary deficiency of vitamin D or inadequate exposure to sunlight—was known. The name "rickets" is assumed by most scholars to be derived from the Greek *rhachitis,* "a disease of the spine" (from the Greek *rhaxis,* "spine," + the suffix *-itis*). This has come to us as **rhachitis,** a synonym for "rickets" and not, as the name might suggest, an inflammatory disease. **Rhachi-** is a combining form that denotes relation to the spine. Prof. H. A. Skinner says, probably rightly, that "rickets" comes from the Anglo-Saxon *wricken,* "to twist." Willard Espy, in *Thou Improper, Thou Uncommon Noun* (Clarkson N. Potter, Inc., New York, 1978), adds still another twist to the story. He points out that the 17th-century gossip John Aubrey asserted:

I will whilst 'tis in my mind insert this Remarque, viz., about 1620 one Ricketts of Newberye, a Practitioner in Physick, was excellent at the Curing of Children with swoln heads, and small legges: and the Disease being new, and without a name, He being so famous for the cure of it, they called the Disease the Ricketts . . . and now 'tis good sport to see how they vex their Lexicons, and fetch it from the Greek.

As Espy says, "Those who vexed their lexicons had the right of it." However, there is another, latter-day Dr. Rickets whose name is properly in the medical lexicon.

Howard Taylor Ricketts (1871–1910), an American pathologist, discovered in 1906 the cause and pathogenesis of Rocky Mountain spotted fever and other typhus-like diseases. The infecting microorganisms are now designated as members of the genus **Rickettsia** and the family Rickettsiaceae. In 1910 Dr. Ricketts died in Mexico City of typhus, the disease he had helped explain.

rigor is the Latin word for "stiffness or numbness" and also for "sternness or severity." This, in turn, is related to the Greek *rhigos,* "shivering or shuddering from cold or from horror." Rigorous chills are those attended not only by a sense of cold but also by visible shaking. **Rigor mortis** (+ Latin *mors, mortis,* "death") is the stiffening of a corpse consequent to depletion of adenosine triphosphate in the muscle fibers.

risus is the Latin word for "laughter," being derived from the verb *ridere,* "to laugh." The **risorius** is "the laughing muscle," so named because when contracted it widens the mouth in a laughing posture. **Risus sardonicus** is a pathologic grin due to spasm of the facial muscles, such as occurs in tetanus. It is so named because of the tradition that a poisonous herb found on the island of Sardinia caused a contorted grin on the face of any person in the throes of having been so poisoned. The adjective "sardonic" has come to refer to bitter or scornful derision.

robust describes whoever or whatever is strong and tough. The word is derived from the Latin *robustus,* "oaken." *Robus* is the Latin name for the oak. Anything robust is "sturdy as an oak." At one time a corroborant was a medicine intended to strengthen a patient. To corroborate a statement is to confirm or to strengthen it.

rodent is derived from the Latin *rodere,* "to gnaw, to corrode." A rodent ulcer was at one time so called because it appeared to eat away at surrounding tissues, with no tendency to heal. This is now recognized as a form of skin cancer.

rouleaux is the plural of the French *rouleau,* "a roll." The term was first used for a cylindrical stack of coins and later, because of the resemblance, for the manner in which agglutinated red blood cells were observed to gather in stacked clumps.

rubella is the feminine form of the Latin adjective *rubellus,* a "reddish" color. Beginning in the 16th century, a form of measles was called "rubella" because of its characteristic red rash. This is now known as "German measles," having been recognized as an entity by German physicians in the mid-18th century. It is also sometimes called "three-day measles" because of the typical duration of the rash. **Rubeola** (the diminutive of the Latin *ruber,* "red") has been adopted as a quasi-scientific name for ordinary measles, wherein the rash usually lasts about seven days. Both forms of measles affect mainly children in populations where most adults are immune, and in children both diseases are relatively benign. Rubella is now more feared because of its teratogenic effect in women who contract the disease early in pregnancy. There is no etymologic difference between the terms "rubella" and "rubeola," but they serve a useful purpose in distinguishing the two similar, yet distinct, contagious diseases. Another disease whose name is taken from the color of its rash is **scarlatina.** The name comes through the Italian *scarlatto* from the Persian *saqalat,* a kind of rich scarlet cloth. Scarlatina is sometimes considered a mild form of scarlet fever, an exanthematous manifestation of streptococcal infection.

rugae literally means "many wrinkles" and is a direct borrowing from the Latin. The **rugal** folds of the stomach lining give a distinctly wrinkled appearance. The singular of the feminine Latin noun is *ruga.* From the same Latin source comes the adjective "corrugated," as it refers to the alternating grooves and ridges of a sheet of paper or metal. Creating a rugous surface is one of nature's ways of increasing the surface area within a limited lumen.

rupture comes from the Latin *ruptus,* "a break or rent," this being the past participle of the verb *rumpere,* "to break down, break open, or burst through." "Rupture" is a common and serviceable word for hernia; both are of classical origin, the difference being that lay persons use "rupture" and doctors use "hernia."

℞ is the symbol used in pharmacy for the Latin *recipe,* this being the imperative of the verb *recipere,* which in this context means "to take." Physicians traditionally write this symbol at the head of a prescription to say, in effect, "Take thou this!" But there is more to it than that. The letter "R" alone could stand for *recipe.* What about the mark that crosses the tail of the "R" to make "℞"? This is said to be significant of the astrological sign of Jupiter: ♃. At one time it was believed that to precede a formula with the Jupiter's sign, as a sort of invocation, would assure a favorable result. Moreover, according to astrologers, the period during the ascendancy of the planet Jupiter was thought to be a good time to gather herbs and concoct medicines.

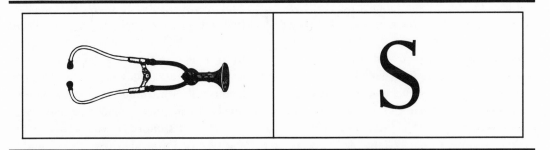

sabot is French for "a boot or shoe." In medical parlance, a **coeur sabot** is a boot-shaped heart and refers to the anteroposterior radiographic silhouette in cases of left ventricular hypertrophy, wherein the cardiac apex extends up and to the left, suggesting the toe of a boot.

sac is an abbreviation of the Latin *saccus,* "a bag or pouch," this being related to the Greek *sakkos,* "a coarse cloth made of hair." Usually this was goat's hair, and when fashioned into a pouch, the cloth could be used for straining a fluid, such as wine. Numerous pouch-like structures in embryology and anatomy are referred to as "sacs." The diminutive **sacculus** is used to designate small pouches, such as the alveolar saccules of the lung.

sacchar- is a combining form taken from the Latin *saccharum* and the Greek *sakcharon,* both meaning "sugar." The Greek term is not native but seems to have come from an oriental source. **Saccharin** is a synthetic coal-tar derivative that is intensely sweet and has been used as a noncaloric substitute for sugar. **Saccharomyces** (+ Greek *mykēs,* "fungus") is the genus constituting yeasts that cause fermentation of sugars and other carbohydrates.

sacrum is derived from the Latin *sacer,* "holy or consecrated." The large, heavy bone at the base of the spine was called *os sacrum* by the Romans and *hieron ostoun* by the Greeks, both meaning "sacred bone." Why sacred? One explanation often given is that the ancients observed that, because of its bulk, the sacrum appeared to be the last of the bones of an interred corpse to decay; hence this bone must be the nidus around which a body would be reassembled in an afterlife. Another explanation is that the Greek *hieron* could also mean "a temple," and that within the concavity of the large bone at the base of the spine lay the sacred organs of procreation. Finally, the shape of the bone may have resembled a vessel used in sacrifice, or the bone itself may have been used in some sort of sacred rite.

sadism is a perverted penchant for inflicting pain, usually in a sexual context. The term is taken from the name of a French writer, Count Donatien Alphonse François de Sade, who lived from 1740 to 1814. During service with the army, he acquired a reputation for being addicted to vicious practices. His literary works were marked by unrelieved obscenity. He was confined to the Bastille as a mentally deranged prisoner. While there he was given to mad harangues and insisted on being addressed as the Marquis de Sade.

Saint Vitus was a Roman lad who suffered martyrdom together with his tutor, Modestus, and his nurse, Crescentia, during the persecutions of the Emperor Diocletian in the 3rd century A.D. During the 15th and 16th centuries, it became the custom, particularly in Germany, for children to dance around statues of Saint Vitus in supplication of good health. The dancing often reached a peak of agitated frenzy. "Saint Vitus's dance" became a name for involuntary writhing movements now known as **athetosis** (Greek *athetos,* "not fixed"), a symptom also called **chorea** (Greek *choreia,* "dance"). There are various choreas of different causes. Most of them are associated with lesions in the caudate nucleus and putamen.

salpinx is an almost direct borrowing of the Greek word for "a trumpet." It was only natural that the term would be applied to anatomic structures of a tubular configuration with a flared, bell-shaped end. There are two such. The better known is the uterine or Fallopian tube, whose flared end embraces the ovary (much as a mute or sordine in the bell of a trumpet). Inflammation of the Fallopian tube is called **salpingitis** (a sort of "hot trumpet"). The second is the auditory or Eustachian tube that connects the pharynx with the tympanic cavity or middle ear. We no longer call this tube a "salpinx," but the term is preserved in the name of the salpingopharyngeal muscle, also called the levator palati. This muscle serves in two helpful ways. It widens and elevates the pharynx as we swallow a bolus of food, and it helps to open the pharyngeal orifice of the Eustachian tube when it is temporarily blocked.

salts owe their collective name to the Latin *sal,* "salt." However, it was not until the 18th century that salts were recognized as compounds formed by an interaction of acids and bases. In 1787 a committee of French chemists, including the famed Antoine Laurent Lavoisier (1743–1794), proposed a nomenclature for salts according to the acids and bases from which they are derived. This is the system we use today.

salve is derived from the Anglo-Saxon *sealf,* "a healing ointment." The German word is *Salbe,* which probably relates to the Gothic *salbōn,* "to anoint." The sense of healing brings to mind the Latin *salvere,* "to be in good health." Incidentally, a "salver" is a small dish on which delicacies are served. This harks back to the dark days of yore when a small portion of a meal was placed on a dish and eaten first by an expendable servant known as a "salver." If the salver survived and showed no ill effect, the food was deemed safe and could be served to the company at large. The name of the servant to whom others owned their salvation was later transferred to the dish.

sanguineous means "bloody" and comes from the Latin *sanguis,* "blood." But many people forget the "e" in "sanguineous." The "e" must be there for both the right spelling and the correct pronunciation. According to ancient humoral pathology, anyone with a preponderance of blood was thought to be of an optimistic temperament, hence our use of "sanguine" as an adjective meaning cheerful or full of hope.

saphenous is a term applied to but one anatomic structure, and that is the saphenous vein, the longest vein in the body, extending in the leg all the way from the foot to the groin. The origin of the term is confusing and somewhat contradictory. The spelling suggests a derivation from the Greek *saphēneia,* "clearness," in the intellectual sense of "the true picture." But this is anything but the true picture of the vein in question. A better explanation is that the name originated in the Arabic *al safin,* "the hidden" (which the vein is, in the tissues of the leg). The Arabic term was then mistakenly given a classical Greek spelling by some benighted scribe.

sapid refers to whatever gives a sensation of taste or flavor. Sapid substances are those which can be perceived by their characteristic taste or smell. The word is derived from the Latin *sapere,* "to have taste, smell, or

flavor." To the Romans, the meaning extended to embrace sensibility generally, and the Latin adjective *sapiens* means "sensible, wise, judicious, and discriminating." Man distinguishes himself (and flatters himself) by referring to his own species as **Homo** (Latin for "person or being") **sapiens.**

sarcoma is from the Greek root *sarko,* "flesh," + *-ōma,* "tumor." A sarcoma is a malignant growth in tissues of mesenchymal origin; hence, most sarcomas are "fleshy tumors," From the same source comes "sarcasm," an utterance intended to "cut the flesh," and "sarcophagus," a box or container intended to "swallow the flesh," i.e., a coffin. **Sarcoid** (+ Greek *eidos,* "like") refers to whatever is "fleshy," but more specifically the term designates a disease characterized by the formation of exuberant granulomas found in the lymph nodes, the liver, the spleen, and other tissues.

sartorius is the name for the long, thin muscle that extends from the anterior superior spine of the ilium to the medial side of the proximal end of the tibia. In contracting it helps to bring the thigh into the cross-legged position assumed by a tailor as he sits at his work. The name of the muscle is taken from the Latin *sartor,* "a tailor."

sassafras is an aromatic substance obtained from the bark of the root of the laurel tree, *Sassafras albidum.* Nowadays, sassafras is used as a flavoring agent in beverages and candy, but formerly it was regarded as a medicinal herb, whence comes its name. "Sassafras" may be a Spanish corruption of the Latin *saxifraga,* this being derived from a combination of *saxum,* "a rock," + *fran-*

gere, "to break into pieces." The presumed explanation is that a decoction of sassafras was supposed to exert a diuretic effect that was thought to be helpful in dislodging calculi in the urinary bladder. Hence, the name means "stone crusher."

saturnine describes a person of a sluggish, gloomy, cold, and taciturn temperament. The mythologic Saturn was a Roman deity, identified with the Greek Kronos (Time), husband of Rhea, who devoured all of his children except Jupiter (Air), Neptune (Water), and Pluto (the Grave)—these Time cannot consume. Astrologers asserted that those born under the sign of Saturn are by nature cold, sluggish, and baleful. In alchemy, Saturn became identified with lead, a heavy, sluggish metal. And in the astronomy of the day, Saturn was given as the name for what was thought to be the outermost planet that "moved slowly in its sullen orbit." In 18th-century Europe and in England there occurred an epidemic of what was called "saturnine gout." Remarkably, this affected only imbibers of port and Madeira, the so-called fortified wines which were imported from Iberia (Spain and Portugal); those who swilled common gin were spared. Fortified wines were those to which brandy was added, the brandy being distilled in apparatus equipped with lead tubing. Another outbreak of "saturnine gout" was noted in the southern U.S., where the local "moonshine" was contaminated with lead. It is now recognized that lead blocks the urinary excretion of uric acid and thus provokes attacks of gouty arthritis in susceptible tipplers.

satyriasis is an excessive venereal impulse in men, the counterpart of **nymphomania** in women. Just as female nymphs seductively cavorted in the mythologic sylvan glades, so male satyrs sought to satisfy what they perceived as a demand for their services. The satyrs, usually depicted in Roman sculpture as hybrids of men and goats, were companions of Bacchus, the god of wine, and were much given to revelry and lasciviousness.

scabies is the Latin word for "the itch" and is related to the verb *scabere,* "to scratch," and, probably, to the Greek verb *skaptein,* "to dig." To the Romans, *scabies* originally meant any itchy, mangy disease of the skin. A common cause of such a condition, the itch mite, was described in the 12th century and is now known as *Sarcoptes scabiei* (the name of the genus being a combination of the Greek *sarx,* "the flesh," + *koptō,* "I smite or cut"). "Scabies" now specifically denotes the skin lesions produced by this mite. **Scab** comes from the Anglo-Saxon *scaeb,* "the crust on a sore." Because sores in the skin often are the consequence of excoriation, doubtless there is a relation to the Latin *scabies.*

scala in Latin means "a ladder or flight of steps." The Romans always used the plural, *scalae.* The scala tympani (Latin *tympanum,* "drum") and the scala vestibuli (Latin *vestibulum,* "entrance or forecourt"), parts of the cochlea, were so named because of their fancied resemblance to a circular staircase.

scald comes through the Italian *scaldare,* "to heat," as a shortened form of the Latin *excaldare,* "to wash in hot water," this being a combination of *ex-,* "out," + *calidus* or *caldus,* "hot."

scalenus is a near borrowing of the Greek *skalēnos,* "uneven or irregular." *Trigōnon skalēnon* was a triangle with uneven sides. The three (sometimes four) scalene muscles extend on either side from the cervical vertebrae to the first and second ribs. As a group they are of irregular triangular shape. The scalenus anticus syndrome involves pain in the shoulder, arm, and neck resulting from compression of nerves and vessels between a cervical rib and a tight anterior scalenus muscle.

scalpel is a slight abbreviation of the Latin *scalpellum,* "a small knife," this being the diminutive of *scalprum,* "a chisel or a knife," and related to the Latin verb *scalpere,* "to carve." The instrument the surgeon uses to cut is simply a small knife, but it takes on a special aura when summoned by the surgeon: "Scalpel!" This is a signal that the operation is to begin.

scaphoid is an adjective derived from the Greek *skaphē,* "anything scooped out, as a trough, a bowl, or a light boat." The root verb is *skaptein,* "to dig." From this same source comes the Latin *scapha* and the English "skiff," both words for a light, open boat. One of the carpal bones is called the "scaphoid" because it has a hollowed surface (to fit the head of an adjacent bone). A thin person, when supine, appears to have a boat-shaped belly that is referred to as a scaphoid abdomen.

scapula was always used by the Romans as the Latin plural *scapulae,* "the shoulder blades" and also "the shoulders or upper part of the back." The term probably relates to the Greek *skaptein,* "to dig," because the broad, flat shape of the shoulder blades suggests a sort of trowel or spade.

schisto-, schizo- are combining forms taken from the Greek *schizō,* "I split or cleave." **Schistocytosis** (+ Greek *kytos,* "cell") is a condition wherein fragments of cleaved erythrocytes are observed in the blood, as in hemolytic anemia. **Schistosomiasis** is an infection by trematodes or blood flukes of the genus *Schistosoma* (+ Greek *sōma,* "body"). The male of this fluke has a deep cleft, the gynecophoric (female-carrying) canal, extending the length of his body; here the slender female is held during copulation. **Schizophrenia** (+ Greek *phrēn,* "the mind") is a term introduced in 1911 by Paul Eugen Bleuler (1857–1939), a Swiss psychiatrist, to characterize a form of dementia praecox in which the afflicted person seems to exhibit a "split personality." It is important to remember that the "sch-" in all terms including "schisto-" or "schizo-," represents the Greek letters sigma and chi (*not* the German "sch-") and always should be pronounced as "sk," not "sh."

sciatic is derived from a Latinized corruption of the Greek *ischiadikos,* "subject to trouble in the hips or loins," this being taken from *ischion,* "the hip joint." The long, thick, sciatic nerve (also known as the *nervus ischiadicus*) extends from the sacrum down the back of the thigh.

scirrhous is an adjective taken from the Greek *skiros* or *skirros,* "hard." The Greek word was used also for gypsum or stucco. Galen is said to have used the term "scirrhus" for an indurated, fixed, painful tumor or swelling, but he distinguished this from "cancer." Today, "scirrhous" describes any lesion of a hard, tough consistency.

sclera is the name for the tough, fibrous, outermost tunic of the eyeball and is taken from the Greek *skleros,* "hard or tough." **Sclero-** is a combining form, similarly derived. **Sclerosis** is a term used in pathology to describe a degenerative process marked by hardening. **Scleredema** (+ Greek *oidēma,* "swelling") is an indurated turgidity of subcutaneous tissues. **Scleroderma** (+ Greek *derma,* "skin") is a systemic disease of connective tissue that results in a hardening or stiffening not only of the skin but also of the viscera. When the disease is widespread it is called "progressive systemic sclerosis." **Sclerotherapy** (+ Greek *therapeia,* "service or care") is the injection of irritant solutions to induce scarring and obliteration of varicose veins, as in hemorrhoids or in the esophagus.

scoliosis is an almost direct borrowing of the Greek *skoliōsis,* "a bending or a curvature." The term appears in Hippocratic writings to denote any sort of curvature, but now it is restricted to a lateral curvature of the spine.

-scope is a combining form, usually a suffix, taken from the Greek *skopein,* which, it is commonly held, means "to see or to view." But more than that, it means observing for a purpose. To the ancient Greeks, *skopein* meant "to look out for, to examine, to monitor." As it turns out, those are the functions of most instruments whose names end in "-scope," even the **stethoscope** (Greek *stethos,* "the chest"), the use of which is to examine or monitor the contents of the chest.

scorbutus is a Medieval Latin term for "scurvy." As such, it is said to have been taken from the Teutonic word *schaarbuyck,* this being a combination of *schaar,* "torn or ruptured," + *buyck,* "belly." This seems a bit farfetched inasmuch as neither rupture nor even swelling of the belly is a symptom of scurvy, now recognized as a manifestation of vitamin C deficiency. Of course, it is possible that in earlier times scurvy may have been confused with other nutritional deficiencies, notably protein deprivation, of which swelling of the belly can be a prominent symptom, especially in children. Whatever cures scurvy is known as an **ascorbutic** agent, hence the name **ascorbic** acid for vitamin C. "Scurvy" is somewhat of a misnomer, too. It is an adjectival derivative of "scurf," a scaly exfoliation of the skin which is not a symptom of vitamin C deficiency as we know it today. Again, when scurvy was so named it may well have been mixed up with other expressions of malnutrition.

scotoma is derived from the Greek *skotos,* "darkness or gloom." The Greeks used the term *skotodinia* to denote dizziness, probably because severe giddiness often is accompanied by ephemeral loss of vision or "dark spots before the eyes." Today, "scotoma" means an area of diminished or suppressed acuity in the visual field. A variant is "scintillating scotoma," wherein there is a luminous appearance before the eyes, sometimes as shining spots and sometimes as a serrated, wall-like outline. The latter is called **teichopsia** from a combination of the Greek *teichos,* "a city wall" of the type that is crenellated as a fortification, + *opsis,* "vision."

scrofula is a now almost archaic term for tuberculous swelling of the cervical lymph glands. It is the diminutive of the Latin *scrofa,* "a breeding sow." Apparently someone fancied that the puffy visage of a patient with cervical lymphadenopathy resembled that of a little pig.

scrotum seems to be a transliterated variant of the Latin adjective *scorteus,* "of leather," the allusion being to a pouch made of leather.

sebum is a direct borrowing of the Latin word for "tallow, suet, or grease." Probably it is related to the Latin *sus,* "hog." The derived adjective is **sebaceous,** as applied to a fatty cyst or to an oil-producing gland in the skin. **Seborrhea** (+ Greek *rhoia,* "a flow") is excessive elaboration of oil by the skin.

secretion is derived from *secretus,* the past participle of the Latin verb *secernere,* "to separate, one from another." It was from *secretus,* "that which is separated," that the name **secretin** was contrived for the first hormone, discovered in 1902 by the English physiologists W. M. Bayliss (1860–1924) and E. H. Starling (1866–1927). Secretin is a potent stimulus to the flow of water and bicarbonate from the pancreas. In strict usage, secretion denotes the elaboration of a substance that acts for a specific purpose within an organism, while excretion denotes the elaboration or separation of a substance intended to be discharged from an organism.

section comes from the Latin *sectio, sectionis,* "a cutting off." To the Romans this often referred to the auctioning off of confiscated property. In anatomy, a section is a slice of tissue cut away for gross or microscopic examination. In surgery, a section or a sectioning is a division of a tissue. A **Caesarean section** is the surgical opening of the uterus for the extraction of a baby.

sedative comes from the Latin *sedare,* "to allay, to calm." In pharmacy, a sedative drug is one that helps a patient to settle down by allaying excessive excitement. From time immemorial, potions have been concocted to induce lethargy or sleep. Among the earliest of the more modern sedative agents were the bromides and chloral hydrate (trichloracetic aldehyde), introduced in the mid-19th century. The popular use of bromides (an effervescent concoction with the trade name "Bromo-Seltzer" was once commonly dispensed at soda fountains) led to the coining of "bromide" to refer to a trite remark uttered by a tiresome person. In the first half of the present century, various derivatives of barbituric acid were the most widely used sedative agents. In recent years it has been more fashionable to use **tranquilizers** (Latin *tranquillare,* "to calm or to make quiet"). **Sediment** comes from a different Latin word, *sedere,* "to sit," and refers to an insoluble substance that settles out or down from a fluid mixture. The **sedimentation rate** measures the extent to which erythrocytes settle out or down from a column of anticoagulated blood.

segment is an abbreviated form of the Latin *segmentum,* "a trimming." To the Romans this meant a flounce or brocade attached to a garment as a trimming. In anatomy, a segment is a defined portion of a larger structure.

sella turcica is Latin for "a Turkish saddle." The Latin *sella* means "a chair or stool." Roman horsemen used no saddle but rode on a cover tied to the back of a horse and called an *ephippium,* "that which is put on a horse." The saddles in which the Turks and Arabs rode had supports, front and rear, and it is from the resemblance to such a saddle that the fossa in the sphenoid bone containing the pituitary gland is named. The anterior and posterior extensions of this fossa are called the **clinoid** processes, from the Greek *klinē,* "a couch or bed," + *eidos,* "like." They look a little like bedposts.

semen is a direct borrowing of the Latin word for "seed or germ" and designates the fluid that conveys the male spermatozoa. From the same Latin source comes the word **disseminate,** literally "to scatter seed," although the scattering may give rise to things as disparate as tumors and knowledge. A **seminar** is a gathering of thinkers where new and fruitful ideas are examined. Those who give rise to original ideas are called **seminal** thinkers.

semester is taken from the Latin *semestris* or *semenstris,* these being composites of *sex,* "six," + *menstruus,* "monthly," thereby denoting a six-month period or whatever occurs at a six-month interval. The "sem-" in the word has nothing to do with "semi-," as in "semiannual," and it is only a coincidence that a six-month period and a semiannual period are the same. A **trimester** is a three-month period. Again, only by coincidence is this one-third of the usual period of human gestation.

semi- is the Latin prefix denoting "a half" and is equivalent to the Greek derivative, *hemi-.* "Semi-" has been attached to various medical terms to indicate half of something. The semicircular canals of the ear are so named because of their shape. Certain structures are described as **semilunar** because they are shaped like a half-moon. The semimembranous and semitendinous muscles of the thigh are composed almost half of connective tissue. Sometimes "semi-" is fallaciously used to mean "sort of" or "not quite," as in "semimalignant." This is as ludicrous as would be "semipregnant."

senile comes from the Latin adjective *senilis,* "aged or old." **Senescent** is taken from the Latin verb *senescere,* "to grow old." The Romans had an exalted view of advanced age, and their *senatus* was "a revered council of elders."

senna is a cathartic substance obtained from the dried leaves or pods of the plant *Cassia acutifolia.* "Senna" comes from the Arabic *sana,* "acute," and refers to the sharply pointed leaves of the plant (as does the Latin *acutifolia*).

sepsis is a derivative of the Greek *sēpsis,* "putrefaction," though the meaning has changed. The Greek term was used by ancient writers to mean the culmination of inflammation in corruption and rottenness. Today, "sepsis" means a condition of illness marked by the noxious effect of toxic products of microbial infection.

septum is a Latin word (sometimes spelled *saeptum*) for "a dividing wall or an enclosure." The related Latin verb is *sepire (saepire),* "to fence in." The Latin noun being neuter, the plural is "septa." The term is used in anatomy and pathology to describe various wall-like or dividing structures, such as the nasal septum and the interventricular septum of the heart. **Septate** describes whatever is divided.

sequestrum is the Latin word for "a thing surrendered or deposited for safekeeping." In skeletal pathology, a sequestrum is a particle of dead bone that has become separated, by injury or disease, from the adjacent healthy bone.

serendipity occasionally accounts for a fortuitous discovery or diagnosis. More than mere luck is implied by serendipity. The encounter is unexpected but is turned to advantage by a prepared mind. The word comes from Horace Walpole's 18th-century version of *The Three Princes of Serendip.* Serendip is an old name for Ceylon, now Sri Lanka. The princes had a knack for making remarkable discoveries they were not seeking.

serpiginous is an adjective derived from the Latin *serpere,* "to creep, to crawl, or to spread slowly." An ulcer that spreads slowly is said to be serpiginous. While the related Latin noun *serpens* means "a creeping thing, as a snake or serpent," the term "serpiginous" refers to the mode of spreading, not to the shape. A structure or lesion that appears shaped like a serpent is properly described as serpentine.

serratus is the Latin word for "notched," taken from the Latin noun *serra,* "a saw." The serratus muscles of the back and thorax have interdigitating slips that resemble the notches on the cutting edge of a saw. Any finely notched border can be referred to as serrated.

serum is the Latin word for "whey." Milk, when it coagulates, as in the making of cheese, separates into solid clumps (curds) and a slightly turbid, watery liquid (whey). It was such a dish that little Miss Muffet was eating when she took offense at the proximity of the spider who sat down beside her. "Whey" is of Anglo-Saxon origin. The Latin *serum* may be related to the Sanskrit *sara,* "flowing." The use of "serum" to designate the watery residue of clotted blood, as analogous to whey, dates back to the 17th century. Serum differs from plasma in that it lacks fibrinogen, which has been consumed in the clotting process.

sesamoid relates to the Greek *sēsamon,* "the sesame plant." The tendons of certain muscles, particularly those in the hands and feet, may be inlaid with small bony nodules which were fancied to resemble sesame seeds; hence they were called sesamoid (*sesam-* + *eidos,* "like") bones.

sex is a word of obscure origin. According to one explanation it is a shortening of the Latin *sexus* (not to be confused with the Latin *sex,* "six"), which is related to the Latin verb *secare,* "to cut or to divide." The word thus denotes a division of living beings into male and female. Another hypothesis has it that "sex" is related to the Latin *secus,* "otherwise." In Latin *secus muliebre* (the second word means "womanly") are females and *secus viriles* (the second word means "manly") are males.

siderosis is a condition marked by an accumulation of excess iron in the tissues of the body. The term is derived from the Greek *sidēros,* "iron." Curiously, we use the Latin *ferrum* as a root for designating iron-containing compounds, but we use the Greek *sidēros* for terms pertaining to abnormalities in iron metabolism. **Sideropenia** (+ Greek *penēs,* "poverty-stricken") is a deficiency of iron in the body. **Sideroblastic** (+ Greek *blastos,* "a bud or germinal form") anemia is characterized by the presence of abnormal, "ringed" sideroblasts in the bone marrow, signifying impaired utilization of iron and, hence, deficient red cells in the circulating blood.

sigmoid is taken from the Greek letter sigma (Σ), equivalent to "S," to which is added *-eidos,* "like." "Sigmoid" describes whatever is Σ-shaped or S-shaped. The best example is the sigmoid segment of the distal colon, which is typically coiled like the letter "S."

sine qua non is a Latin phrase meaning "without which nothing." Whatever is *sine qua non* is indispensable. A feature of a disease that is essential to its diagnosis or to its expression is a *sine qua non.* Gastric acid secretion is a *sine qua non* of peptic ulcer disease.

singultus is medicalese for "hiccup." It is a Latin word meaning "a gasp or a sob," especially occurring in series. *Singultus,* in turn, is related to the Latin adjective *singuli,* "one at a time."

sinister is the Latin word for "left" but, in its English usage, has come to mean "evil or corrupt." This pervasive association of "right" with right and "left" with wrong has been noted in the comment on the word **adroit**. In addition to the tyranny of the majority of right-handed persons exercised over the minority of left-handers, there is another explanation for the ill repute of "left." In Greek augury, the augur faced north, and because on his right was the east with its auspicious connotation, whatever was on his left was deemed unfavored.

sinus is a Latin word meaning "a concave or hollowed-out surface" and also "a pocket, purse, valley, or gulf." The related Latin verb is *sinuare,* "to wind, curve, or arch," from which we derive "sinuous" and "insinuate." In anatomy, "sinus" is used to designate subsidiary cavities which open into larger spaces, e.g., the nasal sinuses. In some instances the term has been extended to refer to widened channels, e.g., venous sinuses. The hybrid term **sinusoid** (+ Greek *eidos,* "like") is similarly used.

Sister Mary Joseph node is a lump or nodule that becomes externally visible or palpable at the umbilicus. It is so called from the name of the nursing nun at Saint Mary's Hospital, in Rochester, Minnesota, who often assisted Dr. William Mayo at operations. It was she who observed the lump when preparing a patient's abdomen for operation, and Dr. Mayo identified the nodule as a metastatic growth from peritoneal carcinomatosis.

skeleton is derived from the Greek *skellō,* "I dry up, parch, or wither." It has been said that the Greeks applied the term to a mummy or a withered corpse, not to the bony framework of the body. So far as the records indicate, it was during the 16th century that "skeleton" was given its modern meaning.

skull is of Scandinavian descent and harks back to such Nordic words as *skál* and *skul,* which meant "bowl or shell." Some say the ultimate origin is in the Teutonic *skal,* "to cleave." The traditional Nordic toast "Skoal!" has been said to derive from the ancient word for skull and the supposed custom of using the inverted dome of the skull to contain ceremonial potions. More likely the call for a toast comes from the Old Norse *skál,* meaning "bowl."

slough comes from the Middle English *slughe,* "the cast-off skin of a snake." In medicine, the term refers to a mass of necrotic tissue that separates, as a result of injury or disease, from a living part or organ.

smegma is the Greek word for "a soap or wax used in cleaning or polishing." The Greek root verb is *smaō,* "I smear or rub." The accretion of fatty discharge under the prepuce from the sebaceous glands at the corona of the penis is called smegma.

solecism is not a medical term, but it is a word worth noting in any book on words and their usage. A solecism is a mistaken use of words or error in grammar, usually for want of knowing better. The inhabitants of the remote Greek colony of Soloi spoke what proper Athenians regarded as atrocious Greek and derided as being *soloikismos,* that is, characteristic of those ignorant oafs of Soloi.

soleus is a masculinized form of the Latin *solea,* which means "the underside or flat of the foot," and also "a sandal" (conforming to the shape of the foot) and "the sole-fish" (shaped similarly). The soleus muscle in the calf of the leg was so named because of its fancied resemblance to the fish.

soma is a direct borrowing of the Greek *sōma,* originally "a corpse" but, later, "a body, dead or living." The Greeks used *sōma* particularly as opposed to *psychē,* "the soul." In like manner we have contrived **psychosomatic** to refer to the interplay between the corporeal substance and the mind.

somnus is the Latin word for "sleep." In Roman mythology, Somnus is the name given to the god of sleep, who, with his brother, Mors (Death), and his father, Nox (Night), lived at the western edge of the world, where the sun is seen to set. A **somnambulist** (+ Latin *ambulare,* "to walk") is one who walks in his sleep, and a **somniloquist** (+ Latin *loqui,* "to speak") is one who talks in his sleep. A **somnifacient** (+ Latin *facere,* "to make or to bring about") is an agent that induces sleep, as employed for the benefit of one who suffers from **insomnia** (Latin *in-,* "lacking"). Another Latin word, *sopor,* means "a deep sleep or stupor," and this, combined with *facere,* gives us **soporific** as a term for a drug that induces sleep.

sound is an English word that can have almost fifty different uses, many of them of different origins and several with medical implications. To be sound in body and mind (or, as some would say today, "to have it all together") relates to the Latin *sanus,* "healthy and rational." Heart sounds, as perceived by means of a stethoscope, relate to the Latin *sonus,* "a noise or tone." A sound used as a probing instrument takes its name from the French *sonder,* "to fathom or to explore." In nautical parlance, a sound (or the French *sonde*) is a weighted line dropped from a boat to measure the depth of the underlying water. This may have been derived from a sort of garbled contraction of the Latin *sub-,* "under," + *unda,* "water or wave."

spasm is taken from the Greek *spasmos,* "a convulsion." Hippocrates used this word in reference to an epileptic fit. The Greek root verb is *spaō,* "I draw out or draw tight." While the Greek word could mean either "to stretch out" or "to tense up," the medical use of the term is usually restricted to the latter sense.

species is a direct borrowing, but with altered meaning, of the Latin word for "view, image, or appearance." The Indo-European root is thought to be *spek-,* "to look keenly." In taxonomy, those entities that have a similar appearance or structure are grouped together as species. An anatomic or pathologic **specimen** is looked at keenly as representative of whatever is being studied. Doctors who have the same particular interest or who perform the same procedures are categorized as specialists.

speculum is the Latin word for "mirror," in which to see a *species* (an image). In medical diagnosis, a speculum is an instrument by which a passage or cavity in the body can be examined. The mirrored instrument that a dentist uses is a true speculum. Most specula used to examine the ear, the nose,

the vagina, or the anus are cylindrical or bivalved tubes that do not have mirrors.

sperm is a slight contraction of the Greek *sperma,* "the seed or germ of anything." The **spermatozoa** (+ Greek *zōon,* "a living animal") are the male seeds of animals. A **spermacide** (+ Latin *caedere,* "to strike down or to slay") is an agent that is destructive to sperm.

sphenoid is the name of a prominent bone at the base of the skull. The name is taken from the Greek *sphēn,* "a wedge," + *eidos,* "like." Galen described the bone as being "like a wedge thrust between the skull and the superior maxilla."

sphincter comes from the name of the Sphinx, which, according to Greek myth, was a monster that had the body of a lion and the head and breast of a woman. The Sphinx was perched on a rock outside Thebes and there posed unanswerable riddles to passing travelers. A wrong answer or no answer at all elicited an asphyxiating embrace by the Sphinx, hence the allusion to the squeezing function of a sphincter muscle. The Sphinx met its match when Oedipus passed by. The challenging riddle: "There is a thing on earth that has four, two, then three feet. Of all the creatures that creep on the earth or move in the air or in the sea, it alone changes its nature—when it moves on the largest number of its feet, the strength in its limbs is the smallest. What is this creature?" Quickly came Oedipus' answer: "Man, who as a helpless babe crawls 'on all fours,' then stands erect on 'his own two feet' as a man, but with age requires a cane or crutch, the third leg." In a fury of frustration, the Sphinx squeezed itself to death.

sphygmomanometer is contrived by combining the Greek *sphygmos,* "the beating of the heart or the pulse," + "manometer," the origin of which is given elsewhere in this book. A sphygmomanometer measures not the frequency of the pulse but, as its name implies, the pulse pressure that is commonly called blood pressure. The instrument, essentially as we know it today, was introduced in 1896 by Scipione Riva-Rocci (1863–1937), an Italian clinician.

spica is the name given to a bandage applied by figure-of-eight turns that overlap in a sort of chevron pattern. The pattern might be thought to resemble the overlapping coverings of an ear of grain; hence, the name is taken from the Latin *spica,* "an ear of grain."

spine comes from the Latin *spina,* "a thorn or a prickly bush." The Romans used this word for the backbone because the series of vertebrae has so many bony protuberances. It was fancied to resemble a thorny twig.

spirochete is a hybrid term wherein the Latin *spira,* "a coil, as of a serpent," is combined with the Greek *chaitē,* "long, flowing hair." The spirochete is an organism that resembles a coil of hair. In 1905 Fritz Schaudinn (1871–1906), a German bacteriologist, discovered the causative organism of syphilis. It was found to be a spirochete (the type having been named earlier), which Schaudinn named *Treponema* (Greek *trepō,* "I turn," + *nēma,* "a thread") *pallida* (Latin for "pale").

splanchnic comes from the Greek *splan*[*n*]*gchna,* "the entrails," and refers to whatever pertains to the viscera. Thus, the splanchnic nerves and vessels serve the internal organs.

spleen is a near borrowing of the Greek *splēn* as the name for the parenchymatous organ, situated high in the left hypochondrium, which serves in the regulation of cellular elements in the blood. The Latin name for the organ, *lien,* appears to be almost the Greek name, with the "sp" lopped off. Possibly they both relate to the Sanskirt *plihan.* An archaic Teutonic term for the spleen is *milt,* preserved in the German *Milz.* This, in turn, may relate to the Icelandic *melta,* "to digest." The ancients had no concept of the function of the spleen. Because it is situated in close company with the stomach, they may have assumed that it served, in some way, in the digestive process.

spondylo- is a combining form taken from the Greek *spondylos,* "a vertebra" or "any round body, such as the weight that twirls a spindle." **Spondylitis** is an inflammation of a vertebra. **Spondylolisthesis** (+ Greek *olisthos,* "slipperiness") is a forward displacement of one vertebra over another, usually of the fifth lumbar vertebra over the sacrum.

sporadic comes from the Greek *sporadikos,* "scattered," this being related to the verb *speirō,* "I sow." A sporadic disease is one that occurs here and there in space or now and then in time, as opposed to a disease that is either endemic or epidemic in a place or in a population. Incidentally, Sporades is the name given to two groups of Greek islands scattered about the Aegean Sea.

spore is derived from the Greek *spora,* "the sowing of seed." Originally the term was applied to plant seeds and to offspring. In the mid-19th century, it was appreciated that certain bacteria could survive unfavorable conditions by developing resistant forms called "spores" that then gave rise to further generations of the organism.

sprain may have come through the Old French *espreindre* or *espraindre,* "to wring out," from the Latin *exprimere,* "to express or to squeeze out." By the same token, **strain** comes through the Middle French *estreindre* or *estraindre,* "to wring hard," from the Latin *stringere,* "to draw tight." In medicine there is a particular distinction between "strain" and "sprain." A strain is an overexertion or an excessive stretching of a muscle; a sprain is a partial rupture of the ligaments supporting a joint. Moreover, there is a distinction between "stress" and "strain" that is not always observed by otherwise careful medical speakers and writers. Stress is the potentially injurious action, while strain is the resulting injury. Twisting one's arm constitutes stress; it may or may not lead to a strain of the arm muscles. An odd and colloquial use of "strain" was by unschooled men to designate gonorrheal urethritis, the painful penile discharge being wrongly attributed to a physical strain such as that of heavy lifting.

sprue is a name for a condition marked by impaired intestinal absorption and consequent malnutrition. There are two types. Tropical sprue occurs in persons who live in or visit for an extended time certain areas of India, Southeast Asia, or the Caribbean islands, and who are subject to an enteric infection that has not yet been precisely defined. "Nontropical sprue" and "idiopathic steatorrhea" are seldom-used synonyms for coeliac disease, particularly that occurring in adults. The term "sprue" comes from the Dutch *spruw* or *sprouw,* which meant "thrush," i.e., the patchy exudative inflammation of the oral and pharyngeal mucosa. Coeliac disease can be marked by redness of the tongue and mouth, but exudation is not a feature unless there is secondary infection. Persons afflicted with coeliac disease, because of their depleted state, may be subject to moniliasis and, hence, thrush.

squamous comes from the Latin *squama,* "the scale of a fish or serpent." The squamal portions of various bones of the skull (frontal, temporal, and occipital) are so called because of their thin, flat, plate-like shape. The squamous cells of the outer layer of the skin (epidermis) are similarly so named. They tend to occur in layers and thereby constitute a stratified squamous epithelium.

squint is a term used to refer to crossed eyes, also known as "strabismus." Ordinarily we think of "squinting" as looking through partly closed eyes, but another and older definition of "squint" is "to look askance or askew." This meaning relates to the Middle Dutch *schuyn,* "oblique or crossways." **Strabismus** is an almost direct borrowing of the Greek *strabismos,* "squinting." Professor H. A. Skinner points out that Strabo, a celebrated geographer and explorer of Alexandria, suffered from a peculiar and noticeable squint. In medicine, Strabo has become immortalized more for his squint than for his geography in that his name gave rise to the Greek verb *strabizein,* "to be like Strabo," and eventually to "strabismus."

stain is ordinarily thought of in the sense of adding color, yet the origin of the word is the opposite. "Stain" is a shortened, Anglicized version of the Old French *desteindre,* "to take away the color," this being derived from a combination of the Latin *dis-,* "apart, away," + *tingere,* "to dye." The idea is that by applying a stain one takes away the original color of an object, albeit by adding another color. A variety of stains have been developed for use in microscopy whereby special features of tissues and cells can be better discerned. Oddly, if we undertake to remove the stain from a section of tissue, we say we "de-stain" it. This is equivalent to "de-de-dye."

stapes is a Late Latin term for "a stirrup." It cannot have been (and was not) a classical Latin word because the Romans rode their horses with neither saddle nor stirrups. The barbarians were cleverer. They hung from a sort of saddle a looped rope by which a man could quickly mount a horse. This was known as a *stigrap* from the Anglo-Saxon *stigan,* "to rise or to mount," + *rap,* "rope." Later, supports for the rider's feet were hung from both sides of the saddle, and these were called *stapes* from combining the Latin *stare,* "to stand," + *pes,* "foot," i.e., "a place for the foot to stand." One of the three small bones in the middle ear is shaped like a tiny stirrup and was given the Late

Latin name. The genitive of *stapes* is *stapedis,* and the little muscle attached to the stapes is thereby called **stapedius.**

starch comes from the Anglo-Saxon *stearc* or *starc,* "stiff or strong," and is related to the German *stark,* "strong." Starch is a substance long known to impart a stiffening to cloth. Starch is a polysaccharide of vegetable origin and has the formula $(C_6H_{10}O_5)_n$.

stasis is a direct borrowing of the Greek word for "the posture of standing," from the verb *histēmi,* "to make stand still." In physiology, stasis is a stoppage in the flow of blood or other body fluid.

steatopygous means just what it would have meant to the Greeks, "having a fat rump." The word combines the Greek *steat-* (from *stear,* "stiff fat or suet") + *pygē,* "the buttocks."

stellate comes from the Latin *stella,* "star," and means "star-shaped." Various anatomic structures with processes radiating from a central point or body are described as being stellate. The stellate (or cervicothoracic) ganglion is situated on the sympathetic trunk anterior to the lowest cervical or first thoracic vertebra.

stenosis comes from the Greek *stenos,* "narrow." Pyloric stenosis is a narrowing of the outlet from the stomach. A stenotic vessel is one in which the lumen is narrowed but not closed.

stent is a supporting device, such as a mold fashioned to hold a graft in place, or a cylinder or tube used to support an anastomosis during the healing process. Tubular stents also can be implanted in the esophagus or biliary ducts to keep open a stenotic lumen.

But "stent" has nothing to do with "stenosis." One might argue that it is related to another "stent," which is a Scottish dialect word for "extend." But, rather, it seems to be taken from the name of Charles Stent, a 19th-century English dentist who fabricated a plastic resinous substance that would set hard and provide a firm impression of the teeth from which a dental prosthesis could be made. The substance became known as Stent's mass and was readily adapted to other uses.

sterco- is a combining form of the Latin *stercus,* "dung." **Stercobilin** is a bile pigment found in feces. A **stercoral** ulcer is the result of erosion of the rectocolic mucosa by a hard, abrasive clump of feces.

stereo- is a combining form taken from the Greek *stereos,* "solid," as a mass having three dimensions. **Stereognosis** (+ Greek *gnōsis,* "knowledge") is the faculty of perceiving the shape and identifying an object by the sense of touch alone. **Steroids** are substances that resemble cholesterol chemically and contain a hydrogenated cyclopentophenanthrene ring in their structural formulas. Included in this group are certain hormones, bile acids, and cardiac glycones. Steroid therapy refers usually to the use of **corticosteroid** hormones, such as cortisone or one of its many kin. The "corti-," of course, indicates an original source in the adrenal cortex.

sterile is a near borrowing of the Latin *sterilis,* "unfruitful, barren, empty, or bare." The related Greek word of the same meaning is *steiros.* The original reference was to a female animal or to a woman who was unable to conceive and bear offspring. This use persists. In medicine, the term has been adopted to mean totally free, or "barren," of bacteria, as surgical paraphernalia must necessarily be.

sternum is a Late Latin term taken from the Greek *sternon,* "the breast or chest." The term was used by some early writers for the chest generally, but this use was soon supplanted by that of "thorax," and "sternum" became the name of the bone in the middle of the anterior chest to which the ribs are attached. Often this is called the breastbone.

stethoscope comes from the Greek *stethos,* "breast or chest," combined with *skopein,* "to view." A prototype of the instrument was invented in 1816 by the French physician René Théophile Hyacinthe Laënnec (1781–1826), who also gave us the word "cirrhosis." The stethoscope was later developed as a binaural device by a New York doctor, George Philip Cammann (1804–1863). One might wonder why the name given to an instrument for listening carries the suffix "-scope," which is usually attached to the names of instruments intended for viewing. Perhaps the stethoscope should have been called a "stethophone." But there is more to the meaning of the Greek verb *skopein* and the Greek noun *skopos.* The former could mean viewing in the broader sense of observing or monitoring; the latter means "a watchman or scout."

-sthenia is a combining form taken from the Greek *sthenos,* "strength, might, or prowess." To be **asthenic** is to lack strength. **Neurasthenia** is a condition marked by nervous exhaustion, less precisely defined as weak nerves. A **hypersthenic** person is well-muscled to the point of being "muscle-bound." In years past, significance was accorded to a person's **habitus** (Latin "condition," from the verb *habere,* "to hold"), i.e., how he "held" himself. A person of the asthenic habitus was slender or frail; a sthenic habitus denoted normal proportions; a person of the hypersthenic habitus was stocky or disproportionately thick.

stigma is a direct borrowing of the Greek word meaning "puncture by a pointed instrument," particularly "a brand mark." The latter is the sense in which "stigma" is used medically as a visible sign of a particular disease. A telangiectasis can be a stigma of cirrhosis.

stimulus is the Latin word for "a pointed stick used as a goad." To the Roman soldier, a *stimulus* was a sharp stake concealed below the ground to injure an unwary enemy. Such a nefarious device has been used as recently as the Vietnam War. The related Greek word is *stigma,* "a puncture." "Stimulus" was used in physiology in the 18th century when it was observed that pricking caused a frog's leg to twitch.

stoma is the Greek word for "the mouth." By extension, the term has long been applied to various mouth-like openings in plants and animals. In medicine, **stomatitis** is inflammation of the oral mucosa. A surgical stoma is an artificial opening in any viscus, created for the purpose of ingress or egress. These are usually specified as gastrostomy, enterostomy, or colostomy, according to their location. Occasionally there is an unwitting confusion between "-stomy" and "-tomy"

(Greek *tomē,* "a cutting"). A gastrotomy is simply an incision in the stomach wall, while a gastrostomy is a mouth-like opening fashioned between the stomach and the anterior abdominal wall to accommodate a feeding tube.

stomach is derived from the Greek *stomachos,* "the throat or gullet," this being related to *stoma,* "mouth." In this sense the gullet was a passage that had a mouth. Through the ages, the assignment of the term "stomach" seems to have gradually descended the alimentary canal: first the throat, then the gullet or esophagus, later the opening into the *ventriculus* (medical Latin for "stomach"), and finally what we now know as the stomach. **Stomachic** is a bygone term for a digestive tonic medicament.

stool probably can be traced to the postulated Indo-European root word *stā,* "that which stands firm," which led to the Anglo-Saxon *stōl,* "a seat." Because of the universal custom of squatting when evacuating the bowel, "to stool" became a euphemism for "to defecate." We still speak of "stooling patterns" when we describe a patient's bowel action. Later, "stool" became a word for the product of "stooling," i.e., for the fecal deposit itself.

stratum is the past participle of the Latin verb *sternere,* "to spread out." The term has been incorporated in a number of anatomic terms for sheetlike structures, particularly those that occur in layers. The stratum corneum (Latin *cornu,* "horn") is the outermost layer of keratinized squamous cells in the skin. The stratum granulosum (Latin *granulum,* "a small grain or seed") of the ovary is the layer of cells lining the theca of an ovarian follicle.

stria is the Latin word for "a groove," especially in architecture, where it means the flute of a column. A series of parallel flutes separated by elevated strips gives the appearance of stripes. **Striated** is used in anatomy to describe structures that are striped, e.g., the striated muscle fibers. The so-called stretch marks on the bellies of some fecund women are known as striae.

stricture is an almost direct borrowing of the Latin *strictura,* "a mass of molten iron," particularly as it is poured into a confining mold. The related Latin verb is *stringere,* "to draw tight or to compress." In pathology, a stricture is an abnormal narrowing caused by a contracting scar, as in the urethra or the esophagus.

stridor is the Latin word for "a shrill sound or a harsh noise." In medicine, "stridor" denotes such a respiratory sound produced by the strenuous effort to inhale through a spastic or constricted larynx and is a sign of respiratory distress. In times when diphtheria was rampant, stridor would send chills to the marrow of parents whose children were stricken with the disease. It meant the diphtheritic membrane in the throat was choking off breath.

stroma is a direct borrowing of the Greek *strōma,* "anything spread out for lying or sitting upon." This, of course, would be a sort of mat. It is in this sense that "stroma" was adopted in anatomy as a term for the matrix in which functional elements of a tissue are supported.

Strongyloides is the name for a genus of roundworms that infect both man and animals. The most notorious species is *Strongyloides stercoralis* (Latin *stercus,* "dung"), which is transmitted by contact with feces expelled by an infected person. Another genus similarly infectious, is **Strongylus.** The names come from the Greek *strongylos,* "round."

struma is the Latin term for "a glandular swelling in the neck" and is related to *strues,* "a pile or heap." (When we construe or misconstrue what someone has said, we build up a heap of belief from what we have heard.) Both "struma" and "scrofula" are old terms used for cervical lymphadenopathy. We have abandoned "scrofula" but have kept "struma," as in struma lymphomatosus, a swelling of the thyroid gland consequent to degeneration of its epithelial components, infiltration by lymphocytes, and proliferation of connective tissue.

Student spelled with a capital "S" is used to designate Student's "t" test, a measure of statistical significance. "Student" was the *nom de plume* of William S. Gossett (1876–1937), a British mathematician who published his exposition of statistical inference in 1908, while he was in the employ of Arthur Guinness & Sons, the brewers.

stupe is a direct borrowing of the Greek *stupē,* "the coarse fiber of flax or hemp." This was woven into cloth that, among its other uses, was soaked in hot water and applied as a therapeutic fomentation or poultice. Thus, a hot stupe is what we would otherwise call a "hot pack."

sty comes from the Anglo-Saxon *stīgend,* "a rising." A sty, which is a swollen, inflamed, sebaceous gland of the eyelid, is a "rising on the eye."

styloid is derived from a combination of the Greek *stylos,* "a pillar or a post," + *eidos,* "like." The Latin *stilus* was a pointed instrument used for writing. The styloid process is a long, slender projection of the temporal bone that serves as a point of attachment for several muscles of the throat and tongue.

styptic comes from the Greek *styptikos,* "an astringent," being related to the Greek verb *styphein,* "to contract or to draw together." A styptic pencil, which can be applied to stop bleeding from minor cuts, contains a core of alum (a double sulfate of aluminum and potassium) that exerts an astringent effect on small blood vessels.

sub- is a combining form, used as a prefix, that is taken from the Latin preposition *sub,* "under, beneath, or to come after." Often it is used, too, in the sense of "less than." **Subacute** (+ Latin *acutus,* "sharp") is an odd word that is generally understood in medicine to mean the duration of a symptom or a disease of some time between acute and chronic. A better word for this purpose would be "subchronic," but it enjoys no currency and probably never will. Another contrived term is **subclinical,** used to describe a disease that is present but not manifest. This is akin to **subliminal** (+ Latin *limen,* "threshold") as used in reference to a stimulus below the threshold of perception. An interesting word is **sublimate,** taken from

the Latin *sublimis* (or a collateral form, *sublimus*), "high or lofty" in the sense of "lifted to a higher plane." In analyzing the Latin *sublimis,* most authorities translate the prefix *sub-* as "up to" and relate "-limis" to *limen,* "threshold," but it would seem as likely to be related to the Latin *lima,* "a polishing or a revision." In any case, "sublimate" has two meanings pertinent to medicine. In chemistry, a sublimate is a substance that can change from a solid to a vapor without intervening liquefaction. In psychology, to sublimate is to divert unacceptable, instinctive drives into personally or socially acceptable channels. **Substantia** is a Latin word meaning "the essence of anything, that of which it is composed"; as such, substantia has been given as a name to various anatomic structures, particularly those in the brain. A **substrate** (+ Latin *stratum,* "a layer") is whatever an enzyme acts on, as if the enzyme were placed over it as a layer. **Subtilis** is Latin for "finely woven or of fine texture" and combines *sub-* + *tela,* "a web." By allusion to whatever was so finely woven as to be almost invisible comes the word "subtle." The microbe *Bacillus subtilis* may have been so named because it is a common contaminant of bacterial cultures, i.e., it often seems to be just lying around, almost invisibly.

succus is the Latin word for "sap or juice" and is related to the verb *sugere,* "to suck." The succus entericus is the digestive juice elaborated by the mucosa of the small intestine. **Succinic** acid was so named because it was originally detected in amber, a fossil resin, called *succinum* by the Romans.

succussion describes the means of eliciting a splash heard in the jostled abdomen of a person whose stomach or fluid-filled bowel fails to empty normally. The term is taken from the Latin *succussus,* "a shaking or a jolt."

sudor is the Latin word for "sweat." The **sudoriferous** (+ Latin *ferre,* "to bring forth") glands in the skin produce sweat. A **sudamen** is a small white vesicle in the skin produced by sweat trapped in a swollen sweat gland. Such vesicles are about the size of millet seeds, and the eruption is sometimes called miliaria.

sulcus is the Latin word for the furrow made by a plow or the rutted track of a wheel. The related Greek word is *holkos,* "track or trail." An almost endless number of grooves, depressions, and wrinkles in anatomic structures have been called a sulcus or, in the Latin plural, *sulci.*

super-, supra- are combining forms, used in English as prefixes. They have been taken from the Latin preposition *super,* "over, above, more than," and the Latin adverb *supra,* "over, above, beyond." As a general rule, "super-" is used with nouns and participles, while "supra-" is affixed to adjectives, but the rule is by no means inflexible.

supine is a near borrowing of the Latin adjective *supinus,* "face up, turned upward." This is almost, but not quite, the opposite of the Latin *pronus,* "leaning, stooping, or bent forward." The supine position is that in which the body is lying on the back with the face up. In the **prone** position, the body lies face and belly down, with the back turned up. This distinction is unknown or forgotten by the careless speaker who says, "He was lying prone on his back," an impossible posture. The terms are also used to describe positions of the arms: supine is with palms up, while prone is with palms down. Thus, a **supinator** muscle turns the arm so that the palms are up, while a **pronator** muscle turns the arm in the opposite direction. The supinators are stronger muscles, thus enabling a right-handed person to more effectively tighten a screw. The fact that most persons are right-handed has determined the angle of the threads on screws and bolts. By the same token, a left-handed person is better at loosening a screw. Derivatives of the Latin *supinus* and *pronus* are also used figuratively. Whoever takes an affront supinely takes it "lying down." Whoever or whatever leans toward something is said to be "prone" to it.

suppository is derived from the Latin *suppositus,* the past participle of *supponere,* "to put something under or next to something else." In pharmacy, a suppository is a fusible or easily melted form of medication that can be inserted in a body orifice, usually the vagina or rectum, there to exert its intended effect.

surgery is an example of a word whose path from Greek to English has been so tortuous as to obscure its origin. It began with the Greek *cheirourgia,* "working with the hands, the practice of a handcraft or art." This was taken into Latin as *chirurgia* and thence into the Old French as *surgerie,* finally becoming the English "surgery." The original Greek word combines *cheir,* "the hand," + *ergon,* "work, a person's employment," and the reference in all derived languages is to manual procedures. To the British, the noun "surgery" also means the place where the work is done, i.e., the room where the doctor performs his manual procedures. An old English spelling of "surgeon" is *chirurgeon,* and a former medical school in Philadelphia was known as the Medico-Chirurgical College.

suspensory is from the Latin *suspendere,* "to hang up or to support," this being derived from the Latin *sub-,* "under," + *pendere,* "to hang down." A support is placed under whatever hangs down to keep it up. Breasts are supported by a brassiere (from the French *bras,* "the arm," + *iere,* a suffix denoting "something connected with"). Some men wear suspenders to keep their pants up. In anatomy, various supporting ligaments are called suspensory ligaments. Closely akin is **sustentaculum,** from the Latin *sustinere,* "to hold up," a term used to denote a supporting structure.

suture is a near borrowing of the Latin *sutura,* "a sewn seam," this being derived from the Latin verb *suere,* "to sew, stitch, or tack together."

sycosis is not to be confused with "psychosis," either in pronunciation or in meaning. Sycosis is an inflammation of the hair follicles, especially of the beard, whereby the surface of the skin becomes rough and irregular. The word comes from the Greek *sykon,* "a fig," a fruit which has an irregular skin.

syn- is a prefix representing the Greek preposition *syn,* "together with, invested or en-dowed with, or in connection with." It can appear also as "sy-" (as in system), "syl-" (as in syllogism), and "sym-" (as in symmetry). This must be the most useful prefix in the language of medicine; it is attached to more words than any other. Only a few examples can be given. **Symbiosis** (+ Greek *bios,* "life") is literally living together, as of two or more organisms, but with the important provision of harmony or, at least, of no harm to each other. (Incidentally, "harmony" and "harm" are of wholly unrelated Greek and Anglo-Saxon origins.) The earliest English use of "symbiosis," in the 17th century, was in a social sense. The term was introduced in biology to denote a friendly relation between host and parasite in the late 19th century. **Sympathetic** (+ Greek *pathos,* "suffering"), as originally used in physiology, was a name given to the whole of the autonomic or involuntary nervous system, and much later was restricted to that portion characterized by adrenergic neuroeffector transmission, the cholinergic component being given the name **parasympathetic** (Greek *para,* "beside"). Presumably because the autonomic tracts serve the viscera, the idea was that the "sympathies" of the organs were thereby aroused. **Sympathomimetic** (+ Greek *mimētikos,* "imitative") became the term of reference for drugs that mimic the effect of adrenergic stimulation (adrenalin was the prototype). **Symphysis** is a direct borrowing of the Greek word for "growing together" and is applied in anatomy to a fixed union of bones, such as that at the pubic symphysis. **Symptom** comes from the Greek *symptōma,* "anything that has befallen one, by chance or mischance" or, literally, "that which falls together with," the related Greek verb being *piptein,* "to fall." **Synapse** as a term for the connection between the processes of two nerve cells was introduced in 1897 by Sir Charles Sherrington (1857–1952), the English physiologist, with the acknowledged help of classical scholars of his acquaintance. The Greek source is *synaptō,* "I join together," this being related to the Greek verb *haptein,* "to fasten upon." **Syncope** is an almost direct borrowing of the Greek *sy-*[*n*]*gkopē,* literally "a cutting into pieces" but also used by the Greeks for "a fainting spell or a swoon," the allusion apparently being to a "cutting off" of strength in a person so afflicted. A **syndrome** (+ Greek *dromos,* "a course, as for running") is a group of symptoms or signs that "run together" as characteristic of a given condition. Sometimes "syndrome" is used rather than "disease" when the full picture of a condition as a true entity has not been yet defined. **Prodrome** comes almost directly from the Greek adjective *prodromos,* an adjective "running ahead (of something else)." This, in turn, comes from a combination of *pro-,* "ahead," + the Greek verb *dramein* "to run." A **prodrome** is a set of symptoms or signs that precedes or "runs ahead" of the full manifestation of a disease. "Prodrome" is usually pronounced in two syllables, while often one hears "syndrome" sounded in three ("syn-dro-me"). The three-syllable pronunciation would seem to be in deference to the origin in the Greek *syndromē,* but *prodromē* is also a Greek word. This is a tempest in a teapot. To insist on different pronunciations of such similar words seems pedantic, and only two syllables will suffice for either of the two words. **Synechia** is a near borrowing of the Greek *synecheia,* "a continuity," related to the Greek verb *synechein,* "to hold or keep together." In medicine today, the term is restricted to an adhesion of the lens of the eye to the cornea or to the iris. **Synovia** is a term contrived by Paracelsus in 1520. He combined *syn-* + Greek *ōon,* "an egg," to come up with a term for various fluids in the body that appeared to resemble the white of an egg. The term has persisted but is now restricted to that slippery fluid found in joint spaces, and sometimes it is used also to refer to the membranes which line the joint spaces, as in "synovitis." **Systole** is a direct borrowing of the Greek *systolē,* "a drawing together or a contraction," the root verb being *systellein,* "to draw together or to pull in, as in shortening a sail." In the 16th century the noun was used to refer to contraction of the heart muscle.

syringe comes from the Greek *syri*[*n*]*gx,* "a shepherd's pipe" such as that played by Pan, the deity of flocks and herds, who also had the reputation of being a lusty lad. In ancient Greek lore, the musical instrument was named for the nymph Syrinx, who was both chaste and, on one fateful occasion, chased. The chaser was the panting Pan. Syrinx took refuge in the River Ladon, where, to escape "a fate worse than death," she prayed to be turned into a clump of reeds. When finally Pan sought to embrace the nymph, he found instead he was clutching only a handful of reeds. Letting out a great sigh, he found that his breath elicited a pleasant note from the hollow reeds. And so it was, if you can believe it, that the shepherd's pipe was invented. Actually, the Greek *syri[n]gx* could be any cylindrical container or conduit, and so became, in English, "syringe." **Syringomyelia** (+ Greek *myelos,* "marrow," i.e., of the spine, as the Greeks conceived the spinal cord to be) was contrived as a reference to abnormal, fluid-filled cavities in the spinal cord consequent to a developmental defect or in association with neoplasia.

syphilis became astonishingly widespread in Europe during the decade following 1495, the year in which Charles VIII of France and his motley army occupied the kingdom of Naples. Rumor had it that the cunning Neapolitans deliberately dispatched prostitutes to infect Charles's troops, who were more than susceptible to dalliance. When the army disbanded, the mercenary soldiers returned to their homelands, where the scourge rapidly became rife.

Charles blamed his troubles on "the Neapolitan disease," while the English and Germans called it "the French disease." In France it was "the Spanish pox" (or "the great pox" to distinguish it from "the small pox"). In Russia it was "the Polish disease," in Persia it was "the Turkish disease," and so on, each nationality reproaching another. The Spanish tried to contend that the disease was imported from the newly discovered West Indies, but it is likely that syphilis was well entrenched in Europe in a less virulent form long before the age of discovery. The term "syphilis" is said to have been coined by Girolamo Fracastoro (1478–1553), a Veronese physician and poet who in 1530 published *Syphilis sive morbus gallicus.* In this poem, Fracastoro concocted a myth wherein the protagonist was a swineherd named Syphilus who was scourged with a disfiguring, debilitating disease because he defied the sun-god. The fellow's name may have been taken from the Greek *sypheos,* "a hog sty."

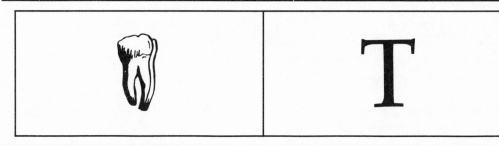

tabagism is a word for any condition resulting from the excess or harmful use of tobacco. It comes from *tabaco,* the Spanish name for the weed, which the Spaniards took from the Carib Indian name for the pipe in which the weed was smoked.

tabes is the Latin word for "decay." This, in turn, is related to the Latin verb *tabere,* "to waste away." Originally the term was applied to any wasting disease. In 1836 the term "tabes dorsalis" was suggested as a name for the disease otherwise known as locomotor ataxia, in the belief that the condition was due to a wastage of the dorsal or posterior columns of the spinal cord. It was not until 1876 that the cause of the disease was identified as syphilis. Later, "tabes" became used as another term for syphilis in its advanced stages.

tachy- is a combining form, usually a prefix, taken from the Greek *tachys,* "quick, swift, or fast." **Tachycardia** (+ Greek *kardia,* "the heart") refers to an abnormally rapid heartbeat, customarily applied to rates in excess of 100 per minute. **Tachypnea** (+ Greek *pnoia,* "a drawn breath"), by the same token, is abnormally rapid breathing. **Tachyphylaxis** (+ Greek *phylaxis,* "a guarding") is a rapid dissipation of the effect of an active substance by its frequently repeated administration. For example, tyramine acts indirectly as a sympathomimetic agent by displacing norepinephrine from binding sites at certain nerve endings; the released norepinephrine then is available to act at receptor sites on effector cells. But the amount of norepinephrine liable to displacement is limited and can be depleted by repeated administration of tyramine.

taenia is Latin for "a ribbon or tape" and is related to the Greek *tainia,* "a band, such as worn around the head in token of victory." In parasitology, *Taenia* is a genus of tapeworms. *Taenia saginata* (Latin *sagina,* "a fattened animal") is found in beef, and *Taenia solium* is found in pork (here *solium* refers to the ring of hooklets around the scolex of the worm and may have been taken either from the Latin *solium,* "a throne," or from the Latin *sol,* "the sun's rays"). The taeniae coli are the three prominent longitudinal bands of muscle in the wall of the colon.

talipes is the Latin word for "clubfoot" and obviously is a combination of the Latin *talus,* "the ankle," + *pes,* "the foot." The deformity is such that, with the foot turned in sharply, the afflicted person appears to be walking on his ankle.

talus is the name of the second largest of the tarsal bones, supporting the tibia above and resting on the calcaneus below. It is also called the **astragulus.** Curiously, both terms once referred to dice, as used in games of chance. The Greek *astragalos* originally meant the upper cervical vertebrae. Soldiers of ancient Greece made their dice from the second cervical vertebrae of sheep, and the word came to refer mainly to the dice. Roman soldiers made their dice (which in the Latin singular, is *taxillus*) from the anklebone or heel bone of the horse. *Taxillus* was later shortened to *talus* and given as a name for the anklebone. Thus, both "talus" and "astragulus" came to be applied to the anklebone—by chance, as it were.

tampon is the French word for "a plug or stopper" and is a sort of nasalized derivative of the French *tapoter,* "to tap," as to open a keg. In medicine, a tampon is a gauze plug inserted in a body cavity to stop or to absorb a flow of fluid. **Tamponade,** from the French *tamponner,* "to plug up," is the procedure of occluding a lumen (as by inflating a balloon in the esophagus or stomach) or applying pressure to a vessel in order to stop bleeding. Cardiac tamponade is a condition wherein pressure is exerted on the beating heart by an accumulation of fluid within the pericardial sac.

tantalum is a rare metallic element (atomic number 73, atomic weight 180.948), often used, because it is malleable and resists corrosion, to fabricate prosthetic appliances, wire sutures, and implantable plates or mesh for covering bony or soft tissue defects. The name comes from that of Tantalus, a mythological king of Lydia. Tantalus presumed on his friendship with the gods and was condemned to everlasting torment in the infernal regions. Plagued by unrelieved hunger and thirst, he could not eat because fruits were held just beyond his reach, and he could not drink because water receded when he stooped to sip—thus, the verb "to tantalize." The derivation for the designation of the metal seems a bit more strained. Probably it was chosen because the element was considered to be beyond the reach of corrosive fluids.

tarsus is a Latinized form of the Greek *tarsos,* "a wicker frame or basket" or any broad, flat surface, such as the flat of the foot. In anatomy, "tarsus" is used also in reference to the plate of connective tissue that serves as a framework for the eyelid.

tartar is a calcareous substance (calcium phosphate and carbonate together with organic matter) that becomes encrusted on teeth. It also is the substance (potassium bitartrate) that becomes encrusted in vats during the fermentation of grape juice as it becomes wine. Just as the process of fermentation harks back to time immemorial, so "tartar" is of ancient lineage. Some scholars have related the word to the Persian *durd* and the Arabic *durdi,* but more clearly it is derived from the Medieval Greek *tartaron* and the Late Latin *tartarum,* all referring to the dregs of wine-making. **Tartaric** acid is so called because it was first obtained from tartar accumulating in wine vats.

taste comes through the Old French *taster,* "to handle, feel, or taste," from the Latin *taxare,* "to appraise." Thus, a discriminating person does not have all of his taste in his mouth. **Tactile,** referring to the sense of touch, comes from the Latin *tactus,* the past participle of *tangere,* "to touch."

technique is a French word derived from the Greek *technikos,* "belonging to the arts." A Greek *tektōn* was "a worker in wood or a carpenter," and the Sanskrit *taksh* meant "to cut wood." This sense is preserved in the scientific use of "technique" to designate a means of accomplishing a procedure, usually by deft use of the hands.

tectum, tegmen are terms taken from the Latin verb *tego, tegere, texi, tectum,* "to cover over, to shelter, or to hide." The mesencephalic tectum is the roof-like covering of the midbrain. The tegmen tympani is the roof of the middle-ear cavity. The Latin **tegmentum** also means "a covering," and this term applies to that part of the cerebral peduncle above the substantia nigra. The **integument** or skin covers the body.

tel- is a combining form, usually a prefix, taken from the Greek *telos,* "the completion or fulfillment of anything" or, adverbially, "at the end, at last." In science, the sense of "tel-" often is "at a distance." **Telangiectasia** (+ Greek *a*[*n*]*ggeion,* "vessel," + *ektasis,* "dilatation") is a condition wherein the end branches of arteries and capillaries are abnormally dilated; a telangiectasis is the spot where telangiectasia has occurred. **Telemetry** (+ Greek *metron,* "a measure") is the means by which measurements are made at a distance from the subject, particularly when the signals are transmitted by radio waves. The **telencephalon** (+ Greek *enkephalon,* "the brain"), sometimes called the endbrain, is made up of the cerebral cortex, the corpus striatum, and the rhinencephalon, all comprising the terminus of higher brain activity. **Telophase** (+ Greek *phasis,* "appearance") is the completing or last of the four stages of mitosis.

tela is the Latin word for "web," particularly the warp, i.e., the threads that run lengthwise in the loom. The term has been applied to numerous weblike anatomic structures, often alternatively with "tunica," as a covering, or with "lamina," as a layer.

temperature comes from the Latin *temperatio,* "a blending, a constitution," related to the Latin verb *temperare,* "to apportion or to regulate." These words can be traced back to the Latin *tempus,* "time," which was early recognized as being regularly apportioned in days, months, seasons, and years. We retain the original idea of "temperament" as the combined attributes or mental cast of an individual being. Presumably the heat of the body was taken to be representative of temperament, hence the temperature. The first **thermometer** (Greek *thermē,* "heat," + *metron,* "a measure") was devised by Galileo in 1592, and shortly thereafter it was discovered that the human body has a relatively constant temperature in health. For many years, body temperature was one of the few objective measurements that could be made, and clinical thermometry became almost a science in itself.

temple is derived from the Latin *tempus,* which means both "time" and "the temple of the head," i.e., the area just behind and lateral to the forehead. To understand the connection, one must go back to the Greek *temnein,* "to cut or to divide." Time was clearly divided into days and nights by the rising and setting of the sun, into months by phases of the moon, and into recurring seasons of the year. Most of these divisions of time were evident by observing the heavens. Ancient augurs would gaze at the sky, mark off a given sector, and study it for signs of things to come or other divine revelations. Such a precinct of the sky or an area of earth marked off for the observation of omens was known by the Greek word *temenos* and the Latin word *templum.* Some say the temple of the head was so called because, by observing the visible subcutaneous vessels and their pulsations, one could divine the temperament of a person. Others have said that the graying of hair at the temple was looked on as a sign of the ravages of time. But the Greek *temnein* also meant "to wound or

maim in battle," and the sides of the head toward the front were early found to be the thinnest part of the skull and, therefore, the most vulnerable to a crippling or lethal blow. A well-aimed blow at the temple surely could cut off one's time on earth. Whatever the origin of the word, we still use **temporal** to refer to the bone, muscle, artery, vein, and nerve that occupy that region of the head.

tendon is derived from the Latin *tendere* and the Greek *teinein,* both meaning "to stretch." The Greek *tenon* is "a sinew or tendon." Both tendons and ligaments are tough, fibrous cords or bands; they differ in that tendons are the fibrous extensions by which muscles are attached to bones, while ligaments bind bone to bone, as at joints. The tendon by which the calf muscles are attached to the calcaneus or heel bone is called the **Achilles tendon** because of the Greek legend that tells of the babe Achilles being dipped in the River Styx by his mother, Thetis. The immersion was intended to make the boy invulnerable. The mother held the dangling infant by his heel. Alas, years later this small, unimmersed area was vulnerable to Paris' well-aimed arrow, which severed the calcaneal tendon of the triceps surae muscle. Thus was felled the hero Achilles. Ever since, any small, unobtrusive point at which an otherwise stalwart person might be subject to attack is referred to as his Achilles' heel. **Tenesmus** is a near borrowing of the Greek *tenesmos,* also from the verb *teinein,* which Hippocrates used for "straining at stool," and so do we. A **tensor** muscle is one that tightens or stretches a part, such as the tensor of the soft palate or the tensor tympani, which stretches the eardrum. **Tentorium** is Latin for "tent," and the tentorium cerebelli is a broad infolding of the dura that covers the cerebellum like a tent. Because this tentorium separates the "thinking" forebrain from the lower "vegetative" portions of the brain, disturbances attributed to psychologic aberration are sometimes referred to as supratentorial. **Tetany,** derived from *teinein*—(the first "n" was lost), is a condition marked by sustained tension of muscles, especially the flexors of the extremities. **Tetanus** is an infectious disease in which the toxin produced by the bacterium *Clostridium tetani* induces muscle spasm, particularly in the masseter, which causes the mandible to clench tightly against the maxilla, hence the colloquial term "lockjaw."

terato- is a combining form taken from the Greek *teras,* "a sign or portent" and also "a monster." The connection is that the ancient Greeks looked upon the appearance of a strange creature, such as a deformed baby, as an omen by which the gods were seeking to deliver a message. We now use **teratogen** (+ Greek *gennaō,* "I produce") as the term for any agent or factor identified as a cause of defects in the developing embryo. **Teratology** (+ Greek *logos,* "a treatise") is the study of congenital defects. A **teratoma** is a true neoplasm composed of aberrant tissues, none of which is indigenous to the area where the tumor occurs.

teres is the Latin word for "smooth and round or cylindrical" and is applied to various ligaments and muscles. The round ligament of the uterus is more formally known as the ligamentum teres uteri. The ligamentum teres hepatis is the smooth cylindrical anterior edge of the falciform ligament that helps support the liver in the upper abdomen.

test comes from the Latin *testa,* "a brick, tile, jug, or crock." An earthenware pot with a lid was a *testum.* Such ceramic utensils were commonly used by alchemists. Substances placed in pots and subjected to heat, so as to see what changes might occur, were said to be tested. Today, many of the tests in a clinical laboratory are done in a flask, dish, or tube.

testis is a direct borrowing of the Latin word for "witness." In ancient times, testimony was validated by the swearer grasping the scrotum, presumably his own, but on occasion someone else's. In Genesis 24:9 it is recorded: "And the servant put his hand under the thigh of Abraham his master, and sware to him concerning that matter."

tetralogy is a series of four related things, the word being derived from the Greek *tetra,* "four," + *logos,* "a statement." In ancient Athens, a *tetralog* was a series of four dramas, three tragic and one satiric, performed consecutively at the festival of Dionysus, the god of wine, whose Roman name was Bacchus. The term is applied, uniquely in medicine, to the tetralogy of Fallot, so called because it was described by Etienne-Louis Fallot (1850–1911), a French physician, and because it has four components: (*a*) stenosis of the pulmonary conus; (*b*) an interventricular septal defect; (*c*) dextroposition of the aorta that overrides the interventricular septum; and (*d*) right ventricular hypertrophy. Fallot's description, in 1888, was preceded, in 1771, by that of Edward Sandifort (1742–1814), a pathologist of Leiden.

thalamus is the Latin name for "an inner chamber," usually a bedroom occupied by the principal married couple in a house—what we would call a master bedroom. How or why Galen gave the name to that solid portion of the diencephalon, which we now know serves as a relay center for sensory impulses to the cerebral cortex, is a bit of a mystery. Perhaps he was referring to the adjacent ventricles of the brain. Nevertheless, the name stuck.

thalassemia is a genetically determined hemolytic anemia that occurs predominantly in persons of Mediterranean stock. The name combines the Greek *thalassa,* "sea," + *haima,* "blood." The *thalassa* best known to the Greeks was the Mediterranean Sea.

theca is a near borrowing of the Greek *thēkē,* "a case to put anything in." The theca folliculi is a fibrous envelope containing an ovarian follicle.

thenar is the Greek word for "that part of the hand with which one strikes," i.e., the flat of the hand. The related Greek verb is *theinō,* "I strike." Originally the term referred to the entire palm of the hand. Later, the thenar eminence was considered to be the area at the base of the thumb, and the **hypothenar** (or lesser) eminence was the area at the base of the little finger.

theophylline is one of three closely related xanthine alkaloids that occur in the leaves and berries of various plants widely distributed in tropical climes throughout the world. The other two are theobromine and caffeine. The alkaloids are best known for their stimulant and antisoporific effects. They have also been used as diuretic agents. The story is told that they were introduced into Western culture by the prior of a convent in Araby who was informed by native shepherds that goats nibbling on the berries of the coffee plant were observed to frolic and gambol through the night rather than to sleep. The prior asked that samples of the berries be brought to him so he might brew a beverage that would enable him to keep awake during the long, nocturnal prayer vigils. Legend would have us believe that this was the first cup of coffee. The alkaloids are readily extracted from tea leaves and from coffee, coca, and cola beans. **Caffeine** comes from the French *café,* "coffee," + *-ine,* denoting a derivative. **Theophylline** combines the Latinized *thea* (taken from the Amoy *t'e,* but *ch'a* in Mandarin Chinese), "tea," + the Greek *phyllon,* "leaf." **Theobromine** incorporates the Greek *brōma,* "food." Some authorities relate the "theo-" to the Greek *theos,* "a god," but a derivation from the word for tea seems more down-to-earth. "Theo-" is not to be confused with the combining form **thio-,** taken from the Greek *theion,* "sulfur." **Aminophylline** is so named because it is a complex of ethylene diamine and theophylline, the former being added to increase the solubility of the xanthine.

therapy is a near borrowing of the Greek *therapeia,* "a service, an attendance," the related Greek verb being *therapeuō,* "I wait upon." **Therapeutics** is that branch of medicine dealing specifically with the treatment of disease. **Chemotherapy** (Greek *chēmeia,* "chemistry") is treatment that employs chemical agents, the term now being usually applied to the use of such agents to combat cancer. One who calls himself a therapist owes his name to the Greek *therapōn,* "a servant," but distinguished from a *doulos,* "a slave," in that a *therapōn* gave his services freely, without bondage or coercion.

thiamine was the first member of the vitamin group to be recognized and often is called vitamin B-1. Beriberi, the disease resulting from a dietary deficiency of thiamine, was not widely known until steam-powered rice mills were introduced in the 19th century. These marvels of technology so refined rice that it was divested of its vitamin-containing husk. In 1882 the Japanese admiral Kanehiro Takaki (1849–1915) found that he could eliminate beriberi in his sailors by adding fish, meat, and vegetables to their regular diet of polished rice. More to the point, Christian Eijkman (1858–1930), a Dutch physician working in Java, demonstrated that feeding the discarded rice husks to victims of beriberi could cure their disease. For this discovery Eijkman was awarded a share of the Nobel prize for medicine in 1929. Thiamine contains one sulfur atom in its pyrimidine-thiazole nucleus, hence its name from the Greek *theion,* "sulfur or brimstone," + *-amine.*

thirst can be traced to the Indo-European root word *ters,* "dry or arid." The Greek *tersomai* means "to become dry or parched."

(However, the Greek *tersainō* means "to dry or wipe up," this being related to the Latin *tersus,* "clean, neat, polished"; hence, a terse lecture is succinct and pithy.) Meanwhile, the Gothic *thaurstei,* "to be dry," from the same Indo-European stem, led to the English "thirsty."

thorax is the Greek word for "a breastplate or cuirass." For added protection to the torso, a double-cuirass was fashioned from a breastplate and a backplate joined with clasps. By extension, the Greek *thōrax* came to refer also to that part of the body thus encased, i.e., the chest.

thrombus comes from the Greek *thrombos,* "a lump or a clump," but also "a curd of milk or a clot of blood." A thrombus is a clot that forms in a blood vessel or chamber of the heart. **Thrombin** is an enzyme that converts fibrinogen to fibrin, thereby promoting the formation of a blood clot. A **thrombocyte** (+ Greek *kytos,* "cell or hollow vessel") is not in itself an actual cell but is a fragment of a **megakaryocyte** (Greek *megas,* "large," + *karyon,* "kernel," + *kytos,* "cell") and is also known as a "blood platelet." Its function is to facilitate the clotting of blood. **Thrombocytopenia** (+ Greek *penēs,* "poverty-stricken") is a deficiency in blood platelets. **Thromboplastin** (+ Greek *plassein,* "to shape") is a factor essential to the production of thrombin and, thus, to the promotion of blood clotting.

thrush is a term, now almost obsolete, for oral infection by *Candida albicans,* also known as "moniliasis." "Thrush" is of murky origin. Possibly it is related to the word "frush," by which farriers referred to the tender hindpart of a horse's foot, just above the hoof. This area was subject to infection and exudation. "Frush," in turn, is said to have been a slurring of the French *fourchette,* as applied to anything shaped like a small fork.

thymus is a fleshy, bilobed lymphoid situated in the anterior mediastinum. The name was given because of its fancied resemblance to a bunch of thyme (which, purists insist, is pronounced "time" because of its French antecedent). Thyme is a member of the mint family of shrubs, and its aromatic leaves are used for seasoning in cooking. The Greek name for the plant is *thymos,* seemingly related to the Greek *thyōma,* "that which is burnt as incense," or, in the plural, "spices." Another Greek word, a homonym, is *thymos,* "the soul," and some people have said the thymus gland was taken to be the seat of the soul, but the Greeks didn't hold such a view.

thyroid is a name first given to the largest cartilage in the larynx and later transferred to the gland that sits in front of the cartilage. The Greek *thyreos* originally was the word for a large stone placed in front of a door to keep it shut. Later it was given as the name of a warrior's oblong shield, with a notch at the top for the chin. The notched laryngeal cartilage resembles such a shield, hence *thyreos + eidos,* "like," became "thyroid." The thyroid gland looks nothing like a shield, but the name serves just as well.

tibia is the Latin word for both the shinbone and a sort of flute. Which bore the name first? No one can be sure. It has been said that primitive flutelike musical instruments were once fashioned from the shinbones of animals.

tincture comes from the Latin *tinctus,* the past participle of *tingere,* "to dip or soak," as one would do in dyeing cloth. In medieval times, various herbal drugs were prepared in alcoholic solutions to which the dissolved substance often imparted a distinct color, which were then used as dyes. An alcoholic solution of a drug is a tincture.

tinea is the Latin name for "a gnawing worm," such as the bookworm or book louse, an insect now classified in the order *Corrodentia.* The book louse is fond of chewing on paper. In figurative usage, a "bookworm" is a person who devours books, too. The name "tinea" was early given to the skin eruption commonly called ringworm. This common term reflects the ringlike shape of the spreading eruption and, presumably, an early belief that the eruption was caused by a worm. It isn't. It is the result of a fungus infection. Calling the disease "tinea" may have been a misunderstood translation of the Arabic *al tin,* a name given to various eruptions of the scalp. In any event, several varieties of tinea have been described: tinea capitis (Latin *caput,* "the head"), tinea barbae (Latin *barba,* "the beard"), and tinea cruris (Latin *crus,* "the leg"). The last form affects the crotch more often than the leg.

tinnitus is Latin for "a ringing or tinkling sound." The word obviously imitates the sound. In medicine, tinnitus (never "tinnitis") is a ringing in the ears.

tissue can be traced, through French, to the Latin verb *texere,* "to weave." This came in turn from the Greek *technē,* "a skill or craft," which can be traced to the Indo-European root *tek, tegh,* "to twine or to build." The Old French word was *tistre,* and from its past participle, *tissu,* came "tissue."

titer is a modification of the French *titre,* "a title or qualification," this being derived from the Latin *titulus,* "an inscription or label." By extension, a *titre* was also proof of the fineness of alloyed gold or silver. When it is important, as it is in knowing the content of a precious metal or of an alcoholic beverage, we insist on a statement of "proof." In chemical or biologic analysis, "titer" has become a term for the dilution of a substance at which a certain reaction is registered.

tongue is said to go back to the Indo-European root word *dnghū,* which referred to that active and useful muscular organ in the floor of the mouth. In early languages there was much confusion between "d," "t," and "l." Thus, the root word led to the archaic Latin *dingua,* which became the classical Latin *lingua;* it led, too, to the Anglo-Saxon *tongue,* which became the English "tongue" (the modern spelling is probably an imitation of the French *langue*). The Greek word for the tongue is *glōssa,* from which we have derived the adjective "glossal" and the combining form **glosso-,** as used in anatomy. This is another example of using a noun derived from one language as the name of a structure, and an adjectival form from another language to describe what pertains to it.

tonsil comes from the Latin plural *tonsillae,* by which the Romans referred to the small glands stuck in the back of the throat. The singular *tonsilla* meant "a pointed pole stuck in the ground, as a mooring stake." The connection between the apparently divergent uses of the singular and plural in Latin is not known. Possibly it relates to the appearance of the glands as being moored to the adjacent pharyngeal folds, looked upon as "pillars" of the throat. It is mere coincidence that the Roman *tonsor* was a barber who cut hair and who later became a surgeon with a proclivity to cut out tonsils.

tonus is taken from the Greek *tonos,* which has a variety of meanings, such as "that which strains or tightens a thing, as a sinew, cord, or brace," "a stretching or tightening, as of the voice in pitching the sound uttered," and "the exertion of force or intensity." Hence, we speak of the tonus or tone of a muscle, as its degree of vigor or tension, and of the tone of voice as its degree of pitch, intensity, or stridency. A **tonic** is a medicine intended to restore or enhance vigor.

tooth can be traced far back to the Indo-European *ed,* "to eat." This led to the Sanskrit *danta,* from which came the Greek *odous, odontos* and the Latin *dens, dentis,* all meaning "the teeth." The Anglo-Saxon *tōth* was "the eating tool" and became the English "tooth." The Latin *dens* provides **dental, dentist,** and **dentistry.** From the Greek *odontos* have been taken the combining form **-dontal,** as in **periodontal** (Greek *peri,* "around"), in reference to the tissues around and supporting the teeth, and **orthodontics** (Greek *orthos,* "straight"), as the practice of straightening irregular or misaligned teeth.

tophus is a Latinization of the Greek *tophos,* "a porous volcanic stone." In medicine, a tophus is a chalklike deposit of urates in tissues, as seen in gout. Such deposits occur in and around joints, particularly that of the big toe, and in cartilage, particularly that of the ear. Such deposits were called tophi long before their content of urate was known.

torso is a direct borrowing of the Italian word for "stump or stalk," this being derived from the Latin *thyrsus,* meaning the same, but more particularly the wand of Bacchus, god of wine. The wand or staff was intertwined with vine tendrils and ivy and capped by a fir cone. With some imagination, this configuration can be likened to that of the main part of the body with its extremities and topped by the head. **Trunk** is often used synonymously with "torso" as a term for the bulk of the body, shorn of the head and extremities. "Trunk" can mean also the main stalk of a tree and, in anatomy, the principal stem of an artery or nerve. The term is derived from the Latin *truncus,* "whatever is stripped of its branches or appendages." The related Latin verb is *truncare,* "to lop off." Hence, whatever is truncated is diminished by having a part chopped off.

torticollis is another name for wryneck and comes from the Latin *tortus,* "twisted," + *collum,* "the neck." From *tortus* also comes tortuous, torture, and even tort, the legal term for a wrongful act. *Collum,* in turn, has yielded accolade, the bestowing of praise, such as might be symbolized by the placing of a wreath around the neck, and *décolleté,* a French word describing a garment cut low at the neck. The Latin *tortus* also gives **torsion** as the term for a twisting, as of a joint anywhere in the body.

tourniquet is a French word meaning "that which turns," such as a turnstile or a swivel. The related French verb is *tourner,* "to turn." The original tourniquets were rather elaborate devices with variations of a screw-type mechanism for constricting a limb in order to stop the flow of blood. Now a simple length of cloth or rubber tubing tied around a digit, arm, or leg suffices. This is a rare, perhaps unique, example of something that has become simpler rather than more complex in its evolution. Being a French word, "tourniquet" should be pronounced with a final "-ay," but no red-blooded American would think of saying anything but "toor'-ni-ket."

toxin is a term introduced to medicine in 1888 by Ludwig Brieger (1849–1909), a Berlin physician, as a name for poisonous substances elaborated by pathogenic organisms. Among the first toxins so recognized were those evolved in decaying meat, but it was soon observed that similar substances were present at the site of bacterial infection of living tissues. **Endotoxins** (Greek *entos,* "within") were contained within bacterial cells, while **exotoxins** (Greek *exo,* "on the outside") were excreted by certain bacterial cells. The term "toxin" was taken from the Latin *toxicum,* "poison." But the Greek *toxon* referred to a stringed bow used for shooting arrows, typically used by the Persians. Some archers took to tipping their arrows with poisonous substances, hence the Latin *toxicum.*

trabecula is the diminutive of the Latin *trabes,* "a beam or plank of wood," such as used in supporting structures. In anatomy, trabeculae are strands of supporting connective tissue, particularly those that extend from the fibrous capsule of an organ into its substance.

trachea is taken from the Greek *traxus,* "rough." The explanation is that ancient anatomists thought that all prominent conduits of the body (other than the alimentary tract) served to conduct air. The Greek *artēria* (combining *aēr,* "air," + *tereō,* "I carry") was the windpipe. Because its wall contained prominent circular cartilaginous ridges, the windpipe was more specifically called *artēria traxeia* (or, in Latin, *arteria aspera*), "the rough artery," to distinguish it from the large afferent vessels of the heart, which were called *artēriai leiai,* "the smooth arteries." About A.D. 1500, the "arteria" was dropped, and the windpipe became known simply as the trachea.

trachoma is an inflammatory eye disease characterized by redness and swelling of the conjunctiva and cornea. The condition was well known to ancient writers as a contagious disease that sometimes led to blindness. It was given the Greek name *trachoma,* "a rough swelling," from the Greek *traxus,* "rough."

tract comes from the Latin *tractus,* "a drawing or dragging out, a trail." The related Latin verb is *trahere,* "to drag or to haul." Applied to anatomy, "tract" refers to a pathway, such as that followed by a bundle of nerve fibers, or to a series of connected organs through which a common substance travels, such as the alimentary tract.

tragus is a near borrowing of the Greek *tragos,* "a he-goat." One of the he-goat's characteristic features is a sort of beard that hangs from his neck. The little projection in front of the ear is called the "tragus" because, at least in elderly men, it often carries a little tuft of hairs. Also, not too surprisingly, the Greek *tragos* and the Latin *tragus* were used to refer to the fetid odor of the armpits.

tranquilizer is a word only recently taken into medicine to designate the newer psychotropic drugs, particularly the benzodiazepines, touted as having a soothing effect on the troubled mind and body. "Tranquilizer" is taken from the Latin *tranquillitas,* "stillness or calmness." These drugs also are sometimes described as being **anxiolytic,** a mongrel term made up of the Latin *anxietas,* "a troubled state," + the Greek *lysis,* "a loosening." So-called tranquilizing drugs act as sedatives. Barbiturates were formerly the most popular sedative agents, but these had gotten a bad name because they were abused. Not surprisingly, the newer tranquilizers have been similarly abused and can be expected to lose their charm.

trans- is a combining form taken directly from the Latin preposition *trans,* "across, over, or beyond." The related Latin verb is *transire,* "to pass over, to cross, or to pass beyond." In anatomy, **transverse** (+ Latin *versus,* "turned so as to face") is applied to anything that lies *crossways.* "Trans-" can also mean "in the wrong direction," a sense conveyed in **transposition** (Latin *positus,* "placed"), as in transposition of the great vessels, a congenital anomaly wherein the aorta arises from the right ventricle of the heart and the pulmonary artery issues from the left ventricle. The first **transfusion,** attempted in the mid-17th century, was "direct," i.e., the donor of blood and the recipient lay side-by-side, their antecubital veins being connected by a tube. This was in accord with the meaning of the Latin *transfusio,* "a transmigration" (*trans-* + *fundere,* "to pour"). When, later, blood was collected from the donor in a flask, then injected into the recipient, the procedure was known as "indirect" transfusion. Today, this is the only way it's done, so there is no need to qualify the term. Whatever is **translucent** (+ Latin *lucere,* "to shine") transmits light but not an image, as would whatever is **transparent** (+ Latin *parere,* "to be visible"). A **transplant** (+ Latin *planta,* "a sprout or a shoot") is the grafting of a tissue from one place to another. An autotransplant occurs in the same individual, while a heterotransplant (Greek *heteros,* "different") involves tissue from one individual engrafted on another. An **orthotopic** (Greek *orthos,* "straight," + *topos,* "a place") transplantation is the grafting of an organ in its customary position, while **heterotopic** transplantation puts the grafted organ in an unaccustomed place. A **transudate** (+ Latin *sudare,* "to sweat") is a fluid that has been generated within a tissue, then passed through a membrane so that it is of watery consistency and relatively devoid of high molecular weight substances or formed cellular elements. This is in contrast to an **exudate** (Latin *exsudare,* "to sweat out"),

which is an outpouring of inflammatory products relatively rich in protein and cellular elements, principally leukocytes.

trapezius comes from the Greek *trapeza,* "a table, especially a dining table or a moneychanger's counter," this being a derived combination of *tetra,* "four," + *peza,* "foot." In geometry, a trapezium is a four-sided plane figure of which no two sides are parallel. "Trapezius" has been given as the name of one of the wrist bones and also of one of the muscles of the back because of their shape.

trauma is a direct borrowing of the Greek word for "a wound" and also for "a damage or a defeat." In medicine, trauma refers to any physically or emotionally inflicted injury.

treatment comes from the French *traitement,* "a handling or a ministration" and also "a salary or stipend." The French noun *traité* means "a compact or agreement" and has been taken into English as "treaty." In medicine, a treatment is a form of handling a problem according to the requirements of a given case. Furthermore, in this modern day, treatment implies an informed consent by the patient, a sort of treaty.

tremor is the Latin adjective that describes "shaking, trembling, or shivering," and it was so used by ancient medical writers. "Tremor" is now an English noun. In physical diagnosis, tremors may be fine or coarse. An intention tremor is one that becomes evident or is intensified when a voluntary or purposeful movement is attempted.

trench foot is a term for the injury to the foot caused by prolonged exposure to moist cold.

It came out of World War I, when the plight of soldiers was to be stuck in cold, damp trenches for days, weeks, and even months on end.

trephine is an instrument with a circular cutting blade or saw (sometimes called a "crown saw") for the purpose of removing a disk of tissue, as from the skull or the cornea. The finding of neatly cut holes in ancient skulls unearthed the world over suggests that operations for cranial decompression may have been among the earliest practiced forms of surgery. Presumably the procedure was intended to allow the escape of evil spirits. The term "trephine" was originally **trepan** (now archaic), from the Greek *trypanon,* "a carpenter's tool, such as an auger or a borer." **Trypanosoma** (+ Greek *sōma,* "body"), members of a genus of sporozoan parasites that can infect man and animals, have a tail (or flagellum) that resembles a borer.

triad is taken through Late Latin from *tria,* the neuter of the Greek *treis,* "three." A triad is a group of three related things and, in medicine, is applied to three component symptoms, signs, or other features that make up a syndrome or a disease entity. The prefix **tri-** comes from the Greek *treis, tria,* and the Latin *tres, tris, tria,* "three." The **triceps** (+ Latin *caput,* "head") muscle that extends the arm has three "heads." **Tricuspid** (+ Latin *cuspis,* "pointed end, as of a spear") describes the valve between the right atrium and ventricle of the heart; it has three pointed leaflets. A tricuspid tooth has three projections on its chewing surface.

trichi-, tricho- are combining forms indicating a relation to hair and taken from the Greek *trichos,* the genitive of *thrix,* "the hair, both of man and beast." **Trichiasis** is, literally, a hairy condition, but in medicine it refers specifically to a condition of ingrown hairs about an orifice, such as ingrowing eyelashes that irritate the cornea. **Trichina** is a worm of the nematode genus **Trichinella**, so called because its members resemble little hairs. **Trichinelliasis** and **trichinosis** are designations of the disease consequent to infection by *Trichinella spiralis* (Latin *spira,* "a coil"), a nematode ingested in raw or undercooked pork. Ambrose Bierce described trichinosis as "the pig's reply to proponents of porcophagy." A **trichobezoar** is a concretion of swallowed hair, typically found lodged in the stomachs of persons given to **trichotillomania** (pulling out one's hair). **Trichomonas** (+ Greek *monas,* "a unit," as a unicellular organism) is a genus of pear-shaped protozoa characterized by hairlike flagella. **Trichuris** (+ Greek *oura,* "tail") is a genus of intestinal nematodes, commonly called "whipworms," so named because of their hairlike tails.

trigeminal is taken from the Latin *trigeminus,* "threefold" (in the plural meaning "triplets"). The trigeminal or fifth cranial nerve is so called because of its three divisions (mandibular, maxillary, and ophthalmic). **Trigeminy** is a disturbance wherein three heartbeats occur in rapid succession, often repetitively.

trigone is a term applied to various triangular areas in anatomy and is derived from the Greek *trigōnon,* a plane figure with three angles, i.e., a triangle. The trigone of the urinary bladder is a triangular portion of the mucosa at the base of that organ. The urogenital trigone or diaphragm is the layer of musculomembranous tissue extending between the ischiopubic rami and surrounding the urogenital ducts.

trimester is commonly used to refer to the equally divided early, middle, and late stages of pregnancy, but the term does not mean a division of time into three periods. "Trimester" means a period of three months and is derived from the Latin *tri-*, "three," + *mestris*, a variant of *menstruus*, "monthly." There are three trimesters in the course of normal human gestation, but an elephant's gestation may occupy six or seven trimesters. Similarly, the meaning of "semester" often is mistaken. This word is a combination of the Latin *sex*, "six," + *menstruus*. The "se-" has nothing to do with "semi-," though again it is a coincidence that six months equal half a year. The average academic semester does not last six months nowadays.

trismus is a near borrowing of the Greek *trismos*, "a squeaking," the related Greek verb being *trizein* "to squeak or creak." Trismus is an inability to open the jaw because of intense muscle spasm. It can be due to a motor disturbance in the trigeminal nerve and, as such, is a frequent symptom of tetanus, commonly known as "lockjaw." The only sound utterable by a patient so afflicted is a squeak.

trocar is a sharply pointed shaft used as an obturator in a cannula with which a body cavity can be pierced, thus permitting the entry of the cannula. Typically a trocar has a three-sided or tribeveled point. The name is an adaptation of the French *trocart,* which is derived from *trois,* "three," + *carré,* "side."

trochanter is a direct borrowing of the Greek word for "a runner" and is related to *trochos,* "a wheel." According to Professor H. A. Skinner, the Greek *trochantēr* originally was used in anatomy as a name for the globular head of the femur, which turns in its socket like a wheel. Later, the usage of the term slipped down the neck of the femoral head and became applied to the lateral process (the greater trochanter) and the medial process (the lesser trochanter), to which the hip and thigh muscles are attached.

trochlea is the Latin word for a pulley block, a device by which heavy loads can be lifted. The related Greek words are *trochilia* and *trochalia,* in turn related to *trochos,* "a wheel." The trochlea of the humerus is an articular cylinder that fits the semilunar notch in the proximal ulna to form the principal joint of the elbow. More like an actual pulley are certain structures through which tendons move so that the direction of pull by a muscle is changed. The best example is the fibrocartilaginous loop in the orbit through which the tendon of the superior oblique muscle passes before it is attached to the eyeball. By this arrangement, contraction of the muscle rotates the eye down and outward. The fourth cranial nerve, whose sole purpose is to supply this one small muscle, is named the trochlear nerve.

-trop- is a combining form that refers to a changing, especially of position or orientation, but also is used in the sense of stimulation and is derived from the Greek *tropos,* "a turning." **Tropism** can be positive (turning toward) or negative (turning away from). **Corticotropin** is a hormone elaborated by the pituitary gland that is directed (or turned toward) the adrenal cortex, wherein it stimulates hormonal activity. Similarly, a **gonadotropin** has a stimulating effect on the gonads or organs of procreation.

-troph- is a combining form that refers to growth and is taken from the Greek *trophē,* "food or nourishment." Thus, **atrophy** is a failure or reversal of growth, and **hypertrophy** is an excessive growth. There is an important distinction between hypertrophy and hyperplasia. Both can result in enlargement of a part or of an organ. When the enlargement is due to an increase in size but not in number of the component cells, the condition is known as "hypertrophy"; when the number but not necessarily the size of the component cells increases, as by proliferation, the condition is known as "hyperplasia." A **trophic** nerve regulates the metabolism and growth of a part. A **trophoblast** (+ Greek *blastos,* "germ or sprout") is the forerunner of the placenta or nourishing organ of the developing embryo. A **trophozoite** (+ Greek *zōon,* "animal") is a unicellular organism in its active, feeding stage, as contrasted to its dormant, encysted stage.

trypsin is a proteolytic enzyme that was so named in 1874 by Willy Kühne (1837–1900), a German physiologist. The name was taken from the Greek *tripsis,* "a rub-

bing," because the substance was first obtained by rubbing or macerating the pancreas. Like pepsin, trypsin, while an enzyme, lacks the customary "-ase" ending. The explanation is that both were named before "-ase" became the conventional suffix denoting an enzyme. **Tryptophan** (+ Greek *phanos,* "bright"), an amino acid obtained by proteolytic enzymatic hydrolysis, is so called because with halogenation it produces a rather bright violet color. **Triturate,** meaning "to rub into a pulp or powder," comes from the Latin *tritura,* "a threshing, as of a grain," which is related to the Greek *tripsis.*

tsutsugamushi disease is another name for scrub typhus. The term is a combination of the Japanese *tsutsuga,* "dangerous," + *mushi,* "bug," which is apt because the causative organism, an Oriental rickettsia, is transmitted by the bite of larval mites or chiggers.

tube comes from the Latin *tuba,* "a trumpet," and is used in anatomy for various structures that might be fancied to resemble a trumpet. The diminutive **tubule,** of course, refers to a little tube.

tubercle is taken from the Latin *tuberculum,* the diminutive of *tuber,* "a lump or bump." Various small anatomic bumps or excrescences are called tubercles. The disease **tuberculosis** is so called because its characteristic lesion is a tiny nodule which, microscopically, is composed of epithelioid and giant cells. This is a granuloma resulting from infection by *Mycobacterium tuberculosis.* These lesions were first called tubercles in 1689 by Richard Morton

(1637–1698), a London physician, in his classic treatise, *Phthisiologia.* The disease, endemic for centuries, was otherwise known as **phthisis** (Greek for "wasting or decay") and **consumption** (because persons so afflicted became wasted, as if they were being consumed by the disease).

tularemia is a disease resembling plague and is the result of infection by the bacterium *Pasteurella tularensis,* which is transmitted among rodents by insect bites. The infection is acquired by man from handling diseased animals. The name for the disease, coined in 1919 by Edward Francis (1872–1957), an American epidemiologist, combines Tulare, the name of a rural county in the central valley of California where the disease was first identified, and the Greek *haima,* "blood," to stress that the disease is bacteremic in animals.

tumor is a Latin word meaning "a swelling, bulging, or elevation" and, figuratively, "excitement, anger, or arrogance." The related Latin verb is *tumere,* "to swell up." In bygone days, "tumor" was used to designate a swelling of any cause (and can still be so used). Celsus included *tumor* as one of the cardinal symptoms of inflammation (the others: *rubor* or redness, *calor* or heat, and *dolor* or pain). In the 19th century, "tumor" tended to be restricted to chronic swellings or lumps and, later, further restricted to the masses caused by neoplastic lesions. To many patients today, "tumor" means cancer, an unfortunate connotation because many tumors are relatively benign.

tunica is the Latin word for "a skin, peel, husk, or other covering." To the Romans it also meant an ordinary sleeved garment (a tunic) worn by men and women. All sorts of coverings and coats in anatomy are called *tunica* (or, in the Latin plural, *tunicae*).

turbinate is taken from the Latin *turbo, turbinis,* "a whorl, an eddy, or a tornado." The related Latin verb is *turbare,* "to throw into confusion." The Latin *turbo* could also refer to a spiral shell, and it is probably in this sense that "turbinate" was given as a name for the curled shelves of bone protruding from the lateral walls of the nasal cavity.

tweezers is the name for the pointed, pronged instrument used at home for picking up minute objects. In medical school the same instrument is called a forceps. It turns out that "tweezers" is or should be a proper medical term. As noted by the Reverend Skeat (*A Concise Etymological Dictionary of the English Language,* 1882), a surgeon's box of instruments was formerly called a tweese, and the delicate tools therein were called tweezes and, later, tweezers. "Tweese" can be traced to the Middle French *estuy,* "a sheath or case."

tympanum is the anatomic name for the cavity of the middle ear, demarcated laterally by the tympanic membrane or eardrum. The Latin *tympanum* and the Greek *tympanon* are words for "a drum," these being related to the Greek verb *typtein,* "to strike or to beat." The Greek *tympanias* referred to a form of dropsy wherein the swollen belly was taut as a drum. In physical diagnosis, **tympany** is the hollow, drumlike sound elicited when a gas-containing cavity, such as the chest or the distended abdomen, is sharply tapped.

typhlitis is an old but still useful term for inflammation of the cecum. In times past, the term was sometimes used for what we now know as appendicitis. It is derived from the Greek *typhlos,* "blind," and thus refers to the cecum as a "blind" pouch, situated where the small and large intestines are joined. The Latin *caecum* also means "blind."

typhoid is a term concocted in 1829 by Pierre Charles Alexandre Louis (1787–1872), a celebrated French physician, as a name for a disease that resembled, but became recognized as distinct from, typhus. Louis simply tucked the Greek *eidos,* "like," onto "typhus." Before the early 19th century the two diseases often were confused. Later it was found that typhoid fever could be further divided, and the term **paratyphoid** (Greek *para,* "beside") was coined.

typhus represents a widespread group of infectious diseases caused by rickettsial organisms. The disease was known to ancient physicians, though probably mixed up with other acute, febrile diseases. Typhus is featured by high, sustained fever, intense headache, and, often, febrile stupor. The Greek *typhos* means "smoke or mist" but was also used in the metaphysical sense of "dullness or stupor."

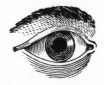

U

ulcer comes through the French *ulcère* from the Latin *ulcus, ulceris,* "a sore or ulcer." The related Greek word is *helkos,* "a wound" and, later, "an ulcer or abscess."

ulna is the Latin word for "the elbow." The related Greek *ōlenē* also means "elbow," but more particularly the arm from the elbow to the wrist, what we call the forearm. Similarly derived is "ell," an archaic unit of linear measure. This was variously taken as the distance from the elbow, the shoulder, or the tip of the nose to the fingertips, so it is not surprising that an ell varied considerably from country to country and from time to time.

ultra- is a combining form directly borrowed from the Latin adverb and preposition meaning "beyond, farther." Thus, **ultraviolet** rays are of a wavelength above and beyond that for visible violet light (and below that for X rays), while **infrared** rays, which convey heat, are of a wavelength just below that for visible red light. Incidentally, a mnemonic device for recalling the order of the visible light spectrum is a man's name: Roy G. Biv (red, orange, yellow, green, blue, indigo, and violet).

Ulysses' syndrome is a term coined by Mercer Rang (*Canad Med Assoc J* 106:122, 1972) in reference to a long and trying journey by a patient and his physician consequent to the discovery of a falsely positive finding on routine screening. Such a spurious finding can initiate a series of wearing diagnostic adventures and misadventures, with ultimate return to the point of departure, as Ulysses returned to Ithaca after his harrowing ten-year odyssey.

umbilicus is the Latin word for the belly button or navel. This is a diminutive of *umbo,* "the boss of a shield," i.e., the ornamental stud at the center of a warrior's shield. The allusion is evident, although the belly button in most people is concave rather than convex. Therefore, in pathology, an indentation or dimple, particularly in an elevated lesion, is called an umbilication.

uncinate comes from the Latin *uncus,* "a hook," and describes any hooklike process or extension. Similarly, **unciform** (+ Latin *forma,* "shape") can refer to anything shaped like a hook, e.g., the unciform bone of the wrist, also called the **hamate** bone (Latin *hamus,* "a hook").

under the weather is a colloquial expression for a state of confining illness. A patient kept from his usual activities because of the 'flu might say, "I've been under the weather these past few days." The phrase has been attributed to seafarers being obliged, in the teeth of a gale, to seek shelter below deck, thus being, literally, "under the weather." The expression can also mean drunk, again presumably because of the refuge sought by a tipsy sailor.

undulant comes from *undula,* the diminutive of the Latin *unda,* "a wave or billow." As another name for brucellosis, undulant fever is so called because of the wave-like pattern of the patient's temperature chart.

ungual is an adjectival form taken from the Latin *unguis,* "a fingernail or a toenail." A **subungual** infection occurs underneath a fingernail or toenail.

unguent is a derivative of the Latin *unguentum* "a salve or ointment." The related Latin verb is *ungere,* "to smear or to anoint."

urachus is the fetal canal that connects the urinary bladder with an outpouching of the hindgut called the **allantois** (Greek *allas,* "sausage," + *eidos,* "like"). "Urachus" combines the Greek *ouron,* "urine," + *cheō,*

"I pour." The urachus persists in the adult as the median umbilical ligament.

urea is taken from the French *urée,* a name for the essential salt of urine. The relation to the Greek *ouron,* "urine," is obvious. **Uremia** (+ Greek *haima,* "blood") is the toxic condition marked by a retention in the blood of nitrogenous substances, notably urea, that normally are excreted with the urine. **Uric** acid is so called because it was first found in urinary bladder stones.

urine is a direct borrowing of the French word that comes from the Latin *urina* and the Greek *ouron,* all meaning "urine" and all traceable to the postulated Indo-European root word *awer,* "wet, or to flow." In Latin there is a curious bifurcation in that, while *urina* means "urine," the verb *urinare* means "to dive," and to the Romans a *urinator* was "a diver." This is a good example of what Prof. Alexander Gode (*JAMA* 199:145, 1967) called "deceptive cognates," i.e., etymologically identical words with riskily divergent meanings. Professor H. A. Skinner points out that Galen thought that urine was excreted directly from the vena cava and that the composition of urine was an indication of the nature of the blood. Consequently, meticulous examination of the urine, or uroscopy, as it was called, has since ancient times been a strong point of diagnosis. Every medieval physician worthy of the name carried a small flask in which to collect, then contemplate, his patient's urine. **Enuresis** incorporates the Greek *en-,* "in," and, of course, means urinating in bed or "wetting the bed." **Ureter** is derived from the Greek *ourein,* "to make water." From the same source comes **urethra**. The ancient writers used the singular of the derived noun for the single urinary duct leading from the bladder to the exterior of the body, and the plural for the paired ducts leading from the kidneys to the bladder.

urticaria comes from the Latin *urtica*, "a nettle," and by extension "a sting or itch." The related Latin verb *urere* means "to burn." The nettle is an herb covered with fine hairs that, when touched, produce a stinging sensation and inflammatory reaction in the skin. *Urticaria* is the Latin term for the sting of a nettle. Today the term applies to a focal, pruritic edema in the skin or mucous membranes signifying an acute allergic reaction to any sort of antigen.

uterus is the Latin word for the womb, but used by the Romans also for the belly or paunch of a man. Presumably the term relates to the Latin *uter,* "a bag or bottle for wine or water" made from the hide of an animal.

uvea is a collective term for the iris, the ciliary body, and the choroid of the eye and is taken from the Latin *uva,* "a grape." If one plucks the stem from a grape, the hole can be imagined as the pupil and the grape as the eyeball. The term is a convenient one in that **uveitis** signifies as inflammation affecting all components of the uveal tract. Unrelated, except in derivation, is **uvula**, the diminutive of the Latin *uva.* The midline appendage at the back of the soft palate must have looked to someone like a little grape.

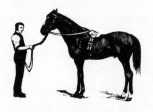

V

vaccine comes from the Latin *vacca,* "a cow," and **vaccinia** is the name of a viral disease of cattle, sometimes called **cowpox.** Edward Jenner, a country physician who practiced in Berkeley, Gloucestershire, England, took seriously the folk belief that dairymaids who contracted a mild reaction to cowpox were thereafter spared the risk of the dreaded smallpox. The idea of protecting against an infectious disease by inoculating one person with pus taken from another person's lesion —a procedure known as variolation—was not new with Jenner. Such attempts to prevent smallpox had been made for many years in the Orient, with varying degrees of success and disaster. In fact, the idea was introduced to England in 1717 by no less a personage than Lady Mary Wortley Montagu, wife of the British ambassador to Turkey. What Jenner contributed was his recognition of the cross-immunity between cowpox and smallpox and the proof, by ex-periment, that persons inoculated with cowpox showed no reaction when later deliberately inoculated with smallpox. It was on 14 May 1796 that Jenner inoculated a young friend, 8-year-old James Phipps, with material taken from a pustule on the hand of Sarah Nelmes, an obliging local dairymaid. On 1 July and again several months later, Jenner demonstrated that material taken from an actual smallpox pustule elicited no reaction when inoculated into James Phipps. In 1797 Jenner submitted a paper describing his observation to the Royal Society. It was rejected with the admonition that Jenner "ought not risk his reputation by presenting to the learned body anything which appeared so much at variance with established knowledge, and withal so incredible." In 1798 Jenner privately published a pamphlet on the subject, bolstered by further evidence. Thereupon Jenner was engulfed by waves of adulation and condemnation, but he was serenely confident that he had conferred a boon on mankind. Originally the term "vaccination" was limited to the inoculation of a preparation derived from cowpox. Later it was extended to the injection of any microbial antigen for the purpose of inducing immunity to a corresponding disease.

vacuole is a diminutive taken from the Latin adjective *vacuus,* "empty," and hence is a term for any little empty space, particularly that apparent in the cytoplasm of cells.

vagina is the Latin word for "a scabbard or a sheath," such as might be used to contain a *gladius,* "a sword." The Romans sometimes used *gladius* as another name for the penis and *vagina* for the female genital introitus.

vagus as a name for the tenth cranial nerve is apt inasmuch as this nerve takes a long and meandering path from its origin in the midbrain to the far reaches of the peritoneal cavity. Thus, it was called "the wanderer," and its name was borrowed directly from the Latin adjective *vagus,* meaning "wandering or inconstant." The medical student, uncertain of the path and purpose of the tenth cranial nerve, will remind us that the Latin *vagus* also gives us our English word "vague." From the same source come vagabond, vagary, and vagrant.

valetudinarian describes a person who, while not necessarily physically ill, is constantly preoccupied by his health and perturbed by his bodily functions. The term comes from the Latin *valetudo,* "state of health," this being related to the Latin verb *valere,* "to be strong." A Roman *valetudinarium* was a hospital.

valgus is the Latin word for "bowlegged" and has been adopted in medicine as an adjective meaning "bent outward." Its ending depends on the gender of the Latin term that is modified, as in **coxa valga** (Latin *coxa,* "hipbone"), in which the thigh is bent outwards; **genu valgum** (Latin *genu,* "knee"), which is an apparent contradiction because to most radiologists and orthopedists this means knock-kneed; **hallux valgus** (Latin *hallux,* "big toe"), a deformity wherein the big toe is bent so as to overlap the adjacent toes; and **talipes valgus** (Latin *talipes,* "clubfoot," from *talus,* "ankle"), in which the heel is turned sharply outward. Deformities the opposite of valgus, i.e., wherein the affected part is bent inwards, are described by forms of the adjective *varus,* the Latin word for "knock-kneed." Again there is a peculiar confusion in that **genu varum** is now customarily taken to be a bowleg. The sense depends on whether one looks at the direction in which the joint is deformed or the direction in which the affected limb is bent. All of this is the subject of an intriguing essay by C. Stuart Houston and Leonard E. Swischuk (*New Eng J Med* 307:471, 1980), who offer the sensible suggestion that, insofar as current usage is confused and confusing, the simple English words "bowlegged" and "knock-kneed" be used in preference to the Latin *genu valgum* and *genu varum,* and that "bunion" be used rather than *hallux valgus.* One would still have to distinguish an inwardly or outwardly bent clubfoot as *talipes varus* or *talipes valgus,* or simply say which way the heel was bent. Referring to the angle between the femoral head and shaft, **coxa vara** means a decrease in the angle, while **coxa valga** means an increase in the angle. In any case, prudence dictates the clear definition of any term used and the choice of the least ambiguous name available.

valve is derived from the Latin *valvae,* used in the plural by the Romans for "a pair of folding or double doors." The valves of the heart and the veins function, in a way, as doors that open to permit traffic in one direction but close to impede traffic in the opposite direction. The **valvulae conniventes** are circular folds in the mucosa of the proximal small intestine. They are so named because they are small (hence the diminutive *valvulae*), and because they tend to come and go as implied by *conniventes* (from the Latin *connivere,* "to wink or blink").

varicose describes veins that are distended and tortuous, such as those that become prominent on the surface of the legs, or those that bulge into the lumen of the esophagus because they are burdened with blood that normally would course through the portal circulation but is blocked by disease in or near the liver. The term is a near borrowing of the Latin *varicosus,* which describes the condition of a *varix,* the Latin name for an overly dilated vein. We still use **varix** and the Latin plural **varices** in the same way today. All these terms are probably related to the Latin *varus,* "crooked."

variola is the Late Latin name for smallpox, having been taken from the classical Latin *varius,* "spotted or variegated." The term "variola" was used generally for mottled rashes as early as the 6th century, but was applied specifically to smallpox when that disease was fully described and differentiated from measles in the 10th century by Abu Bakr Muhammad Ibn Zalariya, the brilliant Persian physician better known to us as Rhazes. Subsequently chickenpox was differentiated as a much milder disease and given the name **varicella,** a diminutive of variola.

vas is the Latin word for "a dish or similar utensil." The term was early applied in anatomy to tubular structures, such as blood vessels, that were identified as carrying fluids. A small blood vessel was called by the diminutive *vasculum,* and from this is derived our adjective **vascular**. Similarly, **vaso-** has come to be a combining form to designate a relationship to blood vessels. **Vasomotor** nerves are those that control the volume of flow through blood vessels by regulating the tone of their muscular walls. Blood vessels themselves must be nourished, and so they are served by fine vascular channels of their own. These are called **vasa vasorum**, a term utilizing both the plural noun and its possessive plural form. The **vas deferens** (or spermatic duct) is so called because it is a vessel that "carries away" (Latin *de-* "away," + *ferre,* "to carry") the sperm-laden fluid from the testis.

vector is the Latin word for "a bearer" and is related to the verb *vehere,* "to convey or transport." In medicine, a vector is an intermediary "vehicle," usually an arthropod, that transfers, by one means or another, an infectious agent from one host to another. The transfer can be from man to man or from animal to man or vice versa. Contagious diseases can sometimes be suppressed by identifying and then eradicating the vector.

vein clearly is derived from the Latin *vena,* but it is interesting to note that the Latin term has a number of meanings other than blood vessel, as does its Greek counterpart, *phleps.* Among these are a spring of water, a course of metal or ore in a mineral deposit, and a distinctive streak of color in a slab of marble. This is carried into English, where a vein can also be a quality, manner, or style. Someone can speak "in a jocular vein" or can write "with a humorous vein coursing through otherwise turgid prose." It seems the use of "vein" as a name for an afferent blood vessel is almost incidental.

velum is the Latin word for "a sail, a curtain, or an awning." In anatomy the term is used for various veil-like coverings or membranes. The soft posterior portion of the palate was once called the *velum palati.*

venereal can be traced to the Sanskrit *wan, van,* "to love, to honor, to desire," which gave rise to a string of more or less related Latin words, including *venus, veneris,* "beauty, pleasure of love, sexual indulgence"; *venari,* "to hunt"; and *venenum,* "a love potion, sorcery, or poison." The ancients were wont to personify concepts and ideas, and so arose the mythological Venus, goddess of beauty and love. Venus figures in all sorts of fascinating tales involving human deities and godlike humans. Alas, a price is exacted for sexual indulgence. Part of the price is the risk of acquiring a *morbus venereus,* or venereal disease, such as syphi-

lis, gonorrhea, or, more recently, herpes. The **mons veneris** is the pubis of a woman or "the mount of Venus."

ventral is taken from the Latin *venter,* "the belly." As a term of anatomic reference, "ventral" means whatever is oriented toward the belly or toward the front of the body. The Latin diminutive *ventriculus,* originally the Latin term for the actual stomach, has become **ventricle** as a word for the bulbous part of a muscle; for the pouch between the true and false vocal cords in the larynx; for the heavy-walled muscular chambers of the heart; and also for the cavities in the brain that connect with the central canal of the spinal cord and contain cerebrospinal fluid.

vermis is the Latin word for "a worm." The vermis cerebelli is the median portion of the cerebellum, which can be fancied in the shape of a worm. Even more wormlike is the **vermiform** (+ Latin *forma,* "shape") **appendix** (Latin for "addition or supplement"), which is stuck on the base of the cecum for no apparent reason in man but to serve as a seat for appendicitis. Out of familiarity, we seldom use the full name of this little organ; we call it simply the appendix. A **vermifuge** (+ Latin *fugare,* "to chase away") is a medicine that expels worms or similar vermin from the gut.

vernix is the Latin word for "varnish." The vernix caseosa is a cheesy or unctuous substance composed of sebum and desquamated epithelial cells that covers the skin of the fetus.

verruca is the Latin term for "a wart." A little boy holds out his finger and says, "Look, I have a wart!" The doctor observes the finger closely and pronounces, "Aha! You have a verruca vulgaris." Both are saying the same thing, though the doctor is identifying the lesion as a common wart (Latin *vulgaris,* "common or usual," from *vulgus,* "the masses or the common herd"). Whatever is **verrucous** is wartlike. **Wart** comes from the Old English *wearte,* used as a term for excrescences of the skin since the 8th century.

vertebra is the Latin word for "a joint or a bone of the spine," being taken from the Latin verb *vertere,* "to turn or to tilt." Altogether there are thirty-three vertebrae making up the spinal column: seven cervical (Latin *cervix,* "neck"); twelve thoracic (Greek *thōrax,* "chest") or dorsal (Latin *dorsum,* "back"); five lumbar (Latin *lumbus,* "loin"); five sacral (Latin *sacrum,* "holy vessel"); and four coccygeal (Greek *kokkyx,* "cuckoo bird"). The sacral and coccygeal vertebrae are fused into two composite bones.

vertex is the Latin word for "a whirlpool, a whirlwind or tornado, the summit of a mountain, or the top of the head," all connected by the sense of spiraling and being related to the Latin *vertere,* "to turn." It is said the top of the head was called the vertex because it is there that the hairs form a whorl. **Vertigo**, also taken from *vertere,* is a hallucination of movement wherein one's surroundings or one's self seems to be whirling around. True vertigo, a rotary phenomenon usually signifying an inner ear disturbance, is not to be confused with simple lightheadedness or giddiness. Patients usually use the term **dizzy** (from the Anglo-

Saxon *dysig,* "foolish," related to the Teutonic form *dwaes,* "a god," hence "god possessed") for both vertigo and giddiness.

verumontanum is an alternative term for the **seminal colliculus** (a diminutive of the Latin *collis,* "a hill," hence "a little mound"), the prominent portion of the urethral crest where join the orifices of the ejaculatory ducts and the sac of the prostate gland. *Verumontanum* is Latin for "the crest or sharp top of a hill or mountain."

vesicle is taken from the Latin *vesiculum,* the diminitive of *vesica,* "a bladder or bag." The anatomic adjective **vesical** is derived directly from *vesica* and does not denote the diminutive but simply refers to whatever pertains to the urinary bladder. A vesicle in anatomy can be any one of a number of small pouches in various organs, while in dermatology a vesicle is a small blister.

vestibule is the Latin term for an entrance or a forecourt, like an enclosed porch. In anatomy, a vestibule is a space or cavity at the entrance of a canal or other sort of channel or vessel. The vestibule of the ear is the oval cavity in the middle of the bony labyrinth.

vestige denotes the nonfunctioning remnant of a structure which, in an antecedent of the species or in a previous stage of individual development, may have had a defined function that no longer pertains. For example, the navel is a vestige of the former entrance of the umbilical cord, vital in the fetus but of no use to the adult. The term is derived from the Latin *vestigium,* "a footprint," as a trace of something that has gone before. But Ambrose Bierce in the *Devil's Dictionary* observed of the ostrich, "The absence of a good working pair of wings is no defect for, as has been ingeniously pointed out, the ostrich does not fly." **Investigation**, essential to medical progress, has a respectable origin in the Latin verb *investigare,* "to track or to search after," this, of course, being related to *vestigium.* Thus, an investigator is one who looks for traces or footprints in quest for whatever is sought.

veterinary refers to whatever pertains to domestic animals, including veterinary medicine, which treats of their diseases. The Latin adjective *veterinus* means "carrying burdens"; the feminine and neuter plural *veterinae* and *veterina* refers to beasts of burden. *Veterinus* is a contraction of *veheterinus,* the related verb being *vehere,* "to carry or to transport."

viable is borrowed from the French and is related to the French *vie,* "life." "Viable," then, means "capable of living." A viable fetus is one that has matured to a stage of development at which it is capable of life independent of the uterus.

Vibrio is a genus of slightly curved, actively motile, gram-negative bacteria. The name comes from the Latin *vibrare,* "to quiver." Among the best known species is the *Vibrio comma,* so designated because it is shaped like the punctuation mark (,). Infection by this organism is the cause of Asiatic cholera, a devastating disease characterized by profuse, often lethal, diarrhea.

villus is the Latin word for "shaggy hair or fleece." The mucosal surface of the small intestine, when looked at with a hand lens, appears to be made up of minute, hairlike projections resembling the nap of a rug.

These are called the intestinal villi. The epithelial cells covering the mucosa, when viewed by electron microscopy, are seen to bear, on their luminal surfaces, even more minute projections of their own cell membranes. These are called **microvilli** (Greek *mikros,* "small"). The busy absorptive surface of the small intestine is thus progressively increased by its corrugated folds, by the villi, and finally by the microvilli. Someone has estimated, taking all these devices into account, that the actual surface area of the human small intestine approximates that of a basketball court.

virus is a Latin word meaning "slime," particularly that which is foul or poisonous. In 16th-century English, "virus" was a synonym for "venom." Later it came to refer to the noxious or infectious essence of pus. After bacteria were discovered in pus and identified as pathogenic microorganisms, it became apparent that even smaller transmitters of disease existed, because certain types of pus could be passed through exceedingly fine filters and still cause infection. Hence it was postulated that there existed filterable viruses. Only much later, with the advent of electron microscopy, were viruses morphologically defined. Viruses have yet to be classified as systematically as bacteria and other pathogenic organisms, but many have been named, some after places (e.g., the **coxsackie virus**, from Coxsackie, New York, the hometown of the patient in whom the virus was first identified), and some as acronyms (e.g., the **echo virus**, from *e*nteric *c*ytopathic *h*uman *o*rphan, the "orphan" referring to the fact that the virus was identified before it could be related to a specific disease). A remarkable concoction is **picornavirus**, whose name makes clear sense to whoever recognizes its components but might, for a while, baffle the uninitiated. The way it is usually pronounced ("pie-korn-uh-virus") seems a deliberate ploy to hide its meaning. Going from aft forward, the "-virus" is easy; the "-rna-" is a set of initials that look familiar when they stand alone as "RNA" (ribonucleic acid); the "pico-," of course, means "small." So, picornaviruses are very small viruses of the RNA-type; they comprise the enteroviruses and the coryzaviruses, and one of their number causes infectious (type A) hepatitis. If the term were pronounced "peeko-RNA-virus," it would be more faithful to the Italian origin of "pico" and easier to understand for the student who hears the term for the first time.

viscus is the Latin word for "an organ of the body," especially one contained within the chest or abdomen. The Latin plural is **viscera**. Probably the term is related to the Latin verb *viscare,* "to make sticky," stickiness being characteristic of the entrails. From this source, too, comes the adjective **viscid**, descriptive of any sticky or glutinous substance.

vision is derived from the Latin *visio,* "an appearance or what is seen," this being related to the Latin verb *videre,* "to see."

vital comes from the Latin *vitalis,* the adjectival derivative of *vita,* "life," related to the Latin verb *vivere,* "to live, to be alive." In biology and medicine, **in vivo** refers to an observation or occurrence within a living organism or tissue; **in vitro** (Latin *vitrum,* "glass"; the neuter plural *vitrea* means glassware) refers to an observation or occurrence outside a living organism, i.e., in a glass receptacle, such as a test tube. Conception in the usual and natural manner is said to occur *in vivo;* the artificial process of uniting a sperm and an ovum in a Petri dish is said to occur *in vitro.* Vital capacity is the maximum volume of gas that can be expelled from the lungs after a maximal inspiration. In only a limited sense is this a measure of one's capacity for life. In vital staining a dye is applied that is compatible with the life of the tissue or cell being examined, thus permitting the study of living cells. **Vivisection** (+ Latin *secare,* "to cut") is the performance of surgical procedures on living animals, especially in the pursuit of medical research. One often hears the triad "Vim, vigor, and vitality." **Vim** is the accusative of the Latin *vis,* "force." **Vigor** is taken from the Latin *vigere,* "to thrive."

vitamin is a term coined by Polish-born Casimir Funk (1884–1967), in 1911, while he was working in England. He had isolated a substance he believed to prevent neuritis in chickens raised on an otherwise deficient diet. Funk spelled the word "vitamine" because the substance he isolated had the chemical characteristics of an amine and because he believed it exerted a protective effect necessary to life. A more general term had been formerly used for such presumed substances: "vital accessory factors." It turned out that the substance found by Funk was an amine of nicotinic acid, the antipellagra factor, rather than the anti-beriberi factor as first supposed. In 1920 J. C. Drummond (1891–1952) suggested dropping the "e" because it was then known that these factors are not necessarily amines. As more vitamins were discovered, and before they were chemically characterized, they were assigned letter-names in alphabetical sequence: A, B, C, D, and so on. An exception is vitamin K, the blood-clotting factor, given its initial, for *Koagulation,* in 1935 by its discoverer, Henrik Dam, a Danish investigator.

volar is taken from the Latin *vola,* "the palm of the hand or the sole of the foot." In anatomy, "volar" describes whatever is related to the palm of the hand, such as the volar surface or the volar artery. The Romans actually used *palma* to refer to the outstretched palm of the hand. The relation of *vola* as a term for the palm might be to the Latin *volens,* "willing," from *volo,* "I wish," perhaps in the sense of the open hand as a gesture of willingness. It has been suggested, too, that *vola* may be related, by transliteration, to the Greek *bolē,* "a throw."

volatile is a near borrowing of the Latin *volatilis,* "flying or fleeting." Whatever is volatile tends to evaporate quickly and seems to "fly away."

volvulus is the Latin word for "rolled up or twisted" and is related to the Latin verb *volvere,* "to roll or to turn about." In medicine, a volvulus is a twisted obstruction in a segment of the gut that is supported by a mesentery (rather than being firmly attached by a peritoneal membrane) and hence liable to twisting on its longitudinal axis. Thus the stomach, the mesenteric small intestine, the cecum, and the sigmoid segment of the colon are all subject to volvulus. The risk is not so much in the twisting alone but more in the consequent constriction of mesenteric blood vessels, which can lead to infarction.

vomit comes from the Latin *vomere,* "to throw up from the stomach." To the Romans a *vomica* was a boil or abscess, the idea being that pus is thrown up by the lesion. *Vomer* is the Latin word for "a plowshare." Presumably the noun is derived from *vomere,* the allusion being to the earth thrown up by the plowshare. The bone in the nasal septum was called the **vomer** because of its fancied resemblance to a plowshare.

vulgaris is the Latin word for "common, general, or usual," and has been incorporated into several medical terms to mean "of the ordinary type" or "common in the population." **Acne vulgaris** is so familiar as to be almost a rite of passage for youngsters. **Lupus vulgaris** is a form of tuberculous dermatitis, once common, now rare.

vulva is a direct borrowing of the Latin word for "a wrapper." It can also be spelled *volva,* which would seem to indicate its origin in the Latin verb *volvere,* "to roll or to turn about." To the Romans, *vulva* also was a word for the womb (a sort of wrapper), particularly that of the sow; the term was later applied to the female genital tract and became restricted to the labia majora, its current designation. Another version has "vulva" related to the Latin *valvae,* "folding or double doors." The sense seems apt but, beyond that, evidence is lacking.

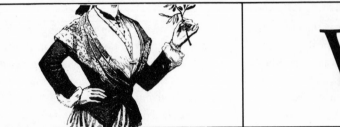

waist refers to that part of the body between the lowest ribs and the hips, usually at the smallest circumference, also known as the **midriff** (Old English *hrif,* "belly"). "Waist" can be traced to the Indo-European *aweg,* "to increase," which became the Anglo-Saxon *weaxan,* "to grow." This, of course, accounts for the "wax" in the phrase "wax and wane." In Middle English, *wast* was "the growth of a man," the part of the body where size and strength were evident. The sense is similar to that of "well girded" or "in fine fettle." Nowadays most people strive for a slim waist, but a thin middle was not always admired.

wean can be traced to the Anglo-Saxon *wenian,* "to accustom." The true meaning of "wean" is to accustom a child to food other than its mother's milk. But often we use the word in a sense of weaning away from the breast, i.e., to deprive or disaccustom, rather than weaning to solid food.

whiplash is a highly descriptive word that conveys a clear meaning, although few persons who use the word have ever held a whip in their hands or felt the sting of a lash. It is a vivid picture-word. The French refer to a sharp wrenching of the neck as a *coup de lapin,* literally a "rabbit punch." To be prepared as food or pelts, rabbits customarily were killed by being held by their hind legs and struck sharply at the nape of the neck by the edge of the hand.

whitlow is a suppurative inflammation or abscess in the nailbed of a finger or toe, also called a felon. According to the Reverend Skeat, "whitlow" is a corruption of "whickflaw," wherein "whick" is a northern pronunciation of "quick," the sensitive part of the finger around and under the nail. "Quick" at one time meant living or lively. The quick of the nailbed and of the dermis generally is so called because of its keen sensitivity. "Flaw" was a crack, a breach, or a sore. **Felon** has two meanings: one in law and one in medicine. Both can possibly be traced to the Latin *fel,* "bile or gall" and, figuratively, "bitterness or animosity." One who is full of fel is likely to be a wicked person. The Old French *felon* was "a traitor." In law, a felony is an offense graver than a misdemeanor and punishable by a loss of citizens' rights and imprisonment, generally, for longer than a year. In medicine, a felon was first an inflamed sore (perhaps as bitterness coming to a head), then was restricted to a sore and swollen finger.

whopper-jawed is a colloquial expression for anything asymmetric or out of line. Originally the term referred to a condition, also known as "lumpy jaw" in cattle, that sometimes produced a grotesque swelling on one side of the mandible. Lumpy jaw is the result of inflammation consequent to infection by actinomyces. Whopper-jawed is a change (some would prefer to call it a mistake) in the spelling of "wapper-jawed." Wapper (or whopper) is of uncertain origin. Possibly the relation is to wap (or to whop), "to throw or to beat violently." A violent stroke to the jaw would certainly induce swelling. Alternatively it could relate to wapper meaning "fatigued or wearied," hence slack-jawed.

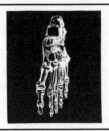

X

xantho- is a combining form taken from the Greek *xanthos,* "yellow." **Xanthine** is a white, amorphous base, 2,6-dioxypurine, and is found in most body tissues; its nitrate is yellow, hence its name. **Xanthinuria** (+ Greek *ouron,* "urine") is a rare genetic disorder in which xanthine oxidase is deficient; consequently xanthines, rather than uric acid, are excreted in the urine as the end products of purine metabolism. A **xanthoma** (+ Greek *-ōma,* "swelling") is a yellow, circumscribed nodule in the skin or mucous membrane that is composed of lipid-laden foamy histiocytes. A **xanthelasma** (+ Greek *elasma,* "a plate") is a flat, plaque-like xanthoma, typically appearing in or near an eyelid.

xero- is a combining form taken from the Greek *xeros,* "dry or parched." **Xeroderma** (+ Greek *derma,* "skin") is a condition marked by a dry, rough, scaly skin. **Xerophthalmia** (+ Greek *ophthalmos,* "eye") is dryness in the conjunctiva (and, in more advanced stages, affecting the cornea), resulting from a deficiency of vitamin A. **Xerostomia** (+ Greek *stoma,* "mouth") is excessive dryness of the mouth due to a lack of saliva from any cause. Dryness in the eyes and mouth is the principal feature of the **sicca** (Latin *siccus,* "dry or thirsty") complex, an early manifestation of Sjögren's syndrome, an immunopathic disorder marked, in part, by degeneration in the lacrimal and salivary glands.

xiphoid is one of the names for the pointed cartilage attached to the lower end of the breastbone or sternum. The name combines the Greek *xiphos,* "a straight sword," + *eidos,* "like." By the same allusion to its shape, the structure also is called the **ensiform** cartilage (Latin *ensis,* "sword," + *forma,* "shape").

X-rays were so named by their discoverer, Wilhelm Konrad Röntgen (1845–1923), a

German physicist, who first observed their remarkable property of penetrating soft tissues on 8 November 1895, at Würzburg. Röntgen called them *X-Strahlen,* naturally using the German word for rays. Röntgen's use of "X" was appropriate because the nature of the phenomenon was then unknown. How "x" came to be a symbol of the unknown is itself unknown or uncertain. According to Professor Alexander Gode (*JAMA* 191:648, 1965), it may have begun with the word used by early Arab mathematicians, *shei,* "a thing," which came to be spelled with an initial "x" by the Spaniards. Descartes, the 17th-century French philosopher and mathematician, seems to have established the systematic use of "x," "y," and "z" as symbols for unknown quantities or qualities.

xyl- is a combining form taken from the Greek *xylon,* "wood." **Xylene,** also called **xylol** (+ Latin *oleum,* "oil"), is a volatile hydrocarbon originally obtained from wood alcohol; it is used in microscopy as a solvent and a clarifier. **Xylose** is a pentose and is sometimes called wood sugar because it can be obtained from certain species of woody plants. The urinary excretion of ingested d-xylose is used as a test of intestinal absorption.

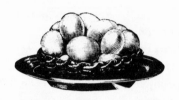

Y

yaws is one name for a tropical infection by a spirochete, *Treponema pertenue,* that is marked by berrylike excrescences, sometimes pustular and ulcerated, in the skin of the face, hands, feet, and genital area. The disease is thought to have originated in Africa, and *yaw* may have been an African word for "berry." Another name for the disease is frambesia tropica, this being related to the French *framboise,* "raspberry."

yellow fever is an acute, systemic, viral infection occurring chiefly in tropical America and Africa, so named because it is characterized, in severe cases, by intense jaundice and high fever, in addition to hemorrhagic lesions in the skin and mucous membranes and tubular necrosis in the kidneys. At one time the disease was a scourge of port cities in the U.S. during the summer months and caused thousands of deaths in New Orleans, Philadelphia, and New York. This was the disease that in Cuba claimed far more victims than did bullets in the Spanish-American War of 1898. Control of the disease was made possible by the valiant investigation of Walter Reed (1851–1902), an American army doctor, who proved that the vector was the mosquito *Aedes aegypti.* In so doing, Reed substantiated the hypothesis advanced by Carlos Juan Finlay (1833–1915), a Cuban physician, whose prior evidence Reed graciously acknowledged.

yolk as the name for the nutritive substance available to an embryo is derived from the Old English *geolca,* from *geolu,* "yellow." The most familiar yolk is that of a hen's egg, which is, indeed, yellow. In Middle English the word became *yolke,* and from that it was a short step to "yolk."

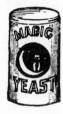

Z

zygomatic describes the quadrilateral bone of the skull that forms the bony prominence of the cheek and the lateral wall of the orbit. The term also describes the bony arch by which a bar-like projection of the temporal bone is joined by a fixed suture to the zygomatic bone. The anatomic adjective is taken from the Greek *zygon,* "a yoke or a crossbar by which two draft animals can be hitched to a plow or a wagon." Also derived from this Greek word is **zygote,** the cell resulting from the fusion (or "yoking together") of two gametes, i.e., the fertilized ovum. An odd-looking and odd-sounding word is **syzygy** (Greek *sy*[*n*], "together"), used to denote a conjunction, as of heavenly bodies when they are aligned in space, or, in biology, to denote a fusion of microorganisms.

zym- is a combining form taken from the Greek *zymē,* "a leavening agent or a fer-ment." **Zymase** (+ suffix *-ase,* denoting an enzyme) was detected in 1897 by Eduard Buchner (1860–1917), a German biochemist, as the active substance in yeast that could produce fermentation in the absence of living yeast cells. For this achievement Buchner was awarded the Nobel prize in chemistry for 1907. Buchner died in 1917 of a wound sustained in World War I. Buchner's discovery was preceded almost forty years by the hypothesis that fermentation could be induced by an inanimate substance, a notion that Louis Pasteur thought preposterous. The hypothesis was advanced in 1858 by Moritz Traube (1826–1894), a Prussian botanist, who went so far as to coin a word for the supposed substance contained in yeast: **enzyme** (Greek *en-,* "within," + *zymē*). It was about the time of Buchner's work that Rudolf Heidenhain (1834–1897), a physiologist at Breslau, observed that a carbohydrate-splitting enzyme was derived from a product of pancreatic acinar cells. This potentially enzymatic ma-terial he called **zymogen** (+ Greek *gennaō*, "I produce") because it is a precursor of the active principle.

INDEX

*Index entries are terms boldfaced within the main entries of the book.
Each is cross-referenced to the main entry in which it appears.*

Index

Index

Index

oxalic, see oxygen, 174
oxyntic, see oxygen, 174

pallor, see appall, 21
palpebral, see palpate, 176
palpitation, see palpate, 176
panarteritis, see pan-, 176
panhysterectomy, see pan-, 176
pantophobia, see phobia, 186
paracentesis, see para-, 177–78
paralysis, see palsy, 176; para-, 177–78
paranoia, see para-, 177–78
paraplegia, see para-, 177–78
parasite, see para-, 177–78
parasympathetic, see syn-, 235
paratyphoid, see typhoid, 254
paregoric, see para-, 177–78
parenchyma, see para-, 177–78
parotid, see para-, 177–78
paroxysm, see para-, 177–78
pathogenesis, see patho-, 179
pathognomonic, see patho-, 179
pathology, see patho-, 179
p.c., see a.c., 2
pectoriloquy, see pectoral, 180
pederasty, see pediatrics, 180
pediatrics, see iatros, 117
pedigree, see pedicle, 180
pelio-, see colors, 58
pemphigoid, see pemphigus, 181
percussion, see per-, 182
perforate, see per-, 182
pericardium, see per-, 182
perineum, see peri-, 182–83
periodontal, see tooth, 246
periosteum, see peri-, 182–83
peristalsis, see peri-, 182–83
peritoneum, see peri-, 182–83
perityphlitis, see cecum, 47
perleche, see per-, 182
pernicious, see per-, 182
pertussis, see per-, 182
phaeo-, see colors, 58
phagedenic, see phage, 184

pharmacopoeia, see pharmacy, 184
phenol, see pheno-, 185
phenomenon, see pheno-, 185
phenotype, see mutation, 158; pheno-, 185
philtrum, see -phil, 185
phlebotomus, see phlebo-, 185
phlebotomy, see phlebo-, 185
phlegmon, see phlegm, 185–86
photophobia, see phobia, 186
phrenic, see dia-, 69
phrenology, see phrenic, 186
phthisis, see tubercle, 252–53
phylogeny, see ontogeny, 171
physician, see iatros, 117
physics, see physician, 187
phytobezoars, see bezoar, 34
picornavirus, see virus, 263–64
pimple, see papule, 177
placenta praevia, see placenta, 189
platyhelminthes, see platy-, 190
platysma, see platy-, 190
pleiotropy, see pleo-, 190
pleomorphic, see pleo-, 190
pleurisy, see pleura, 191
pleurities, see pleura, 191
pleurodynia, see pleura, 191
pneumat-, see pneumo-, 191
pneumaturia, see pneumo-, 191
pneumococcus, see pneumo-, 191
pneumoconiosis, see pneumo-, 191
pneumonia, see pneumo-, 191
podalic version, see podiatry, 192
poikilocytosis, see cyto-, 64
polycythemia, see poly-, 192
polydactyly, see poly-, 192
polydipsia, see poly-, 192
polyp, see poly-, 192–93
polyuria, see poly-, 192
porphyrins, see porphyria, 193
portal, see porta, 193
posthumous, see post-, 193–94
postmortem, see post-, 193
postpartum, see post-, 193
postprandial, see post-, 193

281